2011
YEAR BOOK OF
PULMONARY DISEASE®

The 2011 Year Book Series

Year Book of Anesthesiology and Pain Management™: Drs Chestnut, Abram, Black, Gravlee, Lien, Mathru, and Roizen

Year Book of Cardiology®: Drs Gersh, Cheitlin, Elliott, Gold, Graham, and Thourani

Year Book of Critical Care Medicine®: Drs Dellinger, Parrillo, Balk, Dorman, Dries, and Zanotti-Cavazzoni

Year Book of Dermatology and Dermatologic Surgery™: Dr Del Rosso

Year Book of Diagnostic Radiology®: Drs Osborn, Abbara, Elster, Manaster, Oestreich, Offiah, Rosado de Christenson, Stephens, and Walker

Year Book of Emergency Medicine®: Drs Hamilton, Bruno, Handly, Mullin, Quintana, and Ramoska

Year Book of Endocrinology®: Drs Schott, Apovian, Clarke, Eugster, Ludlam, Meikle, Ovalle, Schinner, Schteingart, and Toth

Year Book of Gastroenterology™: Drs Talley, DeVault, Harnois, Pearson, Picco, Scolapio, Smith, and Vege

Year Book of Hand and Upper Limb Surgery®: Drs Yao and Steinmann

Year Book of Medicine®: Drs Barker, Garrick, Gersh, Khardori, LeRoith, Seo, Talley, and Thigpen

Year Book of Neonatal and Perinatal Medicine®: Drs Fanaroff, Benitz, Donn, Neu, Papile, Polin, and van Marter

Year Book of Neurology and Neurosurgery®: Drs Klimo and Rabinstein

Year Book of Obstetrics, Gynecology, and Women's Health®: Drs Dungan and Shulman

Year Book of Oncology®: Drs Arceci, Bauer, Gordon, Lawton, and Thigpen

Year Book of Ophthalmology®: Drs Rapuano, Cohen, Flanders, Hammersmith, Milman, Myers, Nelson, Penne, Pyfer, Sergott, Shields, and Vander

Year Book of Orthopedics®: Drs Morrey, Beauchamp, Huddleston, Swiontkowski, and Trigg

Year Book of Otolaryngology-Head and Neck Surgery®: Drs Sindwani, Balough, Franco, Gapany, and Mitchell

Year Book of Pathology and Laboratory Medicine®: Drs Raab, Parwani, Bejarano, and Bissell

Year Book of Pediatrics®: Dr Stockman

Year Book of Plastic and Aesthetic Surgery™: Drs Miller, Gosain, Gurtner, Gutowski, Ruberg, Salisbury, and Smith

Year Book of Psychiatry and Applied Mental Health®: Drs Talbott, Ballenger, Buckley, Frances, Krupnick, and Mack

Year Book of Pulmonary Disease®: Drs Barker, Jones, Maurer, Raza, Tanoue, and Willsie

Year Book of Sports Medicine®: Drs Shephard, Cantu, Feldman, Jankowski, Khan, Lebrun, Nieman, Pierrynowski, and Rowland

Year Book of Surgery®: Drs Copeland, Behrns, Daly, Eberlein, Fahey, Huber, Klodell, Jones, Mozingo, and Pruett

Year Book of Urology®: Drs Andriole and Coplen

Year Book of Vascular Surgery®: Drs Moneta, Gillespie, Starnes, and Watkins

2011

The Year Book of PULMONARY DISEASE®

Editor-in-Chief

James A. Barker, MD, FACP, FCCP
Chief, Pulmonary, Critical Care Medicine, and Sleep Internal Medicine, Scott & White Health System; Professor of Medicine, Texas A&M Health Science Center, Temple, Texas

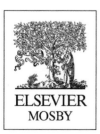

ELSEVIER
MOSBY

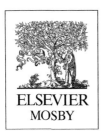

ELSEVIER
MOSBY

Vice President, Continuity: Kimberly Murphy
Developmental Editor: Patrick Manley
Production Supervisor, Electronic Year Books: Donna M. Skelton
Electronic Article Manager: Emily Ogle
Illustrations and Permissions Coordinator: Dawn A. Vohsen

2011 EDITION

Printed and bound by CPI Group (UK) Ltd, Croydon, CR0 4YY
Composition by TNQ Books and Journals Pvt Ltd, India
Transferred to Digital Priting, 2011

Editorial Office:
Elsevier, Inc.
Suite 1800
1600 John F. Kennedy Blvd
Philadelphia, PA 19103-2899

International Standard Serial Number: 8756-3452
International Standard Book Number: 978-0-323-08425-3

Associate Editors

Shirley F. Jones, MD, FCCP, DABSM
Assistant Professor of Internal Medicine, Division of Pulmonary, Critical Care, and Sleep Medicine, Scott & White Memorial Hospital/Texas A&M Health Science Center, Temple, Texas

Janet R. Maurer, MD, MBA
Vice President, Medical Director, Health Dialog Services Corp, Scottsdale, Arizona

Muhammad A. Raza, MD, FCCP, DABSM
Assistant Professor of Medicine, Director, Pulmonary Hypertension Center, Department of Medicine, University of South Carolina, Columbia, South Carolina

Lynn T. Tanoue, MD
Professor of Medicine, Section of Pulmonary and Critical Care Medicine, Yale School of Medicine, Yale University, New Haven, Connecticut

Sandra K. Willsie, DO
Professor of Medicine; Executive Dean, Heartland Health Sciences University, Inc; Dean, College of Osteopathic Medicine, Overland Park, Kansas

Table of Contents

Journal Represented

Journals represented in this YEAR BOOK are listed below.

Academic Emergency Medicine
AJR American Journal of Roentgenology
American Journal of Emergency Medicine
American Journal of Medicine
American Journal of Obstetrics and Gynecology
American Journal of Respiratory and Critical Care Medicine
American Surgeon
Anaesthesia
Anaesthesia and Intensive Care
Anesthesia & Analgesia
Anesthesiology
Annals of Allergy, Asthma & Immunology
Annals of Internal Medicine
Annals of Thoracic Surgery
Archives of Disease in Childhood
Archives of Neurology
Arthritis & Rheumatism
British Journal of Anaesthesia
British Medical Journal
Canadian Journal of Psychiatry
Cancer Journal for Clinicians
Chest
Circulation
Clinical Infectious Diseases
Critical Care Medicine
European Respiratory Journal
Intensive Care Medicine
Journal of Adolescent Health
Journal of Allergy and Clinical Immunology
Journal of Clinical Oncology
Journal of Emergency Medicine
Journal of Heart and Lung Transplantation
Journal of Hypertension
Journal of Rheumatology
Journal of Surgical Research
Journal of the American Medical Association
Journal of Thoracic and Cardiovascular Surgery
Journal of Thoracic Oncology
Journal of Trauma
Journal of Vascular and Interventional Radiology
Lung Cancer
Mayo Clinic Proceedings
Medicine
Medicine and Science in Sports and Exercise
Morbidity and Mortality Weekly Report
Neurology
New England Journal of Medicine

Proceedings of the American Thoracic Society
Obstetrics & Gynecology
Radiology
Respiratory Medicine
Sleep
Spine
Surgery
Thorax
Thrombosis Research
Transplantation

STANDARD ABBREVIATIONS

The following terms are abbreviated in this edition: acquired immunodeficiency syndrome (AIDS), cardiopulmonary resuscitation (CPR), central nervous system (CNS), cerebrospinal fluid (CSF), computed tomography (CT), deoxyribonucleic acid (DNA), electrocardiography (ECG), health maintenance organization (HMO), human immunodeficiency virus (HIV), intensive care unit (ICU), intramuscular (IM), intravenous (IV), magnetic resonance (MR) imaging (MRI), ribonucleic acid (RNA), and ultrasound (US).

NOTE

The YEAR BOOK OF PULMONARY DISEASE is a literature survey service providing abstracts of articles published in the professional literature. Every effort is made to assure the accuracy of the information presented in these pages. Neither the editors nor the publisher of the YEAR BOOK OF PULMONARY DISEASE can be responsible for errors in the original materials. The editors' comments are their own opinions. Mention of specific products within this publication does not constitute endorsement.

To facilitate the use of the YEAR BOOK OF PULMONARY DISEASE as a reference tool, all illustrations and tables included in this publication are now identified as they appear in the original article. This change is meant to help the reader recognize that any illustration or table appearing in the YEAR BOOK OF PULMONARY DISEASE may be only one of many in the original article. For this reason, figure and table numbers will often appear to be out of sequence within the YEAR BOOK OF PULMONARY DISEASE.

1 Asthma and Cystic Fibrosis

Introduction

Again this year, a number of important publications focused on developments in asthma and cystic fibrosis. A larger number of investigations related to asthma therapeutics are highlighted in this volume of the YEAR BOOK OF PULMONARY DISEASE. A randomized placebo-controlled study of IV montelukast in the treatment of acute asthma showed significant improvement in pulmonary function during the first 2 hours of treatment. Reduction in bronchoconstriction was seen in the first 10 minutes, and post hoc analysis showed reduction in the need for hospitalization. Because this study was small, the investigation requires repeating in a larger study before being uniformly applied in the emergency department. Another study evaluated tiotropium bromide added to inhaled corticosteroid (ICS) as step-up therapy as an alternative to doubling of the ICS or the addition of salmeterol to ICS. Tiotropium bromide improved symptoms and lung function in equivalence to the addition of salmeterol to ICS.

In the outpatient setting of chronic pediatric asthma, low-dose fluticasone was shown to be more cost-effective than oral montelukast in children with mild to moderate persistent asthma who demonstrated greater markers of inflammation and increased responsiveness to methacholine. Another investigation evaluated step-up therapy for children with uncontrolled asthma who were receiving ICS. This study involved step-up to one of the following: doubling of the ICS dose; addition of leukotriene-receptor antagonist (LTRA) or addition of a long-acting beta-agonist (LABA). LABA step-up provided the best response, and Hispanics and non-Hispanic white subjects had the best response to LABA step-up therapy and were least likely to respond to ICS doubling. Black subjects had equal likelihood of best response to LABA step-up and ICS doubling and were least likely to have best response to LTRA step-up therapy. This study provides new information on how best to predict response to step-up therapy in children with uncontrolled asthma based on race. An investigation on an experience with 11,849 subjects younger than 18 years who took part in 41 clinical research trials involving formoterol was reported. Eighty-two percent of subjects receiving formoterol in the studies also received ICS. One asthma-related death occurred in 7796 asthmatics treated with formoterol, but no deaths occurred in non-LABA treated subjects. Asthma-related hospitalizations were not different between formoterol-treated subjects and non-LABA–treated subjects, and there was no difference between groups with regard to ethnicity. Supporting previous investigations about the utility of written asthma action plans, Ducharme et al reported their experience with a randomized group of children treated in an emergency department who were assigned to receive usual care or usual care with a written action plan. Adherence to ICS and oral corticosteroids as well as asthma control was significantly improved in the group receiving the action plan.

Finally, two articles evaluate nonprescription therapies in the treatment of asthma. Mendes et al studied the effects of aerobic training on airway inflammation in asthmatics. Utilizing markers of airway inflammation, the investigators showed that aerobic training reduced airway inflammation in asthmatics with moderate or severe asthma, suggesting aerobic training as a potential adjunctive modality for optimizing therapy in asthmatics. As we have discussed previously, many patients utilize complimentary and alternative therapies (CAM) without informing their health care providers. Roy et al surveyed 326 subjects with persistent asthma who were receiving care at inner-city ambulatory clinics and learned that more than 25% were using CAM therapies. In multivariate analysis, herbal use was associated with lower ICS adherence and, predictably, worse outcomes. The health care community must ask about CAM use, inform their patients about the real risks of asthma medications, and the risks of failing to use them. It is time to begin studying CAM therapies that are being used in asthma so that, as health care providers, we have real data on which to base our recommendations to patients.

In the Cystic Fibrosis (CF) section, we highlight 3 investigations, the first centering on a prospective study of an agent (VX 770) that is purported to act to improve function of the CF transmembrane conductance regulator (CFTR). Accurso et al showed within-subject improvements in CFTR and lung function in a study of 39 CF subjects. More studies are needed in larger groups of subjects; however, therapy that targets the genetic defect in this disease in early trials is showing potential promise. Another study of CF patients evaluated whether or not the venue of antibiotic treatment exacerbations is related to pulmonary function deterioration, utilizing data from the US Cystic Fibrosis Twin and Sibling Study care centers between 2000 and 2007. Notably, receipt of IV antibiotics in hospital versus in the home did not significantly impact pulmonary function improvement following exacerbation. Optimal duration of therapy for exacerbations was shown to range from 7 to 10 days, which appears to be shorter than is standard practice in some centers. A study by Aaron et al evaluated outcomes of CF subjects infected with the Liverpool epidemic strain of *Pseudomonas aeruginosa*. CF patients infected with this transmissible strain had a 3-year death rate or rate of transplantation significantly greater ($P = 0.01$) than CF patients infected with other strains.

Sandra K. Willsie, DO

Asthma

A randomized placebo-controlled study of intravenous montelukast for the treatment of acute asthma
Camargo CA Jr, Gurner DM, Smithline HA, et al (Harvard Med School, Boston, MA; Merck Res Laboratories, Rahway, NJ; Tufts Univ School of Medicine, Springfield, MA; et al)
J Allergy Clin Immunol 125:374-380, 2010

Background.—Current treatments for acute asthma provide inadequate benefit for some patients. Intravenous montelukast may complement existent therapies.

Objective.—To evaluate efficacy of intravenous montelukast as adjunctive therapy for acute asthma.

Methods.—A total of 583 adults with acute asthma were treated with standard care during a $\leq$60-minute screening period. Patients with FEV_1 $\leq$50% predicted were randomly allocated to intravenous montelukast 7 mg (n = 291) or placebo (n = 292) in addition to standard care. This double-blind treatment period lasted until a decision for discharge, hospital admission, or discontinuation from the study. The primary efficacy endpoint was the time-weighted average change in FEV_1 during 60 minutes after drug administration. Secondary endpoints included the time-weighted average change in FEV_1 at various intervals (10-120 minutes) and percentage of patients with treatment failure (defined as hospitalization or lack of decision to discharge by 3 hours postadministration).

Results.—Montelukast significantly increased FEV_1 at 60 minutes postdose; the difference between change from baseline for placebo (least-squares mean of 0.22 L; 95% CI, 0.17, 0.27) and montelukast (0.32 L; 95% CI, 0.27, 0.37) was 0.10 L (95% CI, 0.04, 0.16). Similar improvements in FEV_1-related variables were seen at all time points (all P <.05). Although treatment failure did not differ between groups (OR 0.92; 95% CI, 0.63, 1.34), a prespecified subgroup analysis suggests likely benefit for intravenous montelukast at US sites.

Conclusion.—Intravenous montelukast added to standard care in adults with acute asthma produced significant relief of airway obstruction throughout the 2 hours after administration, with an onset of action as early as 10 minutes (Fig 2).

▶ Acute asthma exacerbations are a harbinger of poorly controlled asthma and account for large numbers of emergency department visits annually. Significant hospitalizations result from patients whose acute asthma exacerbations fail to respond to standard asthma therapy in the emergency department setting. Hospitalizations related to acute uncontrolled asthma are associated with significant morbidity and mortality. Montelukast, a leukotriene modifier available for some time as an oral agent, has been reported to have potential efficacy in acute asthma.[1] This investigation used montelukast administered intravenously to patients with acute asthma in this double-blinded, randomized,

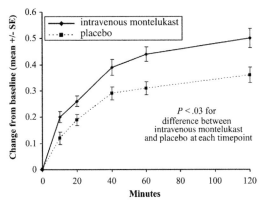

FIGURE 2.—Change from baseline in FEV_1 (L) over time (means ± SEs). (Reprinted from Camargo Jr CA, Gurner DM, Smithline HA, et al. A randomized placebo-controlled study of intravenous montelukast for the treatment of acute asthma. *J Allergy Clin Immunol*. 2010;125:374-380, with permission from American Academy of Allergy, Asthma & Immunology.)

placebo-controlled, multinational study. Demographics of subjects were not statistically different between treated and placebo groups. Fig 2 demonstrates change in forced expiratory volume 1 (FEV_1) over time; statistically significant, although not clinically significant, improvements were seen in FEV_1 over time with intravenous montelukast. Unfortunately, this did not translate to a reduction in hospitalizations. During post hoc analysis, accounting for site of treatment (international vs US sites), the investigators demonstrated that montelukast therapy was associated with a reduction of the need for hospitalization versus placebo. Reduction in bronchoconstriction was seen in as little as 10 minutes following initiation of intravenous montelukast. This therapy deserves further study, particularly as it relates to optimizing patient selection.

S. K. Willsie, DO

Reference

1. Camargo CA Jr, Smithline HA, Malice MP, Green SA, Reiss TF. A randomized controlled trial of intravenous montelukast in acute asthma. *Am J Respir Crit Care Med*. 2003;167:528-533.

Tiotropium Bromide Step-Up Therapy for Adults with Uncontrolled Asthma
Peters SP, for the National Heart, Lung, and Blood Institute Asthma Clinical Research Network (Wake Forest Univ Health Sciences, Winston-Salem, NC; et al)
N Engl J Med 363:1715-1726, 2010

Background.—Long-acting beta-agonist (LABA) therapy improves symptoms in patients whose asthma is poorly controlled by an inhaled glucocorticoid alone. Alternative treatments for adults with uncontrolled asthma are needed.

Methods.—In a three-way, double-blind, triple-dummy crossover trial involving 210 patients with asthma, we evaluated the addition of tiotropium bromide (a long-acting anticholinergic agent approved for the treatment of chronic obstructive pulmonary disease but not asthma) to an inhaled glucocorticoid, as compared with a doubling of the dose of the inhaled glucocorticoid (primary superiority comparison) or the addition of the LABA salmeterol (secondary noninferiority comparison).

Results.—The use of tiotropium resulted in a superior primary outcome, as compared with a doubling of the dose of an inhaled glucocorticoid, as assessed by measuring the morning peak expiratory flow (PEF), with a mean difference of 25.8 liters per minute (P<0.001) and superiority in most secondary outcomes, including evening PEF, with a difference of 35.3 liters per minute (P<0.001); the proportion of asthmacontrol days, with a difference of 0.079 (P = 0.01); the forced expiratory volume in 1 second (FEV_1) before bronchodilation, with a difference of 0.10 liters (P = 0.004); and daily symptom scores, with a difference of −0.11 points (P<0.001). The addition of tiotropium was also noninferior to the addition of salmeterol for all assessed outcomes and increased the prebronchodilator FEV_1 more than did salmeterol, with a difference of 0.11 liters (P = 0.003).

Conclusions.—When added to an inhaled glucocorticoid, tiotropium improved symptoms and lung function in patients with inadequately controlled asthma. Its effects appeared to be equivalent to those with the addition of salmeterol. (Funded by the National Heart, Lung, and Blood Institute; ClinicalTrials.gov number, NCT00565266.)

▶ Since the Salmeterol Multicenter Asthma Research Trial (SMART) was ended prematurely following an interim analysis that showed an increase in asthma-related deaths and respiratory-related deaths in subjects receiving salmeterol, considerable debate ensued that has led the research community to search for additional therapeutic agents with superior or noninferior efficacy to salmeterol in poorly controlled asthmatics.[1,2] This 3-way, double-blinded, triple dummy crossover trial compared the following therapies: addition of tiotropium bromide (T) to beclomethasone (80 µg twice daily); doubling of beclomethasone dose (DB) (160 µg twice daily); and addition of salmeterol (50 µg twice daily) to beclomethasone (SB) (80 µg twice daily). The primary outcome evaluated was morning peak expiratory flow; secondary outcomes evaluated: prebronchodilator forced expiratory volume in 1 second (FEV1) and proportion of asthma-free days. Fig 3 in the original article demonstrates primary and secondary outcomes of the study. Tiotropium added to beclomethasone was superior to doubling of the dose of beclomethasone and was noninferior to salmeterol with beclomethasone. Prebronchodilator FEV1 measurements favored T over SB. Given the small number of subjects studied, the results of this study should not be used to change evidence-based guidelines for asthma. Further, large multicenter trials are warranted to ensure that the findings of this study are generalizable and warrant therapeutic change.

S. K. Willsie, DO

References

1. Nelson HS, Weiss ST, Bleecker ER, Yancey SW, Dorinsky PM, SMART Study Group. The Salmeterol Multicenter Asthma Research Trial: a comparison of usual pharmacotherapy for asthma or usual pharmacotherapy plus salmeterol. *Chest.* 2006;129:15-26.
2. Castle W, Fuller R, Hall J, Palmer J. Serevent nationwide surveillance study: comparison of salmeterol with salbutamol in asthmatic patients who require regular bronchodilator treatment. *BMJ.* 1993;306:1034-1037.

Effect of Pregnancy on Maternal Asthma Symptoms and Medication Use
Belanger K, Hellenbrand ME, Holford TR, et al (Yale Univ School of Public Health, New Haven, CT)
Obstet Gynecol 115:559-567, 2010

Objective.—To examine whether factors related to the patient or her treatment influence asthma severity during pregnancy.

Methods.—Symptom and medication data were collected by in-person and telephone interviews. Women were recruited before 24 weeks of gestation through private obstetricians and hospital clinics. Eight hundred seventy-two women had physician-diagnosed asthma, 686 were active asthmatics, and 641 with complete data were analyzed. The Global Initiative for Asthma measured severity. Cumulative logistic regression models for repeated measures assessed changes in asthma severity during each month of pregnancy.

Results.—Two factors had significant and profound effects on the course of asthma: prepregnancy severity and use of medication according to Global Initiative for Asthma guidelines. Although several factors were analyzed (race, age, atopic status, body mass index, parity, fetal sex, and smoking), none were significant risk factors for changes in asthma severity, measured in a clinically important way as a one-step change in Global Initiative for Asthma category. Women with milder asthma received most benefit from appropriate treatment, 62% decreased risk for worsening asthma among those with intermittent asthma (0.38, 95% confidence interval 0.23–0.64) and 52% decreased risk among those with mild persistent asthma (odds ratio 0.48, 95% confidence interval 0.28–0.84). Month or trimester of gestation was not consistently associated with changes in asthma severity.

Conclusion.—Asthma severity during pregnancy is similar to severity in the year before pregnancy, provided patients continue to use their prescribed medication. If women discontinue medication, even mild asthma is likely to become significantly more severe.

▶ Asthma continues to present a therapeutic challenge for providers caring for asthmatic women during pregnancy. Early investigators evaluating the impact of asthma on pregnancy promoted the prediction rule of thirds: one-third of pregnant asthmatics typically get worse during pregnancy, one-third stay the same, and the remaining one-third of asthmatics get better during pregnancy.[1,2] This prospective study of 741 women evaluated the role of prepregnancy asthma severity, race, body mass index, and use of appropriate evidence-based therapy based on severity of asthma on the impact of asthma during pregnancy. Table 2 in the original article demonstrates that 57.5% of subjects were classified prepregnancy as having intermittent asthma; 20.1%, mild persistent asthma; and 22.5%, moderate persistent asthma. Whites were more likely to have moderate/severe asthma than were blacks and Hispanics. Blacks were more likely to have mild persistent asthma, and Hispanics were more likely to have intermittent asthma prepregnancy. Increasing maternal age was associated with a greater likelihood of having moderate persistent asthma. This investigation showed that the protective effect of evidence-based therapy for asthma was greatest in the intermittent asthmatic group; the protective effect was also seen in the mild persistent asthmatic group. Subjects with moderate persistent asthma who were treated according to evidence-based guidelines enjoyed a protective effect, but this did not reach statistical significance. This investigation showed that prepregnancy asthmatic control (1 year immediately preceding pregnancy) and the use of evidence-based therapy for asthma (Global Initiative for Asthma) are 2 factors with the greatest impact on asthma outcomes during pregnancy. The results of this study shed new light on the contribution of asthma to morbidity during pregnancy. Preconception counseling for the purpose of optimizing asthma control, provision of high-quality patient education, and use of evidence-based therapy for asthma should be made a higher priority by health care providers.

S. K. Willsie, DO

References

1. Schatz M, Harden K, Forsythe A, et al. The course of asthma during pregnancy, post partum, and with successive pregnancies: a prospective analysis. *J Allergy Clin Immunol.* 1988;81:509-517.
2. Juniper EF, Newhouse MT. Effect of pregnancy on asthma: a critical appraisal of the literature. In: Schatz M, Zeiger RS, eds. *Asthma and Allergy in Pregnancy.* New York, NY: Dekker; 1993:223-492.

Written Action Plan in Pediatric Emergency Room Improves Asthma Prescribing, Adherence, and Control

Ducharme FM, Zemek RL, Chalut D, et al (Univ of Montreal, Quebec, Canada; Univ of Ottawa, Ontario, Canada; Montreal Children's Hosp, Quebec, Canada; et al)

Am J Respir Crit Care Med 183:195-203, 2011

Rationale.—An acute-care visit for asthma often signals a management failure. Although a written action plan is effective when combined with self-management education and regular medical review, its independent value remains controversial.

Objectives.—We examined the efficacy of providing a written action plan coupled with a prescription (WAP-P) to improve adherence to medications and other recommendations in a busy emergency department.

Methods.—We randomized 219 children aged 1–17 years to receive WAP-P (n = 109) or unformatted prescription (UP) (n = 110). All received fluticasone and albuterol inhalers, fitted with dose counters, to use at the discretion of the emergency physician. The main outcome was adherence to fluticasone (use/prescribed × 100%) over 28 days. Secondary outcomes included pharmacy dispensation of oral corticosteroids, β_2-agonist use, medical follow-up, asthma education, acute-care visits, and control.

Measurements and Main Results.—Although both groups showed a similar drop in adherence in the initial 14 days, adherence to fluticasone was significantly higher over Days 15–28 in children receiving WAP-P (mean group difference, 16.13% [2.09, 29.91]). More WAP-P than UP patients filled their oral corticosteroid prescription (relative risk, 1.31 [1.07, 1.60]) and were well-controlled at 28 days (1.39 [1.04, 1.86]). Compared with UP, use of WAP-P increased physicians' prescription of maintenance fluticasone (2.47 [1.53, 3.99]) and recommendation for medical follow-up (1.87 [1.48, 2.35]), without group differences in other outcomes.

Conclusions.—Provision of a written action plan significantly increased patient adherence to inhaled and oral corticosteroids and asthma control and physicians' recommendation for maintenance fluticasone and medical follow-up, supporting its independent value in the acute-care setting.

▶ Written asthma action plans have been used to improve patient and family self-knowledge and comanagement of asthma in ambulatory settings. No prior investigation has evaluated the efficacy of a written action plan in the setting of an emergency department. This investigation occurred in the setting of a single emergency department where pediatric asthmatics presented for treatment of an acute exacerbation of asthma were recruited into a study where they were randomized to receive a written action plan plus a prescription for medications compared with usual care without a written action plan. The primary outcome was the use of the inhaled corticosteroids (ICS) over 28 days; additional evaluations included filling prescription for corticosteroids, using β_2-agonists, keeping follow-up appointments, and requiring additional emergency medicine or primary care evaluations/treatment. At follow-up, 40% versus 16% (no written action plan) were still compliant with ICS (odds ratio, 3.61 [95% confidence interval, 1.86-7.02]). Eighty-two percent versus 40% (control group: no written action plan) made arrangements and kept long-term follow-up. These impressive statistics show that taking the time in the emergency department setting to provide a written action plan pays off with improved compliance and follow-up visits for asthma, following an emergency department visit for an asthma exacerbation.

S. K. Willsie, DO

Racial differences in biologic predictors of severe asthma: Data from the Severe Asthma Research Program
Gamble C, Talbott E, Youk A, et al (Univ of Pittsburgh, PA; et al)
J Allergy Clin Immunol 126:1149-1156, 2010

Background.—Biologic factors are known to contribute to asthma severity. It is unknown whether these factors differentially contribute to asthma severity in black compared with white subjects.

Objective.—We sought to assess the extent to which racial disparities between black and white subjects with severe asthma are attributable to physiologic, immunoinflammatory, and sociodemographic variables.

Methods.—Black and white asthmatic adults enrolled in a cross-sectional study focused on severe asthma were evaluated. Severe asthma was identified by using the American Thoracic Society definition. After initial univariable analyses, unconditional logistic regression models were used to estimate the probability of having severe asthma for black and white subjects.

Results.—Differences in severe asthma in black compared with white subjects were observed. In univariable analysis IgE level was not associated with severe asthma in black or white subjects, whereas in multivariable analysis IgE level was significantly associated with severe asthma for black subjects (*P* =.014) but not for white subjects. The odds of having severe asthma more than doubled for black subjects with 2 or more family members with asthma (*P* =.026), whereas the odds of severe asthma for white participants with a strong family history of asthma decreased by almost half (*P* =.05). Atopy was negatively associated with severe asthma in both races in univariable analysis but remained significant only in black subjects, whereas comorbidities were associated with severe asthma in white subjects.

Conclusion.—Biologic factors were distinctly associated with severe asthma only in black subjects. Studies that incorporate comprehensive evaluation of biologic factors associated with asthma might lead to the development of therapies that target biologic abnormalities in black subjects (Fig 1).

▶ Severe asthma in blacks is more likely to be associated with significant morbidity and mortality.[1] Blacks are diagnosed at a younger age (Fig E1 in the original article) and have 4 times the risk of hospitalization and 5 times the risk of mortality compared with whites.[2] This study evaluated whether or not biologic factors contribute to asthma severity in black subjects as compared with white subjects. Black subjects were more likely to enroll in the Severe Asthma Research Program than whites (Fig 1). Logistic regression models estimated that the odds for having severe asthma more than doubled in blacks when there were 2 or more relatives with asthma; this was about half as likely in white subjects. In multivariate, but not univariable, analysis, IgE level was significantly associated with severe asthma in blacks (*P*=.014) but not in whites. Biologic factors were distinctly associated with severe asthma only in

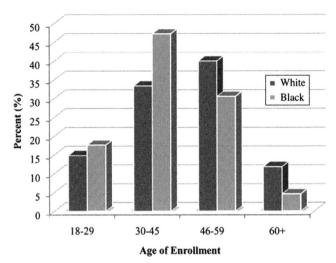

FIGURE 1.—Percentage of black and white participants enrolled into SARP by age at enrollment. Black participants enrolled into SARP at an earlier age compared with white participants (*P* = .011). (Reprinted from Gamble C, Talbott E, Youk A, et al. Racial differences in biologic predictors of severe asthma: Data from the Severe Asthma Research Program. *J Allergy Clin Immunol.* 2010;126:1149-1156, with permission from American Academy of Allergy, Asthma & Immunology.)

black subjects. In summary, severe asthma in black subjects is strongly associated with traditional markers of allergic and genetic patterns of disease. These same patterns were not seen in white subjects.

S. K. Willsie, DO

References

1. Shanawani H. Health disparities and differences in asthma: concepts and controversies. *Clin Chest Med.* 2006;27:17-28.
2. El-Ekiaby A, Brianas L, Skowronski ME, et al. Impact of race on the severity of acute episodes of asthma and adrenergic responsiveness. *Am J Respir Crit Care Med.* 2006;174:508-513.

Oral montelukast in acute asthma exacerbations: a randomised, double-blind, placebo-controlled trial
Ramsay CF, Pearson D, Mildenhall S, et al (Norfolk & Norwich Univ Hosp, UK)
Thorax 66:7-11, 2011

Background.—Although leukotriene receptor antagonists have an established role in the management of patients with chronic asthma, their efficacy in an acute asthma exacerbation is not fully known.

Methods.—87 adults with acute asthma requiring hospitalisation were randomly assigned to receive either montelukast 10 mg or placebo on admission and every evening thereafter for 4 weeks (when they were reviewed as outpatients). All patients were admitted under the care of a consultant chest physician and received full care for acute asthma according to the British Thoracic Society guidelines. The primary end point was the difference in peak expiratory flow (PEF) between active and placebo treatment the morning following admission.

Results.—Primary end point data were analysed for 73 patients. At study entry, patients who received montelukast (n=37) had a mean (±SD) PEF of 227.6 (±56.9) l/min (47.6% predicted) and those who received placebo (n=36) had a PEF of 240.3 (±99.8) l/min (49.6% predicted). The morning after admission, patients who received montelukast achieved a PEF of 389.6 (±109.7) l/min (81.4% predicted) compared with 332.3 (±124.9) l/min (69.8% predicted) for placebo (p=0.046). The mean difference between treatment groups was 57.4 l/min (95% CI of 1.15 to 113.6 l/min or 1.95–21.2% predicted).

Conclusion.—In acute asthma exacerbations the additional administration of oral montelukast results in a significantly higher PEF the morning after admission than that acheivable with current standard treatment.

Clinical Trial Number.—NCT01011452 (Fig 1).

▶ Although leukotriene modifiers have a place within evidence-based algorithms for asthma, relatively little evidence exists to suggest therapeutic efficacy for these agents in the setting of acute asthma exacerbations requiring hospitalizations. Two previous studies have evaluated the role of leukotriene receptor antagonist (LTRA) in the setting of acute asthma.[1,2] This study evaluated the role of LTRA in the setting of acute asthma requiring hospitalization; Montelukast (M) was added

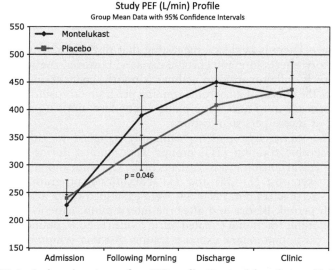

Study PEF (L/min) Profile
Group Mean Data with 95% Confidence Intervals

FIGURE 1.—Study peak expiratory flow (PEF) profile. (Reprinted from Ramsay CF, Pearson D, Mildenhall S, et al Oral montelukast in acute asthma exacerbations: a randomised, double-blind, placebo-controlled trial. *Thorax.* 2011;66:7-11 and reproduced/amended with permission from the BMJ Publishing Group.)

in additional to usual care and was compared with placebo in a randomized, double-blind, placebo-controlled trial. At baseline, 53% of subjects were taking inhaled corticosteroids (ICS). Fig 1 details the change in peak expiratory flow rate (PEFR) (subscript 1) over time; statistically significant improvement was seen in the M group versus placebo at next morning measurement ($P = .046$). There was no difference in the days of hospitalization required between groups, and the difference in PEFR was not statistically significant at hospital discharge or at 4-week follow-up. The investigators suggest that it seems reasonable to use M routinely in the inpatient setting of asthma exacerbation, though the number of subjects enrolled in the trial fell short of recruitment plans, and the P value for next morning peak expiratory flow barely met statistical significance. It seems that this recommendation has not yet met the reasonable standard for efficacy. More studies are needed with larger numbers of patients to determine whether or not reduced hospitalization may result from use of M in addition to usual care.

S. K. Willsie, DO

References

1. Ferreira MB, Santos AS, Pregal AL, et al. Leukotriene receptor antagonists (Montelukast) in the treatment of asthma crisis: preliminary results of a double-blind placebo controlled randomized study. *Allerg Immunol (Paris)*. 2001;33: 315-318.
2. Cýllý A, Kara A, Ozdemir T, Oğüş C, Gülkesen KH. Effects of oral montelukast on airway function in acute asthma. *Respir Med.* 2003;97:533-536.

Effects of Aerobic Training on Airway Inflammation in Asthmatic Patients

Mendes FAR, Almeida FM, Cukier A, et al (Univ of São Paulo, Brazil)
Med Sci Sports Exerc 43:197-203, 2011

Purpose.—There is evidence suggesting that physical activity has anti-inflammatory effects in many chronic diseases; however, the role of exercise in airway inflammation in asthma is poorly understood. We aimed to evaluate the effects of an aerobic training program on eosinophil inflammation (primary aim) and nitric oxide (secondary aim) in patients with moderate or severe persistent asthma.

Methods.—Sixty-eight patients randomly assigned to either control (CG) or aerobic training (TG) groups were studied during the period between medical consultations. Patients in the CG (educational program + breathing exercises; $N = 34$) and TG (educational program + breathing exercises + aerobic training; $N = 34$) were examined twice a week during a 3-month period. Before and after the intervention, patients underwent induced sputum, fractional exhaled nitric oxide (FeNO), pulmonary function, and cardiopulmonary exercise testing. Asthma symptom-free days were quantified monthly, and asthma exacerbation was monitored during 3 months of intervention.

Results.—At 3 months, decreases in the total and eosinophil cell counts in induced sputum ($P = 0.004$) and in the levels of FeNO ($P = 0.009$) were observed after intervention only in the TG. The number of asthma symptom-free days and $\dot{V}O_{2max}$ also significantly improved ($P < 0.001$), and lower asthma exacerbation occurred in the TG ($P < 0.01$). In addition, the TG presented a strong positive relationship between baseline FeNO and eosinophil counts as well as their improvement after training ($r = 0.77$ and $r = 0.9$, respectively).

Conclusions.—Aerobic training reduces sputum eosinophil and FeNO in patients with moderate or severe asthma, and these benefits were more significant in subjects with higher levels of inflammation. These results suggest that aerobic training might be useful as an adjuvant therapy in asthmatic patients under optimized medical treatment.

▶ Limited studies have shown protective effect of aerobic exercise in patients with asthma.[1,2] This provocative study of patients with moderate to severe persistent asthma demonstrated reduced airway inflammation (via sputum cell counts, fractional exhaled nitric oxide [FeNO]) and an increase in symptom-free days in patients with asthma randomized to receive aerobic training in addition to education and respiratory exercises undertaken by the control group. Fig 4 in the original article demonstrates asthma-free days, showing statistically significant increase in symptom-free asthma days after 30, 60, and 90 days of aerobic exercise. Fig 3 in the original article displays FeNO levels in the aerobic exercise group versus control group, demonstrating a statistically significant reduction in the aerobic exercise group versus control group. This is one of the first studies to demonstrate reduced airway inflammation following aerobic exercise. Furthermore, large-scale studies are warranted to confirm this effect in a widely diverse asthmatic population.

S. K. Willsie, DO

References

1. Fanelli A, Cabral AL, Neder JA, Martins MA, Carvalho CR. Exercise training on disease control and quality of life in asthmatic children. *Med Sci Sports Exerc.* 2007;39:1474-1480.
2. Neder JA, Nery LE, Silva AC, Cabral AL, Fernandes AL. Short-term effects of aerobic training in the clinical management of moderate to severe asthma in children. *Thorax.* 1999;54:202-206.

Comparison of the Effect of Low-Dose Ciclesonide and Fixed-Dose Fluticasone Propionate and Salmeterol Combination on Long-Term Asthma Control

Postma DS, O'Byrne PM, Pedersen S (Univ of Groningen, The Netherlands; McMaster Univ, Hamilton, Ontario, Canada; Univ of Odense, Kolping, Denmark)
Chest 139:311-318, 2011

Background.—Patients with mild persistent asthma constitute about 70% of the asthma population; thus, it is important to know which first-line treatment is best for the management of mild asthma. We compared benefits of first-line treatment with ciclesonide and a combination of fluticasone and salmeterol in patients with mild asthma.

Methods.—Patients aged 12 to 75 years with mild persistent asthma were enrolled in a randomized, double-blind, placebo-controlled study. After run-in, patients were randomized to ciclesonide 160 μg once daily (CIC160), fluticasone propionate/salmeterol 100/50 μg bid (FP200/S100), or placebo for 52 weeks. The primary variable was time to first severe asthma exacerbation; the coprimary variable was the percentage of poorly controlled asthma days. Patients recorded asthma symptoms and salbutamol use in electronic diaries and completed a standardized version of the Asthma Quality of Life Questionnaire.

Results.—Compared with placebo, the time to first severe asthma exacerbation was prolonged, and lung function was improved with FP200/S100 treatment ($P = .0002$) but not with CIC160. Both CIC160 and FP200/S100 provided significantly fewer poorly controlled asthma days than placebo ($P \leq .0016$ for both active treatments). Moreover, both active treatments provided significantly more asthma symptom-free days ($P \leq .0001$), rescue medication-free days ($P = .0005$, one-sided), and days with asthma control ($P \leq .0033$). Overall Asthma Quality of Life Questionnaire scores were significantly higher in both active treatment groups than placebo ($P \leq .0017$).

Conclusions.—In mild asthma, FP200/S100 prolonged time to first severe asthma exacerbation, and CIC160 and FP200/S100 were clinically equieffective for most measures of asthma control.

Trial Registry.—ClinicalTrials.gov; No.: NCT00163358; URL: www. clinicaltrials.gov (Table 3).

▶ This is a study of patients with mild persistent asthma, comparing treatment with placebo, fluticasone (F)/salmeterol (S) (100/50 μg twice a day), and ciclesonide (C) (160 μg once daily). Outcomes measured included time to first exacerbation, asthma symptom–free days, and rescue medication–free days. Fig 2 in the original article depicts time to first exacerbation, and Fig 3 in the original article demonstrates asthma symptom–free days; the latter reflects equivalence between F/S and C. Table 3 shows adverse events seen in all 3 groups of subjects (C, F/S, and placebo). Given the status of the current guidelines for asthma care, it seems reasonable that the C represents an equivalent

TABLE 3.—Frequently Reported Adverse Events in the Safety Population (≥5% of Patients in Any Treatment Group)

Adverse Event	CIC160 (n = 210)	FP200/S100 (n = 222)	Placebo (n = 220)
Asthma	61 (29.0)	37 (16.7)	73 (33.2)
Nasopharyngitis	38 (18.1)	29 (13.1)	32 (14.5)
Pharyngitis	16 (7.6)	14 (6.3)	23 (10.5)
Bronchitis acute	14 (6.7)	14 (6.3)	11 (5.0)
Upper respiratory tract infection	14 (6.7)	13 (5.9)	13 (5.9)

Data are presented as No. (%). See Table 1 legend for expansion of abbreviations.

treatment and should be expected to control most asthma-related steps, presuming that the dose prescribed is correct and patient technique is appropriate. When asthma fails to stabilize on monotherapy, it seems reasonable to switch to a combined inhaled corticosteroid and long-acting β-agonist product.

S. K. Willsie, DO

Safety of formoterol in children and adolescents: experience from asthma clinical trials
Price JF, Radner F, Lenney W, et al (King's College Hosp, London, UK; AstraZeneca R&D, Lund, Sweden; Univ Hosp of North Staffordshire, Stoke on Trent, UK)
Arch Dis Child 95:1047-1053, 2010

Background.—The safety of long-acting β_2 agonist (LABA) therapy in asthma remains controversial but no large scale analyses have been published of LABA safety in children.

Methods.—The frequency of asthma-related deaths and hospitalisations following formoterol use in children (4–11 years) and adolescents (12–17 years), compared with non-LABA treatment, was assessed in all AstraZeneca-sponsored, randomised, controlled, parallel-group trials (≥3 months) where formoterol was used as maintenance and/or as reliever therapy.

Results.—11 849 children and adolescents under the age of 18 years from 41 trials were identified, 82% of whom used an inhaled corticosteroid (ICS) as concomitant medication. The number of asthma-related deaths (one 13-year-old boy among 7796 formoterol-treated patients, and none among 4053 non-LABA-treated patients) was too low to allow any between-group comparison. The frequency of patients with asthma-related hospitalisations was not different in formoterol-treated versus non-LABA-treated patients, either in children (1.16% (38/3263) vs 1.11% (24/2165)) or in adolescents (0.51% (23/4533) vs 0.85% (16/1888)). Asthma-related hospitalisations based on daily dose of formoterol were: (A) 4.5 or 9 µg: 1.9% (18/980); (B) 18 µg: 0.5% (14/2870); (C) 36 µg: 0% (0/67); and (D) variable dosing: 0.75% (29/3879). There was no difference between formoterol-treated and non-LABA-treated patients as regards ethnicity.

Conclusions.—Formoterol use in children and adolescents (4–17 years) with asthma in this large study where the majority are prescribed concomitant ICS is not associated with any increased risk of asthma-related hospitalisations. The results are not influenced by dose or ethnicity (Table 4).

▶ This is a compilation of all Astra-Zeneca trials comparing formoterol (F) use in children aged 4 to 11 years and 12 to 17 years with non–long-acting β-agonist (non-LABA) treatment in which F was used as a maintenance and/or reliever therapy. Nearly 12 000 children and adolescents were identified; 82% of these children received concomitant treatment with an inhaled

TABLE 4.—Incidence of Adverse Events (Serious and Non-Serious) Belonging to the System Organ Classes 'Cardiac Disorders' and 'Vascular Disorders' and of the Preferred Term 'Tremor' in Trials with LABA as well as Non-LABA Treatment Arms (Mantel–Haenszel Dataset)

Preferred Term	Number (%) of Patients Reporting at Least One AE	
	FORM (N=5354)	Non-LABA (N=4053)
Arrhythmia	0	1 (0.02)
Arrhythmia, supraventricular	0	1 (0.02)
Atrioventricular block, second degree	1 (0.02)	0
Palpitations	7 (0.13)	2 (0.05)
Rheumatic heart disease	0	1 (0.02)
Sinus arrhythmia	1 (0.02)	0
Sinus tachycardia	0	1 (0.02)
Supraventricular extrasystoles	1 (0.02)	0
Tachycardia	6 (0.11)	4 (0.10)
Ventricular extrasystoles	1 (0.02)	1 (0.02)
Ventricular hypertrophy	1 (0.02)	1 (0.02)
Ventricular tachycardia	0	1 (0.02)
Wolff–Parkinson–White syndrome	2 (0.04)	0
Hypotension	1 (0.02)	1 (0.02)
Vasoconstriction	1 (0.02)	0
Tremor	35 (0.65)	9 (0.22)

AE, adverse event; FORM, formoterol; LABA, long-lasting β antagonist.

corticosteroid (ICS). There was no difference in asthma-related deaths between F and non-LABA groups (1 vs 0). Adverse events in both groups are detailed in Table 4. Use of F in this group of children and adolescents did not appear to be associated with increased risk of asthma-related hospitalizations. It must be noted that 82% of subjects were receiving concomitant therapy with ICS. Results did not appear to be influenced by race or ethnicity.

S. K. Willsie, DO

Factors predicting inhaled corticosteroid responsiveness in African American patients with asthma

Gould W, Peterson EL, Karungi G, et al (Henry Ford Health System, Detroit, MI; et al)
J Allergy Clin Immunol 126:1131-1138, 2010

Background.—African American patients disproportionately experience uncontrolled asthma. Treatment with an inhaled corticosteroid (ICS) is considered first-line therapy for persistent asthma.

Objective.—We sought to determine the degree to which African American patients respond to ICS medication and whether the level of response is influenced by other factors, including genetic ancestry.

Methods.—Patients aged 12 to 56 years who received care from a large health system in southeast Michigan and who resided in Detroit were recruited to participate if they had a diagnosis of asthma. Patients were treated with 6 weeks of inhaled beclomethasone dipropionate, and pulmonary function was remeasured after treatment. Ancestry was determined by genotyping ancestry-informative markers. The main outcome measure was ICS responsiveness defined as the change in prebronchodilator FEV_1 over the 6-week course of treatment.

Results.—Among 147 participating African American patients with asthma, average improvement in FEV_1 after 6 weeks of ICS treatment was 11.6%. The mean proportion of African ancestry in this group was 78.4%. The degree of baseline bronchodilator reversibility was the only factor consistently associated with ICS responsiveness, as measured by both an improvement in FEV_1 and patient-reported asthma control ($P = .001$ and $P = .021$, respectively). The proportion of African ancestry was not significantly associated with ICS responsiveness.

Conclusions.—Although baseline pulmonary function parameters appear to be associated with the likelihood to respond to ICS treatment, the proportion of genetic African ancestry does not. This study suggests that genetic ancestry might not contribute to differences in ICS controller response among African American patients with asthma (Fig 1).

▶ African Americans with asthma are more likely to have poorly controlled asthma as evidenced by higher rates of asthma-related emergency department visits, hospitalizations, and deaths than their white counterparts.[1] A wide variety of reasons[2-5] have been hypothesized as accounting for racial disparities in asthma, including reduced responsiveness to inhaled corticosteroids (ICSs).[6] This investigation sought to evaluate responsiveness to ICS therapy and the factors responsive to the treatment, including the role played by genetic

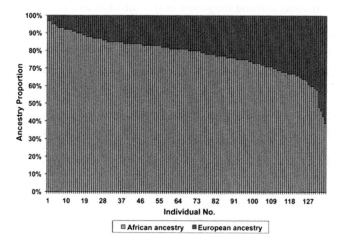

FIGURE 1.—Distribution of African *(blue)* and European *(purple)* ancestry for African American patients with asthma who completed 6 weeks of ICS therapy. Genetic ancestry was estimated in 135 of the 147 participants who completed therapy. For interpretation of the references to color in this figure legend, the reader is referred to web version of this article. (Reprinted from Gould W, Peterson EL, Karungi G, et al. Factors predicting inhaled corticosteroid responsiveness in African American patients with asthma. *J Allergy Clin Immunol.* 2010;126:1131-1138, with permission from American Academy of Allergy, Asthma & Immunology.)

ancestry. Fig 1 demonstrates the contribution of African and European ancestry in African American subjects with asthma who completed 6 weeks of ICS therapy in this study. The proportion of African ancestry was not associated with response to ICS. A consistent relationship was observed between baseline bronchodilator responsiveness and ICS responsiveness. The investigators hypothesize that there are other important determinants of ICS responsibility in these asthmatic subjects. Further trials of minority subjects are needed to determine key factors responsible for racial variations in responsiveness to ICS.

S. K. Willsie, DO

References

1. Moorman JE, Rudd RA, Johnson CA, et al. National surveillance for asthma—United States, 1980-2004. *MMWR Surveill Summ.* 2007;56:1-54.
2. Yang JJ, Burchard EG, Choudhry S, et al. Differences in allergic sensitization by self-reported race and genetic ancestry. *J Allergy Clin Immunol.* 2008;122:820-827.
3. Joseph CL, Ownby DR, Peterson EL, Johnson CC. Racial differences in physiologic parameters related to asthma among middle-class children. *Chest.* 2000; 117:1336-1344.
4. Gelber LE, Seltzer LH, Bouzoukis JK, Pollart SM, Chapman MD, Platts-Mills TA. Sensitization and exposure to indoor allergens as risk factors for asthma among patients presenting to hospital. *Am Rev Respir Dis.* 1993;147:573-578.
5. Rosenstreich DL, Eggleston P, Kattan M, et al. The role of cockroach allergy and exposure to cockroach allergen in causing morbidity among inner-city children with asthma. *N Engl J Med.* 1997;336:1356-1363.
6. Federico MJ, Covar RA, Brown EE, Leung DY, Spahn JD. Racial differences in T-lymphocyte response to glucocorticoids. *Chest.* 2005;127:571-578.

Advances in adult asthma diagnosis and treatment and HEDQ in 2010

Apter AJ (Univ of Pennsylvania, Philadelphia)
J Allergy Clin Immunol 127:116-122, 2011

This summary reviews research published over the past year on asthma and through the prism of health care delivery and quality. Special attention is given to management, therapeutics, and the role of environmental exposures and their interactions with genetics. The discussion is framed around the 3 stages of translational research: from bench to first studies in human subjects, then to larger efficacy studies in well-defined patient populations, and finally into practice through effectiveness research in real-world settings (Fig 1).

▶ This is a must-read just published in the *Journal of Allergy and Clinical Immunology*. The template upon which a discussion of recent literature is reviewed is outlined in Fig 1; this review is focused on the role of bench to bedside research, translation of bench research to patients, and application of research to real world medicine, inclusive of best evidence. Key highlights include the Food and Drug Administration's more restrictive labeling of long-acting β-agonists' (LABAs) use in asthma. LABAs are to be used with anti-inflammatory therapy but not necessarily inhaled corticosteroids (ICSs).[1,2] Focus on the potential

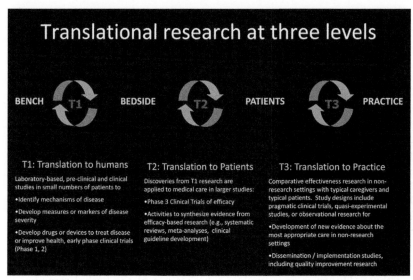

FIGURE 1.—Translational research trajectory along 3 continuous and overlapping levels: *T1*, the translation of knowledge from the laboratory to initial studies in patients; *T2*, larger studies, including clinical trials examining efficacy in patients under tightly controlled conditions; and *T3*, research, including CER, investigating how the findings of efficacy are disseminated and implemented in real-world and varied practice settings.[12,14] (Courtesy of Jerry A. Krishnan, MD, PhD.) *Editor's Note*: Please refer to original journal article for full references. (Reprinted from Apter AJ. Advances in adult asthma diagnosis and treatment and HEDQ in 2010. *J Allergy Clin Immunol*. 2011;127:116-122.)

risks of using LABAs has brought about increased study of alternative agents. A crossover study of the long-acting anticholinergic agent, tiotropium (T), with low-dose ICS versus double dosing of the low-dose ICS was favorable to T and showed noninferiority versus addition of salmeterol (LABA) to the low-dose ICS.[3] Evaluation of the role of statins[4] showed that addition of simvastatin to placebo demonstrated statin-treated sputum eosinophil counts were reduced, the steroid effect on interleukin 10 was enhanced, and some of the corticosteroid-inhibiting effects on inflammatory markers were increased. More research is needed to demonstrate safety and improved efficacy of statins in the setting of asthma, particularly given the morbidity seen with use in the general population. Of considerable interest and relevance is a study showing that lowered levels of vitamin D are associated with higher odds of any hospitalization or emergency department visit.[5] In addition, a number of environmental and socioeconomic studies are reviewed. This is a must-read for any clinician caring for patients with asthma.

S. K. Willsie, DO

References

1. Chowdhury BA, Dal Pan G. The FDA and safe use of long-acting beta-agonists in the treatment of asthma. *N Engl J Med*. 2010;362:1169-1171.
2. Riley K, Jefferson E. FDA Announces New Safety Controls for Long-Acting Beta Agonists, Medications Used to Treat Asthma, http://www.fda.gov/NewsEvents/Newsroom/PressAnnouncements/ucm200931.htm. Accessed March 15, 2011.

3. Peters SP, Kunselman SJ, Icitovic N, et al. Tiotropium bromide step-up therapy for adults with uncontrolled asthma. *N Engl J Med.* 2010;363:1715-1726.
4. Maneechotesuwan K, Ekjiratrakul W, Kasetsinsombat K, Wongkajornsilp A, Barnes PJ. Statins enhance the anti-inflammatory effects of inhaled corticosteroids in asthmatic patients through increased induction of indoleamine 2, 3-dioxygenase. *J Allergy Clin Immunol.* 2010;126:754-762.
5. Brehm JM, Schuemann B, Fuhlbigger AL, et al. Serum Vitamin D levels and severe asthma exacerbations in the Childhood Asthma Management Program Study. *J Allergy Clin Immunol.* 2010;126:52-58.

Use of herbal remedies and adherence to inhaled corticosteroids among inner-city asthmatic patients

Roy A, Lurslurchachai L, Halm EA, et al (Mount Sinai School of Medicine, NY; Univ of Texas Southwestern Med Ctr, Dallas; et al)
Ann Allergy Asthma Immunol 104:132-138, 2010

Background.—Complementary and alternative medicines (CAM), such as herbal remedies, are widely used by patients with chronic diseases, such as asthma. However, it is unclear whether use of the herbal remedies is associated with decreased adherence to inhaled corticosteroids (ICSs), a key component of asthma management.

Objective.—To examine the association among use of herbal remedies, adherence to prescribed ICSs, and medication and disease beliefs.

Methods.—We surveyed 326 adults with persistent asthma who received care at 2 inner-city outpatient clinics. Patients were asked about CAM use (teas, herbs, and rubs) for the treatment of asthma in the prior 6 months. Medication adherence was assessed using the Medication Adherence Report Scale, a validated self-report measure. Univariate and multiple regression analyses were used to assess the relationship among herbal remedy use, adherence to ICSs, and medication and disease beliefs.

Results.—Overall, 25.4% (95% confidence interval, 20%–30%) of patients reported herbal remedy use. Univariate analyses showed that herbal remedy use was associated with decreased ICS adherence and increased asthma morbidity. In multivariable analysis, herbal remedy use was associated with lower ICS adherence (odds ratio, 0.4; 95% confidence interval, 0.2–0.8) after adjusting for confounders. Herbal remedy users were also more likely to worry about the adverse effects of ICSs ($P = .01$).

Conclusions.—The use of herbal remedies was associated with lower adherence to ICSs and worse outcomes among inner-city asthmatic patients. Medication beliefs, such as worry about ICS adverse effects, may in part mediate this relationship. Physicians should routinely ask patients with asthma about CAM use, especially those whose asthma is poorly controlled (Table 2).

▶ Poor adherence to medication regimens has been associated with worsened morbidity in asthmatics.[1,2] This investigation surveyed persistent asthmatics receiving care in 2 inner-city ambulatory care centers about use of complementary

TABLE 2.—Results of Multivariable Analyses of Predictors of Adherence to Inhaled Corticosteroids

Variable	Odds Ratio (95% Confidence Interval)
Use of herbal remedies	0.4 (0.2–0.8)
Age	1.0 (0.9–1.0)
Female sex	1.4 (0.7–2.9)
Race	
White	Reference
Black	0.5 (0.2–1.4)
Latino	0.3 (0.1–0.9)
Other	0.5 (0.1–2.2)
High school graduate	2.3 (1.3–4.1)
Time with asthma	1.0 (0.9–1.0)
History of oral steroid use	1.0 (0.5–2.0)
History of intubation	1.6 (0.7–3.7)
English as a native language	0.6 (0.3–1.2)
Comorbidities	
Sinusitis	1.1 (0.6–2.1)
Allergies	1.1 (0.6–1.9)
Depression	0.8 (0.4–1.5)
Anxiety	0.9 (0.4–1.6)

and alternative medicines (CAM). Quality of life and adherence to inhaled corticosteroid (ICS) therapy were also assessed. Of the patients surveyed, 25.4% reported use of CAM; less than 40% had disclosed their use of CAM to their medical provider. CAM use was associated with lower quality of life and difficulty following medication regimens ($P = .001$), and morbidity was increased in CAM users ($P = .01$). Most individuals reporting use of CAM expressed concerns about the effects of ICS ($P = .001$). Table 2 displays a multivariate analysis of predictors of adherence to ICS treatment. The adjusted odds of ICS adherence among herbal remedy users were less than half of those of nonusers (odds ratio, 0.4; 95% confidence interval, 0.2-0.8). All health care providers should inquire about the use of CAM therapies and explore ways to reduce barriers to adherence to medical regimens.

As an aside, adaptive use of selected concepts of appreciative inquiry, traditionally considered an organizational technique for fostering collaborative relationships, may assist providers in removing barriers to open patient-provider communication and foster collaborative care planning. Appreciative inquiry has been shown to assist in reducing critical and problem-focused inquiries.[3]

S. K. Willsie, DO

References

1. Halm EA, Mora P, Leventhal H. No symptoms, no asthma: the acute episodic disease belief is associated with poor self-management among inner-city adults with persistent asthma. *Chest.* 2006;129:573-580.
2. Horne R. Compliance, adherence, and concordance: implications for asthma treatment. *Chest.* 2006;130:65S-72S.
3. Ludema J. *From Deficit Discourse to Vocabularies of Hope: The Power of Appreciation. Appreciative Inquiry: An Emerging Direction for Organization Development.* 1st ed. Champaign, IL: Stipes Publishing L.L.C., 2001.

Step-up Therapy for Children with Uncontrolled Asthma Receiving Inhaled Corticosteroids

Lemanske RF Jr, for the Childhood Asthma Research and Education (CARE) Network of the National Heart, Lung, and Blood Institute (Univ of Wisconsin School of Medicine and Public Health, Madison; et al)
N Engl J Med 362:975-985, 2010

Background.—For children who have uncontrolled asthma despite the use of low-dose inhaled corticosteroids (ICS), evidence to guide step-up therapy is lacking.

Methods.—We randomly assigned 182 children (6 to 17 years of age), who had uncontrolled asthma while receiving 100 μg of fluticasone twice daily, to receive each of three blinded step-up therapies in random order for 16 weeks: 250 μg of fluticasone twice daily (ICS step-up), 100 μg of fluticasone plus 50 μg of a long-acting beta-agonist twice daily (LABA step-up), or 100 μg of fluticasone twice daily plus 5 or 10 mg of a leukotriene-receptor antagonist daily (LTRA step-up). We used a triple-cross-over design and a composite of three outcomes (exacerbations, asthma-control days, and the forced expiratory volume in 1 second) to determine whether the frequency of a differential response to the step-up regimens was more than 25%.

Results.—A differential response occurred in 161 of 165 patients who were evaluated (P<0.001). The response to LABA step-up therapy was most likely to be the best response, as compared with responses to LTRA step-up (relative probability, 1.6; 95% confidence interval [CI], 1.1 to 2.3; P = 0.004) and ICS step-up (relative probability, 1.7; 95% CI, 1.2 to 2.4; P = 0.002). Higher scores on the Asthma Control Test before randomization (indicating better control at baseline) predicted a better response to LABA step-up (P = 0.009). White race predicted a better response to LABA step-up, whereas black patients were least likely to have a best response to LTRA step-up (P = 0.005).

Conclusions.—Nearly all the children had a differential response to each step-up therapy. LABA step-up was significantly more likely to provide the best response than either ICS or LTRA step-up. However, many children had a best response to ICS or LTRA step-up therapy, highlighting the need to regularly monitor and appropriately adjust each child's asthma therapy. (ClinicalTrials.gov number, NCT00395304.)

▶ This is a multicenter, 3-way crossover, placebo-controlled trial in children with uncontrolled asthma (on 100 μg of fluticasone twice a day) evaluating response to 3 different step-up treatments: higher dose fluticasone (250 μg twice a day) (inhaled corticosteroids [ICS]); long-acting beta-agonist (LABA) group (50 μg salmeterol twice a day) + ICS (100 μg twice a day); and leukotriene-receptor antagonist (LTRA) group (5-10 mg montelukast daily) + ICS (100 μg fluticasone twice a day). Primary outcome evaluated was the differential response to each of the 3 different step-up treatment groups based on need for oral prednisone to treat acute asthma exacerbations, number of asthma-control days, and forced expiratory volume in 1 second. Fig 2 in the original article demonstrates pairwise comparison to different step-up treatments according to randomization group. Fig 4 in the original article demonstrates that race was a significant predictor of best response to treatment ($P = .005$). Hispanics and non-Hispanic whites had the best response to the LABA step-up treatment and were least likely to respond to the ICS step-up. Blacks were equally likely to have best response to LABA and ICS step-up treatments and least likely to have best response to LTRA step-up therapy. Subjects who lacked eczema and those with higher response to the Asthma Control Tests were most likely to have best response to LABA step-up treatment. Interestingly, genotype did not correlate with pattern of response to step-up treatment. The results of this study add considerably to the literature's evidence base assisting providers with choice of therapy for asthmatic children who remain uncontrolled on low-dose ICS.

S. K. Willsie, DO

Cost-effectiveness analysis of fluticasone versus montelukast in children with mild-to-moderate persistent asthma in the Pediatric Asthma Controller Trial
Wang L, Hollenbeak CS, Mauger DT, et al (Pennsylvania State Univ College of Medicine, Hershey; et al)
J Allergy Clin Immunol 127:161-166, 2011

Background.—Cost-effectiveness analyses of asthma controller regimens for adults exist, but similar evaluations exclusively for children are few.

Objective.—We sought to compare the cost-effectiveness of 2 commonly used asthma controllers, fluticasone and montelukast, with data from the Pediatric Asthma Controller Trial.

Methods.—We compared the cost-effectiveness of low-dose fluticasone with that of montelukast in a randomized, controlled, multicenter clinical trial in children with mild-to-moderate persistent asthma. Analyses were also conducted on subgroups based on phenotypic factors. Effectiveness measures included (1) the number of asthma-control days, (2) the percentage of participants with an increase over baseline of FEV_1 of 12% or greater, and (3) the number of exacerbations avoided. Costs were analyzed from both a US health care payer's perspective and a societal perspective.

Results.—For all cost-effectiveness measures studied, fluticasone cost less and was more effective than montelukast. For example, fluticasone treatment cost \$430 less in mean direct cost ($P < .01$) and resulted in 40 more asthma-control days ($P < .01$) during the 48-week study period. Considering sampling uncertainty, fluticasone cost less and was more effective at least 95% of the time. For the high exhaled nitric oxide (eNO) phenotypic subgroup (eNO ≥ 25 ppb) and more responsive PC_{20} subgroup (PC_{20} <2 mg/mL), fluticasone was cost-effective compared

TABLE 2.—Comparison of Demographic and Outcome Features Between Fluticasone and Montelukast

Variable	Fluticasone (n = 79)	Montelukast (n = 75)	P value
Age (y), mean ± SD	9.7 ± 2.2	9.7 ± 2.2	.94*
Sex, no. (%)			
Male	47 (59)	48 (64)	.57†
Female	32 (41)	27 (36)	
Height increase in cm, mean ± SD	5.4 ± 1.8	5.8 ± 1.9	.16*
Baseline FEV_1, mean ± SD	1.86 ± 0.56	1.96 ± 0.536	.24*
Baseline eNO (ppb), median (quartile 1-quartile 3)	24.5 (13.0-48.5)	29.4 (12.7-55.4)	.82‡
Baseline methacholine PC_{20} (mg/mL), median (quartile 1-quartile 3)	0.76 (0.27-2.81)	0.85 (0.28-2.57)	.95‡
Outcomes (mean ± SD)			
Treatment exposure days	336 ± 17.6	338 ± 19.8	.49*
ACDs during study period	210 ± 97	170 ± 90	.009*
Percentage with an increase of FEV_1 ≥12%	73	41	<.001†
No. of exacerbations	0.66 ± 0.9	1.13 ± 1.1	.002§
Emergency department visits	0.10 ± 0.3	0.35 ± 0.6	.002§
Physician's office visits	2.19 ± 1.9	2.08 ± 1.8	.64§
Hospital days	0	0	NA
Missed school days	1.4 ± 2.5	2.1 ± 3.1	<.001§
Missed work days	0.6 ± 1.5	0.8 ± 1.9	.06§

*Two-sample t tests for difference in mean.
†Two-sample z tests for proportions.
‡Mann-Whitney U test for difference in median.
§Simple Poisson regression with the treatment group as the predictor.

with montelukast for all cost-effectiveness measures, whereas not all the effectiveness measures were statistically different for the other 2 phenotypic subgroups.

Conclusion.—For children with mild-to-moderate persistent asthma, low-dose fluticasone had lower cost and higher effectiveness compared with montelukast, especially in those with more airway inflammation, as indicated by increased levels of eNO and more responsivity to methacholine (Table 2).

▶ This is a cost-effectiveness study comparing Montelukast with inhaled fluticasone (IF) in children with mild to moderate persistent asthma, particularly those with greater inflammation (as reflected by increased nitric oxide levels). IF led to more asthma-controlled days, greater improvements in forced expiratory volume in the first second of expiration, and less asthma exacerbations (Table 2) at lower direct costs and reduced societal costs (less missed work and school). This study supports tenets of the National Asthma Education and Prevention Program, which supports inhaled corticosteroids as the preferred asthma controller therapy for mild to moderate persistent asthma in children.

S. K. Willsie, DO

Efficacy and safety of ciclesonide in the treatment of 24,037 asthmatic patients in routine medical care

Vogelmeier CF, Hering T, Lewin T, et al (Univ of Marburg, Baldingerstraße, Germany; Pneumology Practice, Schloßstr, Berlin (Tegel), Germany; Nycomed Deutschland GmbH, Moltkestraße, Konstanz, Germany)
Respir Med 105:186-194, 2011

Background.—The efficacy and safety profile of ciclesonide (CIC) in the treatment of asthma was evaluated in a large patient population in a real-life setting in Germany.

Methods.—24,037 patients with persistent mild/moderate bronchial asthma were enrolled into three observational studies with identical design. Data were pooled and analyzed. Patients received ciclesonide (160 µg/day) and were observed for 3 months. FEV_1, PEF, NO, asthma episodes, use of rescue medication and adverse drug reactions (ADR) were recorded.

Results.—Mean (95% CI) FEV_1 significantly increased from 80.7 [80.5; 80.9]% of predicted at baseline to 90.1 [89.9; 90.2]% after 3 months ($n = 20,297$), mean PEF significantly increased from 338 [335; 340] l/min to 392 [390; 395] l/min ($n = 8100$). NO was significantly reduced from 53.6 [51.8; 55.4] ppb to 26.2 [25.2; 27.1] ppb ($n = 971$). The percentage of patients with daily symptoms declined from 24.3% to 1.9%, night-time symptoms from 13.3% to 1.3%, and β_2-agonists use from 26.9% to 8.8%. ADRs were reported by 51 patients (0.2%). Most frequent ADRs were: dysphonia ($n = 11$), cough ($n = 10$), dyspnoea, throat irritation, and oral candidiasis ($n = 5$ each). 46 patients terminated the study prematurely, 41 due to ADR and 5 due to unknown/missing reason. One patient died due to cardiac failure (no causal relation).

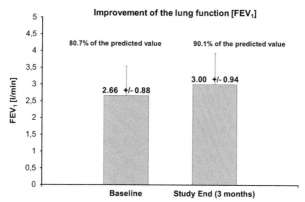

FIGURE 1.—Improvement of the lung function with once daily 160 µg ciclesonide. Data presented are mean values (standard deviation) of FEV1 [l] (*N* = 19,953) and % of the predicted value (*N* = 20,297) from patients with complete data at both visits. (Reprinted from Vogelmeier CF, Hering T, Lewin T, et al. Efficacy and safety of ciclesonide in the treatment of 24,037 asthmatic patients in routine medical care. *Respir Med.* 2011;105:186-194, with permission from Elsevier.)

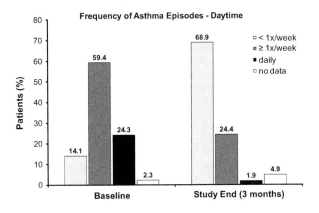

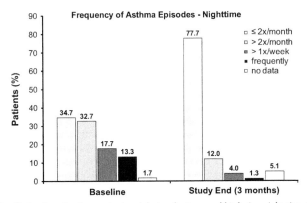

FIGURE 2.—Reduction of asthma episodes a) during daytime, and b) during night-time ($N = 24,037$). (Reprinted from Vogelmeier CF, Hering T, Lewin T, et al. Efficacy and safety of ciclesonide in the treatment of 24,037 asthmatic patients in routine medical care. *Respir Med*. 2011;105:186-194, with permission from Elsevier.)

Conclusion.—These observational studies under real-life conditions support findings from controlled clinical studies regarding efficacy and tolerability of ciclesonide in patients with mild to moderate bronchial asthma. No unexpected ADRs were detected (Figs 1 and 2).

▶ The results of pooling of 3 prospective, open-label, observational trials of 160 μg of ciclesonide inhaled daily for 3 months in > 24 000 patients with mild to moderate asthma are presented. Fig 1 demonstrates improvement in baseline forced expiratory volume in the first second of expiration from 80.7% to 90.1% following 3 months of therapy. Fig 2 details the occurrence of asthma episodes during the daytime and nighttime hours, showing a statistically significant reduction in asthmatic episodes on treatment with ciclesonide. The proportion of patients with asthma who had daily daytime asthma episodes dropped from 24.3% to 1.9%. Subjects experiencing nighttime asthma episodes reduced from 13.3% to 1.3%. Importantly, only 0.2% demonstrated any adverse events (AEs) compared with 4% of subjects in randomized trials who experienced AEs. The 2 most commonly reported AEs were dysphonia and cough. Oral candidiasis was noted in 5 of > 24 000 subjects. Forty-six subjects discontinued ciclesonide because of a probably or definite causal relation of symptoms related to ciclesonide (< 0.2% of subjects). The investigators state in their conclusion that ciclesonide is appropriate for first-line treatment of asthma.

S. K. Willsie, DO

Efficacy and Safety of Subcutaneous Omalizumab vs Placebo as Add-on Therapy to Corticosteroids for Children and Adults With Asthma: A Systematic Review
Rodrigo GJ, Neffen H, Castro-Rodriguez JA (Hosp Central de las Fuerzas Armadas, Montevideo, Uruguay; Hosp de Niños "O. Allassia," Santa Fe, Argentina; Pontificia Universidad Católica de Chile, Santiago, Chile)
Chest 139:28-35, 2011

Background.—Omalizumab is a humanized monoclonal anti-IgE for the treatment of severe allergic asthma. Because omalizumab targets an immune system molecule, there has been particular interest in the drug's safety.

Methods.—To establish the efficacy and safety of subcutaneous omalizumab as add-on therapy to corticosteroids, a systematic review of placebo-controlled studies was performed. Primary outcomes were reduction of steroid use and asthma exacerbations. Secondary outcome measures included lung function, rescue medication use, asthma symptoms, health-related quality of life, and adverse effects.

Results.—Eight trials (3,429 participants) fulfilled the selection criteria. At the end of the steroid-reduction phase, patients taking omalizumab were more likely to be able to withdraw from corticosteroids completely compared with those taking placebo (relative risk [RR] = 1.80; 95% CI, 1.42-2.28; $P = .00001$). Omalizumab patients showed a decreased risk of asthma exacerbations at the end of the stable (RR = 0.57; 95% CI, 0.48-0.66; $P = .0001$) and adjustable-steroid phases (RR = 0.55; 95% CI, 0.47-0.64; $P = .0001$); post-hoc analysis suggests this effect was independent of duration of treatment, age, severity of asthma, and risk of bias. The frequency of serious adverse effects was similar in the omalizumab (3.8%) and placebo (5.3%) groups. However, injection site reactions were more frequent in the omalizumab patients (19.9% vs 13.2%). There were no indications of increased risk of hypersensitivity reactions, cardiovascular effects, or malignant neoplasms.

Conclusions.—Data indicate that the efficacy of add-on omalizumab in patients with moderate-to-severe allergic asthma is accompanied by an acceptable safety profile.

▶ Systematic review of placebo-controlled trials of subcutaneous omalizumab (O) add-on therapy in the setting of corticosteroids in patients with moderate to severe allergic asthma was undertaken. Following a rigorous evaluation process (Fig 1 in the original article), 8 total studies were selected; primary outcomes evaluated were reduction of steroid use and asthma exacerbations. Secondary outcomes measured included asthma symptoms, health-related quality of life, adverse effects, lung function, and rescue medication needs. Following the steroid-reduction phase, subjects receiving O were more likely to be able to withdraw completely from corticosteroids compared with those randomized to placebo (relative risk [RR] = 1.80; 95% confidence interval [CI], 1.42-2.28; $P = .00001$). Asthma exacerbation rate per 100 patient-years was 37.6 in the O group and 69.9 in the placebo group (RR = 0.57; 95% CI, 0.48-0.66 and number needed to treat for benefit = 10; 95% CI, 7-13, respectively) (Fig 2 in the original article). With regard to safety, there was no difference in the number of subject withdrawals between the O group and placebo-treated subjects. No significant adverse effects were seen in subjects taking O in studies less than 1-year duration. Longer clinical studies are required for evaluation of long-term efficacy and safety of 0 in patients with moderate-to-severe asthma.

S. K. Willsie, DO

Cystic Fibrosis

Location and Duration of Treatment of Cystic Fibrosis Respiratory Exacerbations Do Not Affect Outcomes
Collaco JM, Green DM, Cutting GR, et al (Johns Hopkins Univ, Baltimore, MD)
Am J Respir Crit Care Med 182:1137-1143, 2010

Rationale.—Individuals with cystic fibrosis (CF) are subject to recurrent respiratory infections (exacerbations) that often require intravenous antibiotic treatment and may result in permanent loss of lung function. The optimal means of delivering therapy remains unclear.

Objectives.—To determine whether duration or venue of intravenous antibiotic administration affect lung function.

Methods.—Data were retrospectively collected on 1,535 subjects recruited by the US CF Twin and Sibling Study from US CF care centers between 2000 and 2007.

Measurements and Main Results.—Long-term decline in FEV_1 after exacerbation was observed regardless of whether antibiotics were administered in the hospital (mean, -3.3 percentage points [95% confidence interval, -3.9 to -2.6]; n = 602 courses of therapy) or at home (mean, -3.5 percentage points [95% confidence interval, -4.5 to -2.5]; n = 232 courses of therapy); this decline was not different by venue using t tests ($P = 0.69$) or regression ($P = 0.91$). No difference in intervals between courses of antibiotics was observed between hospital (median, 119 d [interquartile range, 166]; n = 602) and home (median, 98 d [interquartile range, 155]; n = 232) ($P = 0.29$). Patients with greater drops in FEV_1 with exacerbations had worse long-term decline even if lung function initially recovered with treatment ($P < 0.001$). Examination of FEV_1

TABLE 1.—Demographics

	All	Hospital Only	Home Only	Combination: Hospital and Home	P Value (Hospital vs. Home)*
Data by Subject					
Number of subjects	479	261	114	248	—
Mean courses of antibiotics per subject in dataset	2.7 ± 2.4	—	—	—	—
Age at most recent FEV$_1$ (yr) (mean ± SD)	19.4 ± 8.3	18.2 ± 6.5	22.3 ± 9.4	20.4 ± 9.0	<0.0001
Sex (% male)	47.4	49	34.2	44	0.01
CFTR (% F508del homozygotes)	49.2 (n = 478)	51.2 (n = 260)	43	48.6 (n = 247)	0.35
Data by Therapy Course					
Number of courses	1,278	602	232	444	—
Age at start of therapy (yr) (mean ± SD)	17.8 ± 8.0	16.2 ± 6.1	22.0 ± 10.0	17.8 ± 8.2	<0.0001
P. aeruginosa (% positive)	96.4	95.7	97.8	96.6	0.14
B. cepacia (% positive)	10.6	11.5	9.9	9.9	0.52
Days treated in hospital (mean ± SD)	—	12.7 ± 5.3	—	6.0 ± 4.3	—
Days treated at home (mean ± SD)	—	—	18.9 ± 7.4	12.5 ± 5.7	—
Total days of treatment (mean ± SD)	15.8 ± 6.7	12.7 ± 5.3	18.9 ± 7.4	18.5 ± 6.0	<0.0001
Baseline FEV$_1$ (mean ± SD)	68.4 ± 22.0	67.4 ± 22.4	65.1 ± 22.1	71.4 ± 21.2	0.17
Pretherapy FEV$_1$ (mean ± SD)	60.4 ± 22.0	58.8 ± 22.0	59.5 ± 22.3	63.0 ± 21.5	0.68
Posttherapy FEV$_1$ (mean ± SD)	68.7 ± 23.4	67.9 ± 23.3	64.4 ± 23.5	72.0 ± 23.0	0.05
New baseline FEV$_1$ (mean ± SD)	64.9 ± 23.3	64.1 ± 23.1	61.5 ± 23.5	67.8 ± 23.3	0.15

*These P values reflect the difference between the hospital and home categories. P values were determined using Student t and chi-square tests.

measures obtained during treatment for exacerbations indicated that improvement in FEV_1 plateaus after 7–10 days of therapy.

Conclusions.—Intravenous antibiotic therapy for CF respiratory exacerbations administered in the hospital and in the home was found to be equivalent in terms of long-term FEV_1 change and interval between courses of antibiotics. Optimal duration of therapy (7–10 d) may be shorter than current practice. Large prospective studies are needed to answer these essential questions for CF respiratory management (Table 1).

▶ Retrospective data collection from the US Cystic Fibrosis Twin and Sibling study from US cystic fibrosis care centers between 2000 and 2007. Table 1 demonstrates numbers of subjects, numbers treated within the hospital, home, and combination of both; P values are given comparing hospital with home. There was no statistical difference in the numbers of exacerbations, which were because of *Pseudomonas aeruginosa* or *Burkholderia cepacia* ($P > .05$). Baseline forced expiratory volume in the first second of expiration (FEV_1), pretherapy FEV_1, posttherapy FEV_1, and new baseline FEV_1 did not vary significantly between groups. Fig 4 in the original article details improvement of FEV_1 by day of therapy. Pulmonary function tests obtained during therapy demonstrates that improvement occurred until approximately 8 to 10 days of therapy at which time the FEV_1 plateaus. Beyond this time period, there was no significant improvement, and actually, there was deterioration of FEV_1, despite continued treatment. The venue for intravenous antibiotic therapy for clinician-defined respiratory exacerbation does not affect long-term decline in FEV_1; most improvement in lung function appears to occur within the first 8 to 10 days following the initiation of antibiotic therapy.

S. K. Willsie, DO

Effect of VX-770 in Persons with Cystic Fibrosis and the G551D-*CFTR* Mutation

Accurso FJ, Rowe SM, Clancy JP, et al (Univ of Colorado Denver and Children's Hosp, Aurora; Univ of Alabama at Birmingham, AL; et al)
N Engl J Med 363:1991-2003, 2010

Background.—A new approach in the treatment of cystic fibrosis involves improving the function of mutant cystic fibrosis transmembrane conductance regulator (CFTR). VX-770, a CFTR potentiator, has been shown to increase the activity of wild-type and defective cell-surface CFTR in vitro.

Methods.—We randomly assigned 39 adults with cystic fibrosis and at least one G551D-*CFTR* allele to receive oral VX-770 every 12 hours at a dose of 25, 75, or 150 mg or placebo for 14 days (in part 1 of the study) or VX-770 every 12 hours at a dose of 150 or 250 mg or placebo for 28 days (in part 2 of the study).

Results.—At day 28, in the group of subjects who received 150 mg of VX-770, the median change in the nasal potential difference (in response to the administration of a chloride-free isoproterenol solution) from baseline was −3.5 mV (range, −8.3 to 0.5; P = 0.02 for the within-subject comparison, P = 0.13 vs. placebo), and the median change in the level of sweat chloride was −59.5 mmol per liter (range, −66.0 to −19.0; P = 0.008 within-subject, P = 0.02 vs. placebo). The median change from baseline in the percent of predicted forced expiratory volume in 1 second was 8.7% (range, 2.3 to 31.3; P = 0.008 for the within-subject comparison, P = 0.56 vs. placebo). None of the subjects withdrew from the study. Six severe adverse events occurred in two subjects (diffuse macular rash in one subject and five incidents of elevated blood and urine glucose levels in one subject with diabetes). All severe adverse events resolved without the discontinuation of VX-770.

Conclusions.—This study to evaluate the safety and adverse-event profile of VX-770 showed that VX-770 was associated with within-subject improvements in CFTR and lung function. These findings provide support for further studies of pharmacologic potentiation of CFTR as a means to treat cystic fibrosis. (Funded by Vertex Pharmaceuticals and others; ClinicalTrials.gov number, NCT00457821.)

▶ Despite advances in antibiotic therapy and improved rescue therapy for subjects with cystic fibrosis with chest infections, this multisystem disease continues to cause considerable morbidity and mortality.[1] One of the newer approaches to this disease involves direct targeting of the genetic defect in order to improve the function of the cystic fibrosis transmembrane conductance regulator (CFTR).[2,3] VX-770, known to be a CFTR potentiator,[4] was studied in a randomized, double-blind, placebo-controlled, multicenter study involving patients with cystic fibrosis who had at least on G551D-*CFTR* allele. Subjects took oral VX-770 every 12 hours at doses that ranged from 25 to 150 mg versus placebo for 14 days or doses of 150 or 250 mg versus placebo for 28 days. Fig 2 in the original article demonstrates changes in sweat chloride by dose and days of treatment, and Fig 3 in the original article delineates changes in pulmonary function with treatment. Though no significant differences were seen between VX-770 and placebo groups, significant within-subject improvement was seen, particularly related to respiratory (nasal potential difference), nonrespiratory (sweat chloride concentrations), and improved pulmonary function. In general, the investigational agent was well tolerated in comparison to placebo. Further studies are needed to evaluate VX-770 as a viable therapeutic option for patients with cystic fibrosis.

S. K. Willsie, DO

References

1. Sawicki GS, Sellers DE, Robinson WM. High treatment burden in adults with cystic fibrosis: challenges to disease self-management. *J Cyst Fibros.* 2009;8:91-96.
2. Amaral MD, Kunzelmann K. Molecular targeting of CFTR as a therapeutic approach to cystic fibrosis. *Trends Pharmacol Sci.* 2007;28:334-341.
3. Yang Y, Devor DC, Engelhardt JF, et al. Molecular basis of defective anion transport in L cells expressing recombinant forms of CFTR. *Hum Mol Genet.* 1993;2: 1253-1261.

4. Van Goor F, Hadida S, Grootenhuis PD, et al. Rescue of CF airway epithelial cell function in vitro by a CFTR potentiator, VX-770. *Proc Natl Acad Sci U S A*. 2009; 106:18825-18830.

Infection With Transmissible Strains of *Pseudomonas aeruginosa* and Clinical Outcomes in Adults With Cystic Fibrosis

Aaron SD, Vandemheen KL, Ramotar K, et al (Univ of Ottawa, Ontario, Canada; et al)
JAMA 304:2145-2153, 2010

Context.—Studies from Australia and the United Kingdom have shown that some patients with cystic fibrosis are infected with common transmissible strains of *Pseudomonas aeruginosa*.

Objectives.—To determine the prevalence and incidence of infection with transmissible strains of *P aeruginosa* and whether presence of the organism was associated with adverse clinical outcomes in Canada.

Design, Setting, and Participants.—Prospective observational cohort study of adult patients cared for at cystic fibrosis clinics in Ontario, Canada, with enrollment from September 2005 to September 2008. Sputum was collected at baseline, 3 months, and yearly thereafter for 3 years; and retrieved *P aeruginosa* isolates were genotyped. Vital status (death or lung transplant) was assessed for all enrolled patients until December 31, 2009.

Main Outcome Measures.—Incidence and prevalence of *P aeruginosa* isolation, rates of decline in lung function, and time to death or lung transplantation.

Results.—Of the 446 patients with cystic fibrosis studied, 102 were discovered to be infected with 1 of 2 common transmissible strains of *P aeruginosa* at study entry. Sixty-seven patients were infected with strain A (15%), 32 were infected with strain B (7%), and 3 were simultaneously infected with both strains (0.6%). Strain A was found to be genetically identical to the Liverpool epidemic strain but strain B has not been previously described as an epidemic strain. The incidence rate of new infections with these 2 transmissible strains was relatively low (7.0 per 1000 person-years; 95% confidence interval [CI], 1.8-12.2 per 1000 person-years). Compared with patients infected with unique strains of *P aeruginosa*, patients infected with the Liverpool epidemic strain (strain A) and strain B had similar declines in lung function (difference in decline in percent predicted forced expiratory volume in the first second of expiration of 0.64% per year [95% CI, -1.52% to 2.80% per year] and 1.66% per year [95% CI, -1.00% to 4.30%], respectively). However, the 3-year rate of death or lung transplantation was greater in those infected with the Liverpool epidemic strain (18.6%) compared with those infected with unique strains (8.7%) (adjusted hazard ratio, 3.26 [95% CI, 1.41 to 7.54]; $P=.01$).

Conclusions.—A common strain of *P aeruginosa* (Liverpool epidemic strain/strain A) infects patients with cystic fibrosis in Canada and the

United Kingdom. Infection with this strain in adult Canadian patients with cystic fibrosis was associated with a greater risk of death or lung transplantation.

▶ This prospective observational study monitored patients with cystic fibrosis over time to determine whether or not their sputum contained *Pseudomonas aeruginosa* isolates that were considered to be common transmissible strains. Outcomes measures included *P aeruginosa* isolation, rate of lung function decline, time to death, or lung transplantation. Of the 446 patients, 102 were infected with 1 of 2 common transmissible strains of *P aeruginosa* at study entry. Of the 102, 67 (15%) were infected with strain A, 32 (7%) were infected with strain B, and 3 were simultaneously infected with both strain A and strain B (0.6%). The 3-year death rate or rate of lung transplantation (Fig 3 in the original article) was greater in those infected with strain A (also known as the Liverpool epidemic strain) compared with those infected with other strains (adjusted hazard ratio, 3.26; 95% CI, 1.41-7.54; $P = .01$).

S. K. Willsie, DO

2 Chronic Obstructive Pulmonary Disease

Introduction

Chronic obstructive pulmonary disease (COPD) remains one of the most common chronic diseases and the fourth-leading cause of death in the United States, according to the most recent morbidity and mortality data.[1] While chronic lung disease is a much smaller fraction of the overall mortality rate than the top 3 causes (heart disease, cancer, and cerebrovascular disease), it is not declining as a cause of death like heart and cerebrovascular disease have.

A major concern is that probably up to half of people who have COPD are undiagnosed and therefore unaware of the potential impact of their disease. A number of investigators have focused on ways to better "find" or better characterize this population. Two articles relate to this issue. Eisner et al present data on a survey tool designed to measure COPD and its severity on a population basis without doing pulmonary function tests. The tool is promising but requires more validation. A second study by Kalhan et al suggests that pulmonary functions done as a screening in an asymptomatic cohort of young adults will identify a number with obstructive defects that persist. Whether this has implications for the current recommendation against screening spirometry remains to be determined.

In doing population studies to "find" asymptomatic disease as well as in assessment of known disease, it is important to be certain that the measurements accurately identify and quantify disease. This has been problematic in populations such as the very elderly where generally accepted "normal" values do not exist. Vaz Fragosso et al address the issue of false-positive diagnoses of obstructive disease in the elderly and suggest a better methodology for this population. O'Donnell et al challenge the dogma that helium-dilution volumes are inaccurate in obstructive disease and, in fact, suggest that plethysmographically determined volumes are often overestimates. In a final paper in the measurement section, Hannink et al measured dynamic hyperinflation in a spectrum of COPD patients and found that it is a significant functional limitation factor in relatively early disease.

Articles chosen for the medication management section of this chapter focus primarily on corticosteroid use. The longstanding controversy over use of antibiotics in conjunction with corticosteroids for exacerbations has recently swung toward more use of antibiotics. Rothberg et al reported on a large retrospective hospitalized cohort of COPD patients with exacerbations and concluded that patients who received antibiotics in the first 2 days had better outcomes; however, the controversy continues as Daniels et al report a prospective randomized trial in which outcomes were similar with or without the use of antibiotics. As the use of inhaled corticosteroids (ICS) becomes more ubiquitous in the maintenance management of COPD patients, so has the reporting of complications related to their use. One of the reported complications has been an increased rate of pneumonia. Malo de Molina et al followed ICS-treated COPD patients who developed pneumonia to determine mortality impact. The results might be surprising to you! A study by Shu et al reports that tuberculosis, especially in geographic areas where the disease is common, is also a complication of the use of ICS. A final study in the medication section (Ogale et al) addresses the controversy about increased cardiovascular events with the use of ipratropium bromide.

Much of the success in management of patients with chronic diseases has to do not with the management specific to the disease itself, but to the overall management of the patient and his or her ability to cope with and self-manage symptoms. Several articles address various aspects of this "whole patient" management. Slatore et al address the importance of the type of communication that occurs between patient and physician. Omachi et al studied a patient's level of feeling helpless in dealing with his disease and found correlation with exacerbations; however, Rice et al demonstrate improved self-management and reduced utilization by COPD patients through a well-designed but simple disease management program. Panic attacks are common in COPD patients and greatly impair their quality of life. Livermore et al studied a simple but effective approach to managing these attacks.

An article by Terada et al reports a relatively small but provocative study that suggests aspiration is related to COPD exacerbations. Incalzi et al point out that nearly half of COPD patients older than 64 years have some degree of chronic renal failure, a rarely mentioned but potentially significant comorbidity than can greatly complicate management. The final study is one documenting trends and burdens of bronchiectasis in the United States. This study by Seitz et al serves to remind us that bronchiectasis is still an important, albeit somewhat neglected, disease.

Janet R. Maurer, MD, MBA

Reference

1. http://www.cdc.gov/NCHS/data/nvsr/nvsr58/nvsr58_19.pdf. Accessed February 27, 2011.

Abnormal Swallowing Reflex and COPD Exacerbations

Terada K, Muro S, Ohara T, et al (Kyoto Univ, Japan)
Chest 137:326-332, 2010

Background.—It is unclear whether an abnormal swallowing reflex affects COPD exacerbations. This study investigated the prevalence of abnormal swallowing reflexes and its relationship with COPD exacerbation prospectively. We also clarified its association with gastroesophageal reflux disease (GERD) and airway bacterial colonization.

Methods.—Swallowing reflex and serum C-reactive protein (CRP) levels were examined in subjects with stable COPD and in control subjects. Concurrently, GERD symptoms were assessed using a self-reported questionnaire, and sputum bacterial cultures were investigated in the same subjects. Exacerbations were counted prospectively during the following 12 months.

Results.—The study group comprised 67 subjects with COPD and 19 controls. The prevalence of abnormal swallowing reflex was significantly higher in subjects with COPD (22/67) than controls (1/19; $P = .02$). Among subjects with COPD, the serum CRP level, GERD symptoms, isolation of sputum bacteria, and the frequency of exacerbations were significantly increased in those with abnormal swallowing reflexes compared with controls (2.72 vs 1.04 mg/L, $P = .04$, for serum CRP level; 6.75 vs 4.10 points, $P = .04$, for GERD symptoms; 5/11 vs 3/22, $P = .04$, for the isolation of sputum bacteria; and 2.82 vs 1.56/y, $P = .007$, for the annual frequency of exacerbations). Multivariable analysis confirmed that abnormal swallowing reflex was significantly associated with frequent exacerbations ($\geq 3/y$; $P = 0.01$).

Conclusions.—Abnormal swallowing reflexes frequently occurred in subjects with COPD and predisposed them to exacerbations. Abnormal swallowing reflexes in COPD might be affected by the comorbidity of GERD, and cause bacterial colonization.

▶ Several observational studies have documented a higher rate of gastroesophageal reflux in patients with chronic obstructive pulmonary disease (COPD) and swallowing abnormalities associated with gastroesophageal reflux.[1-3] Gastroesophageal reflux is associated with aspiration syndromes and recently has been shown to have an important association with bronchiolitis obliterans in lung transplant recipients. Abnormal swallowing mechanisms are associated both with oropharyngeal and gastric contents aspiration. In this study, patients with abnormal swallowing had a higher rate of airway colonization possibly related to aspiration episodes. It is not surprising to find a correlation between reflux and COPD exacerbations. What is perhaps surprising is that this is the first study to prospectively look at abnormal swallowing reflexes and reflux in a cohort of patients with COPD and correlate those findings with colonization and exacerbations. While this is a relatively small study, it is provocative and suggests the need for a larger prospective study with a longer follow-up period. If a portion of exacerbations is related to the aspiration of oropharyngeal or gastric contents, it certainly makes sense to use relatively simple preventive approaches to reducing the risk of microaspiration, for example, elevating the head of the bed, etc.

J. R. Maurer, MD, MBA

References

1. Marik PE. Aspiration pneumonitis and pneumonia. *N Engl J Med.* 2001;344: 665-672.
2. Teramoto S, Kume H, Ouchi Y. Altered swallowing physiology and aspiration in COPD. *Chest.* 2002;122:1104-1105.
3. Kobayashi S, Kubo H, Yanai M. Impairment of the swallowing reflex in exacerbations of COPD. *Thorax.* 2007;62:1017.

The COPD Helplessness Index: A New Tool to Measure Factors Affecting Patient Self-Management
Omachi TA, Katz PP, Yelin EH, et al (Univ of California, San Francisco; et al)
Chest 137:823-830, 2010

Background.—Psychologic factors affect how patients with COPD respond to attempts to improve their self-management skills. Learned helplessness may be one such factor, but there is no validated measure of helplessness in COPD.

Methods.—We administered a new COPD Helplessness Index (CHI) to 1,202 patients with COPD. Concurrent validity was assessed through association of the CHI with established psychosocial measures and COPD severity. The association of helplessness with incident COPD exacerbations was then examined by following subjects over a median 2.1 years, defining COPD exacerbations as COPD-related hospitalizations or ED visits.

Results.—The CHI demonstrated internal consistency (Cronbach $\alpha = 0.75$); factor analysis was consistent with the CHI representing a single construct. Greater CHI-measured helplessness correlated with greater COPD severity assessed by the BODE (Body-mass, Obstruction, Dyspnea, Exercise) Index ($r = 0.34$; $P < .001$). Higher CHI scores were associated with worse generic (Short Form-12, Physical Component Summary Score) and respiratory-specific (Airways Questionnaire 20) health-related quality of life, greater depressive symptoms, and higher anxiety (all $P < .001$). Controlling for sociodemographics and smoking status, helplessness was prospectively associated with incident COPD exacerbations (hazard ratio = 1.31; $P < .001$). After also controlling for the BODE Index, helplessness remained predictive of COPD exacerbations among subjects with BODE Index ≤ median (hazard ratio = 1.35; $P = .01$), but not among subjects with higher BODE Index values (hazard ratio = 0.93; $P = .34$).

Conclusions.—The CHI is an internally consistent and valid measure, concurrently associated with health status and predictively associated with COPD exacerbations. The CHI may prove a useful tool in analyzing differential clinical responses mediated by patient-centered attributes.

► As health care costs continue to spiral out of control, the federal government and others have emphasized better understanding of and increased self-management by sufferers of chronic disease as an important element in containing those costs. This requires the patient to take ownership of the disease and actively self-commit to management strategies that are likely to reduce hospitalizations and possibly even limit the ravages of the disease. In chronic obstructive pulmonary disease (COPD), this might include stopping smoking, participating in rehabilitation, using medications and oxygen correctly, etc. However, it is clear that only a minority of patients with chronic conditions take an active role in their own management. Why is that? This very interesting article addresses the issue of learned helplessness, a mindset of passive resignation that patients may adopt when they feel they have no control over important aspects of their disease, eg, an acute exacerbation in COPD. This can lead to loss of motivation and an inability to actively participate in self-management. The authors developed a COPD Helplessness Index based on a similar tool designed for arthritis patients and were able to demonstrate internal consistency.[1] Higher levels of feelings of helplessness on the 13-question survey correlated well with more severe disease but helplessness itself also appeared to worsen disease when measured by some indices, for example, the Body-mass, Obstruction, Dyspnea, Exercise Index. Most interestingly, in patients with milder COPD, increased emergency health care use was correlated with higher degrees of helplessness. While this measure certainly needs further validation, it could prove to be a very useful tool in identifying patients who are likely to do poorly based on their mindsets with respect to their disease. This type of identification could also lead to individualized psychological support aimed at developing improved coping skills and improved capability of self-management.

J. R. Maurer, MD, MBA

Reference

1. Nicassio PM, Wallston KA, Callahan LF, Herbert M, Pincus T. The measurement of helplessness in rheumatoid arthritis. The development of the arthritis helplessness index. *J Rheumatol.* 1985;12:462-467.

Dynamic Hyperinflation During Daily Activities: Does COPD Global Initiative for Chronic Obstructive Lung Disease Stage Matter?
Hannink JDC, van Helvoort HAC, Dekhuijzen PNR, et al (Radboud Univ Nijmegen Med Centre, The Netherlands)
Chest 137:1116-1121, 2010

Background.—One of the contributors to exercise limitation in COPD is dynamic hyperinflation. Although dynamic hyperinflation appears to occur during several exercise protocols in COPD and seems to increase with increasing disease severity, it is unknown whether dynamic hyperinflation occurs at different severity stages according to the Global Initiative for Chronic Obstructive Lung Disease (GOLD) in daily life. The present study, therefore, aimed to compare dynamic hyperinflation between COPD GOLD stages II-IV during daily activities.

Methods.—Thirty-two clinically stable patients with COPD GOLD II (n = 10), III (n = 12), and IV (n = 10) participated in this study. Respiratory physiology during a daily activity was measured at patients' homes with Oxycon Mobile. Inspiratory capacity maneuvers were performed at rest, at 2-min intervals during the activity, and at the end of the activity. Change in inspiratory capacity is commonly used to reflect change in end-expiratory lung volume ($\triangle$EELV) and, therefore, dynamic hyperinflation. The combination of static and dynamic hyperinflation was reflected by inspiratory reserve volume (IRV) during the activity.

Results.—Overall, increase in EELV occurred in GOLD II-IV without significant difference between the groups. There was a tendency for a smaller $\triangle$EELV in GOLD IV. $\triangle$EELV was inversely related to static hyperinflation. IRV during the daily activity was related to the level of airflow obstruction.

Conclusions.—Dynamic hyperinflation occurs independent of GOLD stage during real-life daily activities. The combination of static and dynamic hyperinflation, however, increases with increasing airflow obstruction.

▶ O'Donnell[1] and others have shown that one of the limiting factors in exercise tolerance of patients with severe chronic obstructive pulmonary disease (COPD) is the development of dynamic hyperinflation. Increased air trapping occurs as expiratory time is decreased when the patient struggles to breathe more rapidly. The resulting decrease in inspiratory reserve volume is felt as dyspnea by the patient. The early reports of dynamic hyperinflation were in patients with severe or very severe disease. In this study, the authors found that dynamic hyperinflation occurs in patients with much less severe disease and that it occurs during normal activities of daily living. Patients experiencing more severity actually had less dynamic hyperinflation but, when combined with their larger static hyperinflation, were more functionally limited. What is not clear from this study is how significant the finding of dynamic hyperinflation is in less severe degrees of COPD since most of the patients with less severe disease studied were not dyspnea limited. It would be useful to follow these patients longitudinally to determine if the degree of dynamic hyperinflation in earlier stage disease has any predictive value for future exercise limitation.

J. R. Maurer, MD, MBA

Reference

1. O'Donnell DE, Revill SM, Webb KA. Dynamic hyperinflation and exercise intolerance in chronic obstructive pulmonary disease. *Am J Respir Crit Care Med.* 2001;164:770-777.

Chronic Renal Failure: A Neglected Comorbidity of COPD

Incalzi RA, on behalf of the Extrapulmonary Consequences of COPD in the Elderly Study Investigators (University Campus BioMedico, Rome, Italy; et al)
Chest 137:831-837, 2010

Background.—To the best of our knowledge, the association between COPD and chronic renal failure (CRF) has never been assessed. Lean mass is frequently reduced in COPD, and the glomerular filtration rate (GFR) might be depressed in spite of normal serum creatinine (concealed CRF). We investigated the prevalence and correlates of both concealed and overt CRF in elderly patients with COPD.

Methods.—We evaluated 356 consecutive elderly outpatients with COPD enrolled in the Extrapulmonary Consequences of COPD in the Elderly Study and 290 age-matched outpatients free from COPD. The GFR was estimated using the Modification of Diet in Renal Disease Study Group equation. Patients were categorized as having normal renal function (GFR $\geq$ 60 mL/min/1.73 m^2), concealed CRF (normal serum creatinine and reduced GFR), or overt CRF (increased serum creatinine and reduced GFR). Independent correlates of CRF were investigated by logistic regression analysis.

Results.—The prevalence of concealed and overt CRF in patients with COPD was 20.8% and 22.2%, respectively. Corresponding figures in controls were 10.0% and 13.4%, respectively. COPD and age were significantly associated with both concealed CRF (COPD: odds ratio [OR] = 2.19, 95% CI = 1.17-4.12; age: OR = 1.06, 95% CI = 1.04-1.09) and overt CRF (COPD: OR = 1.94, 95% CI = 1.01-4.66; age: OR = 1.06, 95% CI = 1.04-1.10). Diabetes (OR = 1.96, 95% CI = 1.02-3.76), hypoalbuminemia (OR = 2.83, 95% CI = 1.70-4.73), and muscle-skeletal diseases (OR = 1.78, 95% CI = 1.01-3.16) were significant correlates of concealed CRF. BMI (OR = 1.05, 95% CI = 1.01-1.10) and diabetes (OR = 2.25, 95% CI = 1.26-4.03) were significantly associated with overt CRF.

Conclusions.—CRF is highly prevalent in patients with COPD, even with normal serum creatinine, and might contribute to explaining selected conditions such as anemia that are frequent complications of COPD.

▶ Chronic renal failure is not one of the common comorbidities that come to mind when we think of chronic obstructive pulmonary disease (COPD). However, this study suggests that nearly half of COPD patients older than 64 years have either overt (creatinine of at least 2 mg/dL) or concealed (creatinine normal, but glomerular filtration rate less than 60 mL/min/1.73 m^2) chronic renal failure. It is not surprising that concealed chronic renal failure is seen in COPD because these patients often have decreased lean body mass, a determinant of the creatinine level. When little creatinine is being turned over, serum creatinine may be normal, inaccurately suggesting normal renal function. Why should we care about renal function in COPD patients? Abnormal renal function as a comorbidity of cardiovascular disease, diabetes, or other chronic conditions portends a poorer prognosis; that may be true in COPD as well. Abnormal renal function is associated with hypertension, coronary disease, anemia, hypoalbuminemia, and other metabolic derangements. While this study did not follow patients prospectively to determine the impact of renal dysfunction on survival, that certainly would be a very interesting future study.

J. R. Maurer, MD, MBA

Comparison of Plethysmographic and Helium Dilution Lung Volumes: Which Is Best for COPD?

O'Donnell CR, Bankier AA, Stiebellehner L, et al (Beth Israel Deaconess Med Ctr, Boston, MA; Med Univ of Vienna, Austria; et al)
Chest 137:1108-1115, 2010

Background.—Theoretical considerations and limited scientific evidence suggest that whole-body plethysmography overestimates lung volume in patients with severe airflow obstruction. We sought to compare plethysmography (Pleth)-, helium dilution (He)- and CT scan-derived lung volume measurements in a sample containing many patients with severe airflow obstruction.

Methods.—We measured total lung capacity (TLC) in 132 patients at three hospitals, with monitored application of recommended techniques for Pleth and He measurements of lung volume and by thoracic CT scans obtained during breath hold at full inspiration.

Results.—Average TLC among 132 subjects was 6.18 L ($\pm$ 1.69 L) by Pleth-derived TLC, 5.55 L ($\pm$ 1.39 L) by He-derived TLC, and 5.31 L ($\pm$ 1.47) by CT scan-derived TLC. Pleth-derived TLC was significantly greater than either He-derived TLC or CT scan-derived TLC ($P \leq .001$), whereas there was no significant difference between He-derived and CT scan-derived values. When examined separately, there were significant within-subject differences in TLC by measurement technique among subjects with airflow obstruction, but not among those without airflow obstruction. Plethysmographic overestimation of TLC was greatest among subjects with FEV_1 <30% of predicted.

Conclusions.—In the setting of airflow obstruction, Pleth systematically overestimates lung volume relative to He or thoracic imaging despite adherence to current recommendations for proper measurement technique.

▶ Conventional wisdom is that to get accurate lung volume values in patients with chronic obstructive pulmonary disease, measurement with a plethysmograph is necessary. This article challenges that conventional wisdom and suggests in fact that the much maligned helium dilution technique is actually more accurate. The theory supporting a body box approach over helium dilution in these patients has to do with the assumed differences in airflow in different lung regions. Low ventilation perfusion ratio areas of lung (poorly ventilated) are assumed to equilibrate slowly and would therefore result in an underestimation of the volumes in these areas. On the other hand, in using the pressure/volume relationships that are calculated in plethysmographic measurements, the assumption is that all gas-filled areas are equally compressed and decompressed, thereby giving a more accurate estimate of the air volume in the chest. In this study, computed tomography at full inspiration, helium dilution, and plethysmography were all used in each subject to compute total lung capacity. Though computed tomography at full inspiration has several possible potential sources of error, it likely is the most accurate of the 3 methods to measure volume. In this study, these volumes correlated closely with helium dilution values but not with plethysmographic volumes, especially in patients with severe obstruction. A helium dilution technique that allowed a greater period of time for equilibration than traditional methods was used and likely contributed to a more accurate measurement of volume by this technique. But why would plethysmography overestimate lung volumes? The authors review several possible reasons: (1) high panting frequency may interfere with equilibration of mouth and alveolar pressures; (2) there may be heterogeneity of alveolar pressure swings during panting; and (3) excessive compliance of the extrathoracic airway. Accurate measurement of volumes in patients with severe disease has important implications for management, so establishing the best measurement approach should be a priority.

J. R. Maurer, MD, MBA

Prevention of panic attacks and panic disorder in COPD
Livermore N, Sharpe L, McKenzie D (Prince of Wales Hosp, New South Wales, Australia; Univ of Sydney, New South Wales, Australia)
Eur Respir J 35:557-563, 2010

This study examined whether cognitive behavioural therapy (CBT) could prevent the development or worsening of panic-spectrum psychopathology and anxiety symptoms in chronic obstructive pulmonary disease (COPD).

41 patients with COPD, who had undergone pulmonary rehabilitation, were randomised to either a four-session CBT intervention condition (n=21) or a routine care condition (n=20). Assessments were at baseline, post-intervention, and at 6-, 12- and 18-month follow-ups. Primary outcomes were the rates of panic attacks, panic disorder and anxiety symptoms. Secondary outcomes were depressive symptoms, catastrophic cognitions about breathing difficulties, disease-specific quality of life and hospital admission rates.

There were no significant differences between the groups on outcome measures at baseline. By the 18-month follow-up assessment, 12 (60%) routine care group participants had experienced at least one panic attack in the previous 6 months, with two (17%) of these being diagnosed with panic disorder, while no CBT group participants experienced any panic attacks during the follow-up phase. There were also significant reductions in anxiety symptoms and catastrophic cognitions in the CBT group at all three follow-ups and a lower number of hospital admissions between the 6- and 12-month follow-ups.

The study provides evidence that a brief, specifically targeted CBT intervention can treat panic attacks in COPD patients and prevent the development and worsening of panic-spectrum psychopathology and anxiety symptoms.

▶ Panic attacks, an extreme form of anxiety, are common in patients with chronic obstructive pulmonary disease (COPD) and are related to a diminished quality of life.[1] Yet even when the symptoms are relayed to his/her physician, little is often done to address the issue. This is likely because physicians consider anxiety an integral part of the disease or simply do not know how to address it appropriately. This is unfortunate because panic disorder has been estimated to occur in up to 35% of COPD sufferers.[2] Another possible reason that physicians caring for patients with COPD may shy away from treating panic symptoms is that they feel the problem requires ongoing long-term psychotherapy or medications that may be detrimental to the patient's respiratory status. In this study, significant improvement, not only in panic symptoms but also in hospitalizations, was achieved in a population treated with a cognitive behavioral therapy (CBT) approach to prevention and treatment of panic disorder that had been adapted for a COPD population. The CBT consisted of four 1-hour sessions done as an outpatient once a week. This approach could easily be administered by a trained nurse or other health care professional as part of rehabilitation programs or through outpatient office visits. Not only does this have potential for much improved quality of life for a subset of patients with COPD but also possibly significantly less use of urgent care.

J. R. Maurer, MD, MBA

References

1. Halbert RJ, Natoli JL, Gano A, Badamgarav E, Buist AS, Mannino DM. Global burden of COPD: systematic review and meta-analysis. *Eur Respir J.* 2006;28: 523-532.
2. Smoller JW, Pollack MH, Otto MW, Rosenbaum JF, Kradin RL. Panic anxiety, dyspnea, and respiratory disease. Theoretical and clinical considerations. *Am J Respir Crit Care Med.* 1996;154:6-17.

Chronic obstructive pulmonary disease in older persons: A comparison of two spirometric definitions
Vaz Fragoso CA, Concato J, McAvay G, et al (Yale Univ School of Medicine, New Haven, CT)
Respir Med 104:1189-1196, 2010

Background.—Among older persons, we previously endorsed a two-step spirometric definition of chronic obstructive pulmonary disease (COPD) that requires a ratio of forced expiratory volume in 1 sec to forced vital capacity (FEV_1/FVC) below .70, and an FEV_1 below the 5th or 10th standardized residual percentile ("SR-tile strategy").

Objective.—To evaluate the clinical validity of an SR-tile strategy, compared to a current definition of COPD, as published by the Global Initiative for Obstructive Lung Disease (GOLDCOPD), in older persons.

Methods.—We assessed national data from 2480 persons aged 65–80 years. In separate analyses, we evaluated the association of an SR-tile strategy with mortality and respiratory symptoms, relative to GOLD-COPD. As per convention, GOLD-COPD was defined solely by an FEV_1/FVC < .70, with severity staged according to FEV_1 cut-points at 80 and 50 percent predicted (%Pred).

Results.—Among 831 participants with GOLD-COPD, the risk of death was elevated only in 179 (21.5%) of those who also had an FEV_1 < 5th SR-tile; and the odds of having respiratory symptoms were elevated only in 310 (37.4%) of those who also had an FEV_1 < 10th SR-tile. In contrast, GOLD-COPD staged at an FEV_1 50–79%Pred led to misclassification (overestimation) in terms of 209 (66.4%) and 77 (24.6%) participants, respectively, not having an increased risk of death or likelihood of respiratory symptoms.

Conclusion.—Relative to an SR-tile strategy, the majority of older persons with GOLD-COPD had neither an increased risk of death nor an increased likelihood of respiratory symptoms. These results raise concerns about the clinical validity of GOLD guidelines in older persons.

▶ This group has previously reported that current spirometric definitions of obstructive disease, when applied to the elderly, overdiagnose and wrongly diagnose a number of these patients. In particular, the authors argue that if one uses the Global Initiative for Obstructive Lung Disease (GOLD) guideline recommendation of forced expiratory volume in the first 1 second (FEV_1)/ forced vital capacity of the lungs ratio < 0.7 to diagnose chronic obstructive pulmonary disease, a number of elderly and especially very elderly patients, who have normal age-related loss of lung function will be given a pathological diagnosis. However, these elderly patients may not have the small airways disease and parenchymal destruction typical of the pathology of obstructive disease. In previous studies, the authors have proposed a mechanism by which to reduce the likelihood of false diagnoses in this population. That method is to use the GOLD guideline cutoff value as a type of screen for patients with potential obstructive disease and then apply a secondary measure called a standardized residual (SR)-tile.[1] An SR-tile expresses the FEV_1 as an SR calculated as: (measured minus predicted)/(standard deviation of the residuals). A residual is the difference between a measured and the predicted value, and the standard deviation is a constant that quantifies the spread of the reference data (based on age, sex, height, and ethnicity). A percentile based on the SR is then computed with a scale of 1 to 100. This approach basically sorts those.

The purpose of this article was to provide further validation/comparison of this approach by comparing the pulmonary function results of a single large population using GOLD as the authors' approach. The results show significant differences in identification between the 2 approaches that seem to favor the SR-tile approach. This approach should be evaluated with a large prospective trial. The number of elderly patients is increasing dramatically and misdiagnosis could result in the unnecessary use of health care resources and cause significant distress for many patients.

J. R. Maurer, MD, MBA

Reference

1. Vaz Fragoso CA, Concato J, McAvay G, et al. Defining chronic obstructive pulmonary disease in older persons. *Respir Med.* 2009;103:1468-1476.

Use of High-Dose Inhaled Corticosteroids is Associated With Pulmonary Tuberculosis in Patients With Chronic Obstructive Pulmonary Disease

Shu C-C, the Taiwan Anti-Mycobacteria Investigation (TAMI) Group (Natl Taiwan Univ Hosp, Taipei; et al)
Medicine 89:53-61, 2010

The use of high-dose inhaled corticosteroids (ICS) in patients with chronic obstructive pulmonary disease (COPD) has recently been shown to increase the incidence of pneumonia. However, to our knowledge, the impact of high-dose ICS on pulmonary tuberculosis (TB) has never been investigated. To study that impact, we conducted a retrospective study including patients aged more than 40 years old with irreversible airflow limitation between August 2000 and July 2008 in a medical center in Taiwan.

Of the 36,684 patients who underwent pulmonary function testing, we included 554 patients. Among them, patients using high-dose ICS (equivalent to >500 µg/d of fluticasone) were more likely to have more severe COPD and receive oral corticosteroids than those using medium-dose, low-dose, or no ICS. Sixteen (3%) patients developed active pulmonary TB within a follow-up of 25,544 person-months. Multivariate Cox regression analysis revealed that the use of high-dose ICS, the use of 10 mg or more of prednisolone per day, and prior pulmonary TB were independent risk factors for the development of active pulmonary TB. Chest radiography and sputum smear/culture for *Mycobacterium tuberculosis* should be performed before initiating high-dose ICS and regularly thereafter.

▶ Since inhaled corticosteroids (ICS) were shown to decrease exacerbations in patients with severe chronic obstructive pulmonary disease (COPD), their use as a maintenance treatment has increased dramatically. In fact, the most widely used clinical practice guideline around the management of COPD, the Global Obstructive Lung Disease guideline, recommends a combination of inhaled corticosteroid therapy and inhaled bronchodilator therapy for patients with COPD with severe disease and repeated exacerbations.[1] This approach, while potentially decreasing the morbidity from exacerbations, is not without its side effects. Already, articles have been published documenting, mostly incidentally, increases in the rates of pneumonia in patients treated chronically with ICS. Recently, it has been documented that this risk occurs even in newly diagnosed patients placed on ICS.[2] Since corticosteroids are immunosuppressive, this should not be a surprise. In this study, 3% of 554 patients with fixed airflow obstruction in a Taiwanese clinic developed active tuberculosis over a period of follow-up of at least 6 months (but a mean of 40-50 months); those on oral steroids or high-dose ICS were at greatest risk and developed the disease at a median of about 20 months. The authors make a general recommendation that patients being placed on high-dose ICS have routine chest X-ray and sputum smear/culture before being started on the drug and regularly thereafter. This may be reasonable in populations with high rates of tuberculosis, but it is not a cost-effective approach in general. However, it is important for clinicians caring for COPD patients on ICS to be aware of this risk and to consider tuberculosis in any atypical presentation of pneumonia.

J. R. Maurer, MD, MBA

References

1. Guidelines and Resources. Available at: <http://www.goldcopd.com>. Accessed August 15, 2010.
2. Joo MJ, Au DH, Fitzgibbon ML, Lee TA. Inhaled corticosteroids and risk of pneumonia in newly diagnosed COPD. *Respir Med.* 2010;104:246-252.

Cardiovascular Events Associated With Ipratropium Bromide in COPD
Ogale SS, Lee TA, Au DH, et al (Univ of Washington, Seattle; Hines VA Hosp, IL)
Chest 137:13-19, 2010

Background.—Studies have suggested an increased risk of cardiovascular morbidity and mortality associated with the use of ipratropium bromide. We sought to examine the association between ipratropium bromide use and the risk of cardiovascular events (CVEs).

Methods.—We performed a cohort study of 82,717 US veterans with a new diagnosis of COPD between 1999 and 2002. Subjects were followed until they had their first hospitalization for a CVE (acute coronary syndrome, heart failure, or cardiac dysrhythmia), they died, or the end of the study period (September 30, 2004). Cumulative anticholinergic exposure was calculated as the number of 30-day equivalents (ipratropium bromide) within the past year. We used Cox regression models with time-dependent covariates to estimate the risk of CVE associated with anticholinergic exposure and to adjust for potential confounders, including markers of COPD severity and cardiovascular risk.

Results.—We identified 6,234 CVEs (44% heart failure, 28% acute coronary syndrome, 28% dysrhythmia). Compared with subjects not exposed to anticholinergics within the past year, any exposure to anticholinergics within the past 6 months was associated with an increased risk of CVE (hazard ratio [95% CI] for ≤ four and > four 30-day equivalents: 1.40 [1.30-1.51] and 1.23 [1.13-1.36], respectively). Among subjects who received anticholinergics more than 6 months prior, there did not appear to be elevated risk of a CVE.

Conclusions.—We found an increased risk of CVEs associated with the use of ipratropium bromide within the past 6 months. These findings are consistent with previous concerns raised about the cardiovascular safety of ipratropium bromide.

▶ Over the past few years there has been an ongoing controversy about the safety of inhaled anticholinergics with respect to cardiovascular events and deaths. In 2008, an important meta-analysis by Singh et al,[1] included 17 randomized controlled trials using inhaled anticholinergics. This analysis was designed to look for cardiovascular risks, including myocardial infarction, death, and stroke. The authors concluded that inhaled anticholinergics in general have an increased cardiovascular risk in all domains studied. In 2009, a meta-analysis focusing specifically on tiotropium challenged this conclusion. In that analysis, Rodrigo et al analyzed 19 randomized controlled trials involving more than 18 000 patients with chronic obstructive pulmonary disease (COPD). Studies compared tiotropium use with either a β agonist or placebo; no increase in cardiovascular risk was found in the tiotropium group.[2] Another overlapping report by Celli et al published in 2010 that looked at studies involving almost 19 500 patients supported these findings.[3] However, the article by Ogale et al abstracted here supports the finding of increased cardiovascular events in patients using the short-acting drug, ipratropium bromide. While the controversy is surely not yet over and the reported increased cardiovascular risk is modest at best, the prudent approach at present appears to be to opt for tiotropium when possible.

J. R. Maurer, MD, MBA

References

1. Singh S, Loke YK, Furberg CD. Inhaled anticholinergics and risk of major adverse cardiovascular events in patients with chronic obstructive pulmonary disease: a systematic review and meta-analysis. *JAMA.* 2008;300:1439-1450.
2. Rodrigo GJ, Castro-Rodriguez JA, Nannini LJ, Plaza Moral V, Schiavi EA. Tiotropium and risk for fatal and nonfatal cardiovascular events in patients with chronic obstructive pulmonary disease: systematic review with meta-analysis. *Respir Med.* 2009;103:1421-1429.
3. Celli B, Decramer M, Leimer I, Vogel U, Kesten S, Tashkin DP. Cardiovascular safety of tiotropium in patients with COPD. *Chest.* 2010;137:20-30.

Antibiotics in Addition to Systemic Corticosteroids for Acute Exacerbations of Chronic Obstructive Pulmonary Disease

Daniels JMA, Snijders D, de Graaff CS, et al (Med Ctr Alkmaar, The Netherlands; et al)
Am J Respir Crit Care Med 181:150-157, 2010

Rationale.—The role of antibiotics in acute exacerbations is controversial and their efficacy when added to systemic corticosteroids is unknown.

Objectives.—We conducted a randomized, placebo-controlled trial to determine the effects of doxycycline in addition to corticosteroids on clinical outcome, microbiological outcome, lung function, and systemic inflammation in patients hospitalized with an acute exacerbation of chronic obstructive pulmonary disease.

Methods.—Of 223 patients, we enrolled 265 exacerbations defined on the basis of increased dyspnea and increased sputum volume with or without increased sputum purulence. Patients received 200 mg of oral doxycycline or matching placebo for 7 days in addition to systemic corticosteroids. Clinical and microbiological response, time to treatment failure, lung function, symptom scores, and serum C-reactive protein were assessed.

Measurements and Main Results.—On Day 30, clinical success was similar in intention-to-treat patients (odds ratio, 1.3; 95% confidence interval, 0.8 to 2.0) and per-protocol patients. Doxycycline showed superiority over placebo in terms of clinical success on Day 10 in intention-to-treat patients (odds ratio, 1.9; 95% confidence interval, 1.1 to 3.2), but not in per-protocol patients. Doxycycline was also superior in terms of clinical cure on Day 10, microbiological outcome, use of open label antibiotics, and symptoms. There was no interaction between the treatment effect and any of the subgroup variables (lung function, type of exacerbation, serum C-reactive protein, and bacterial presence).

Conclusions.—Although equivalent to placebo in terms of clinical success on Day 30, doxycycline showed superiority in terms of clinical success and clinical cure on Day 10, microbiological success, the use of open label antibiotics, and symptoms.

Clinical trial registered with www.clinicaltrials.gov (NCT00170222).

▶ It is often difficult to determine the underlying cause of acute exacerbations of chronic obstructive pulmonary disease (COPD). Nevertheless, a recent meta-analysis supported the use of antibiotics[1] (presuming a bacterial cause), and they are now in common use for exacerbations, especially if the patient has increased purulent sputum. However, controversy still exists over the widespread use of antibiotics in exacerbations, especially because the routine use of systemic corticosteroids typically results in significant symptom improvement. Prospective studies that evaluated antibiotic use against placebo were primarily done before the routine use of systemic corticosteroids as part of the management. The authors of this well-designed study sought to determine if antibiotics (doxycycline) added anything to systemic corticosteroids in the contemporary management of acute exacerbations. While there was some early improvement in symptoms in the group with antibiotic at day 10, by day 30, clinical outcomes were essentially the same. It is of note that patients included in the study were hospitalized, though care was taken to exclude any from the study who had fever or radiological signs of pneumonia, and may have represented patients for whom doxycycline was not an ideal antibiotic choice. Nevertheless, this is the first prospective randomized trial of antibiotics in COPD exacerbations in which systemic steroids were commonly also used. The findings suggest a need for reassessment of the routine role of antibiotics, particularly when increasing resistance and side effects are considered.

J. R. Maurer, MD, MBA

Reference

1. Ram FS, Rodriguez-Roisin R, Granados-Navarrete A, Garcia-Aymerich J, Barnes NC. Antibiotics for exacerbations of chronic obstructive pulmonary disease. *Cochrane Database Syst Rev.* 2006;2. CD004403.

Lung Function in Young Adults Predicts Airflow Obstruction 20 Years Later
Kalhan R, Arynchyn A, Colangelo LA, et al (Northwestern Univ, Chicago, IL; Univ of Alabama at Birmingham; et al)
Am J Med 123:468.e1-468.e7, 2010

Objective.—The burden of obstructive lung disease is increasing, yet there are limited data on its natural history in young adults. To determine in a prospective cohort of generally healthy young adults the influence of early adult lung function on the presence of airflow obstruction in middle age.

Methods.—A longitudinal study was performed of 2496 adults who were 18 to 30 years of age at entry, did not report having asthma, and returned at year 20. Airflow obstruction was defined as a forced expiratory volume in 1 second/forced vital capacity ratio less than the lower limit of normal.

Results.—Airflow obstruction was present in 6.9% and 7.8% of participants at years 0 and 20, respectively. Less than 10% of participants with airflow obstruction self-reported chronic obstructive pulmonary disease. In cross-sectional analyses, airflow obstruction was associated with less education, smoking, and self-reported chronic obstructive pulmonary disease. Low forced expiratory volume in 1 second, forced expiratory volume in 1 second/forced vital capacity ratio, and airflow obstruction in young adults were associated with low lung function and airflow obstruction 20 years later. Of those with airflow obstruction at year 0, 52% had airflow obstruction 20 years later. The forced expiratory volume in 1 second/forced vital capacity at year 0 was highly predictive of airflow obstruction 20 years later (c-statistic 0.91; 95% confidence interval, 0.89-0.93). The effect of cigarette smoking on lung function decline with age was most evident in young adults with preexisting airflow obstruction.

Conclusion.—Airflow obstruction is mostly unrecognized in young and middle-aged adults. Low forced expiratory volume in 1 second, low forced expiratory volume in 1 second/forced vital capacity ratio, airflow obstruction in young adults, and smoking are highly predictive of low lung function and airflow obstruction in middle age.

▶ The population used for this report is from the Coronary Artery Risk Development in Young Adults longitudinal study that in 1985 to 1986 enrolled healthy young adults who did not have known asthma or other airway disease.[1] Lung function was measured at entry, during the study, and after 20 years. Most of the studies of lung function done to date in young adults have either had relatively short follow-up times or have just been cross-sectional. While a correlation has been shown between pulmonary symptoms in early adult life and later development of obstructive airways disease,[2] the long-term outcome or predictive value of asymptomatic obstruction detected early in life has not been previously reported. Currently, spirometry screening for patients who do not report symptoms suggestive of lung disease is not recommended, as it is not cost-effective. However, this study is provocative in that it suggests that lung function abnormalities picked up in early adult life tend to persist. This information would be very valuable for patients to know as they could be counseled to avoid behaviors or occupations that might exacerbate their underlying lung disease.

J. R. Maurer, MD, MBA

References

1. Friedman GD, Cutter GR, Donahue RP, et al. CARDIA: study design, recruitment, and some characteristics of the examined subjects. *J Clin Epidemiol.* 1988;41:1105-1116.
2. de Marco R, Accordini S, Cerveri I, et al. Incidence of chronic obstructive pulmonary disease in a cohort of young adults according to the presence of chronic cough and phlegm. *Am J Respir Crit Care Med.* 2007;175:32-39.

Measurement of COPD Severity Using a Survey-Based Score: Validation in a Clinically and Physiologically Characterized Cohort
Eisner MD, Omachi TA, Katz PP, et al (Univ of California-San Francisco; et al)
Chest 137:846-851, 2010

Background.—A comprehensive survey-based COPD severity score has usefulness for epidemiologic and health outcomes research. We previously developed and validated the survey-based COPD Severity Score without using lung function or other physiologic measurements. In this study, we aimed to further validate the severity score in a different COPD cohort and using a combination of patient-reported and objective physiologic measurements.

Methods.—Using data from the Function, Living, Outcomes, and Work cohort study of COPD, we evaluated the concurrent and predictive validity of the COPD Severity Score among 1,202 subjects. The survey instrument is a 35-point score based on symptoms, medication and oxygen use, and prior hospitalization or intubation for COPD. Subjects were systemically assessed using structured telephone survey, spirometry, and 6-min walk testing.

Results.—We found evidence to support concurrent validity of the score. Higher COPD Severity Score values were associated with poorer FEV_1 ($r = -0.38$), $FEV_1\%$ predicted ($r = -0.40$), Body mass, Obstruction, Dyspnea, Exercise Index ($r = 0.57$), and distance walked in 6 min ($r = -0.43$) ($P < .0001$ in all cases). Greater COPD severity was also related to poorer generic physical health status ($r = -0.49$) and disease-specific health-related quality of life ($r = 0.57$) ($P < .0001$). The score also demonstrated predictive validity. It was also associated with a greater prospective risk of acute exacerbation of COPD defined as ED visits (hazard ratio [HR], 1.31; 95% CI, 1.24-1.39), hospitalizations (HR, 1.59; 95% CI, 1.44-1.75), and either measure of hospital-based care for COPD (HR, 1.34; 95% CI, 1.26-1.41) ($P < .0001$ in all cases).

Conclusion.—The COPD Severity Score is a valid survey-based measure of disease-specific severity, both in terms of concurrent and predictive validity. The score is a psychometrically sound instrument for use in epidemiologic and outcomes research in COPD.

▶ This study is essentially further validation of a tool that is designed to characterize chronic obstructive pulmonary disease (COPD) severity in large populations in the absence of lung function studies and other measures. The authors previously developed and preliminarily validated this tool, called the COPD Severity Score.[1] This study differs from the authors' previous validation in that rather than actual measurements made on a subset of patients, a large number of measurements were made on an entire large cohort of patients with COPD. These measurements included all data needed to calculate the Body Mass, Obstruction, Dyspnea, Exercise Index, quality of life measurements, and a functional limitation questionnaire that included additional functional questions from the Short Form 36 questionnaire.

The authors state that the idea was to concurrently validate the COPD Severity Score by assessing its association with pulmonary function and other physical measurement, health-related quality of life, and functional limitations.

The COPD cohort used in the current validation study was from a large health plan, included a broad spectrum of COPD, and the population was demographically diverse. The COPD Severity Score itself asks about respiratory symptoms, use of corticosteroids, use of other COPD medications, hospitalizations/intubations, and home oxygen use. A weighted scoring system is used that results in a score of 0 to 35.

This tool appears to have high correlation with actual measured parameters that we typically use to assess the impact on an individual of COPD; hopefully, it can help us better understand the impact of COPD on population health.

J. R. Maurer, MD, MBA

Reference

1. Eisner MD, Trupin L, Katz PP, et al. Development and validation of a survey-based COPD severity score. *Chest.* 2005;127:1890-1897.

Antibiotic Therapy and Treatment Failure in Patients Hospitalized for Acute Exacerbations of Chronic Obstructive Pulmonary Disease
Rothberg MB, Pekow PS, Lahti M, et al (Baystate Med Ctr, Springfield, MA; Univ of Massachusetts School of Public Health, Amherst)
JAMA 303:2035-2042, 2010

Context.—Guidelines recommend antibiotic therapy for acute exacerbations of chronic obstructive pulmonary disease (COPD), but the evidence is based on small, heterogeneous trials, few of which include hospitalized patients.

Objective.—To compare the outcomes of patients treated with antibiotics in the first 2 hospital days with those treated later or not at all.

Design, Setting, and Patients.—Retrospective cohort of patients aged 40 years or older who were hospitalized from January 1, 2006, through December 31, 2007, for acute exacerbations of COPD at 413 acute care facilities throughout the United States.

Main Outcome Measures.—A composite measure of treatment failure, defined as the initiation of mechanical ventilation after the second hospital day, inpatient mortality, or readmission for acute exacerbations of COPD within 30 days of discharge; length of stay, and hospital costs.

Results.—Of 84 621 patients, 79% received at least 2 consecutive days of antibiotic treatment. Treated patients were less likely than nontreated patients to receive mechanical ventilation after the second hospital day (1.07%; 95% confidence interval [CI], 1.06%-1.08% vs 1.80%; 95% CI, 1.78%-1.82%), had lower rates of inpatient mortality (1.04%; 95% CI, 1.03%-1.05% vs 1.59%; 95% CI, 1.57%-1.61%), and had lower rates of readmission for acute exacerbations of COPD (7.91%; 95% CI, 7.89%-7.94% vs 8.79%; 95% CI, 8.74%-8.83%). Patients treated with antibiotic agents had a higher rate of readmissions for *Clostridium difficile* (0.19%; 95% CI, 0.187%-0.193%) than those who were not treated (0.09%; 95% CI, 0.086%-0.094%). After multivariable adjustment, including the propensity for antibiotic treatment, the risk of treatment failure was lower in antibiotic-treated patients (odds ratio, 0.87; 95% CI, 0.82-0.92). A grouped treatment approach and hierarchical modeling to account for potential confounding of hospital effects yielded similar results. Analysis stratified by risk of treatment failure found similar magnitudes of benefit across all subgroups.

Conclusion.—Early antibiotic administration was associated with improved outcomes among patients hospitalized for acute exacerbations of COPD regardless of the risk of treatment failure.

▶ The role of antibiotics in acute exacerbations of chronic obstructive pulmonary disease (COPD) has been controversial over the years and has never been really well defined. As the authors note, current recommendations to use antibiotics come from a relatively small number of randomized trials incorporating only 917 patients and that looked only at short-term outcomes and treatment failure. In addition, the bulk of the studies were done before 1992. In the current era, large databases of patients with different types of diagnoses and in different settings are available and can be mined for various purposes. While studies done from these databases are typically retrospective, they have the benefit of looking at the treatments and outcomes of large numbers of patients, especially if the parameters for entry into the database are standardized. In this study, the authors looked at a database, Premier's Perspective, (a database developed for measuring quality and utilization). The data came from more than 400 hospitals across the country and included more than 84 000 hospitalizations of patients for COPD exacerbations. Approximately 79% of patients received antibiotics in this study, and in those who received antibiotics, there was a 13% decrease in the risk of treatment failure (defined as initiation of mechanical ventilation after hospital day 2, in-hospital mortality, or readmission for COPD within 30 days of discharge). The major negative effect of antibiotic use was readmission due to *Clostridium difficile* infection/diarrhea. While the methodology of this study is not as robust as that of a prospective trial, its findings are compelling. Certainly the findings beg for a large randomized trial of patients with COPD exacerbations; however, as we know from multiple other attempts at large randomized trials, they are very hard to recruit to and complete, and it is not clear whether such a trial will ever be done. In the absence of that level of evidence, the authors' conclusions that generally antibiotics are indicated in patients with COPD exacerbations should be heeded—at least until definitive markers are identified that predict good outcomes without antibiotic treatment.

J. R. Maurer, MD, MBA

Patient-Clinician Communication: Associations With Important Health Outcomes Among Veterans With COPD

Slatore CG, Cecere LM, Reinke LF, et al (Portland Veterans Affairs Med Ctr, OR; Univ of Washington, Seattle)
Chest 138:628-634, 2010

Background.—High quality patient-clinician communication is widely advocated, but little is known about which health outcomes are associated with communication for patients with COPD.

Methods.—Using a cross-sectional study of 342 veterans enrolled in a randomized controlled trial, we evaluated the association of communication, measured with the quality of communication (QOC) instrument, with subject-reported quality of clinician care, breathing problem confidence, and general self-rated health. We measured these associations using general estimating equations and adjusted odds ratios (OR) of patient-reported outcomes associated with one-point changes in QOC scores.

Results.—Nearly one-half of the subjects reported receiving the best imaginable care (47%), whereas fewer reported being confident with their breathing problems all the time (29%) or in very good or excellent health (15%). General communication was associated with best-imagined quality of care (OR, 4.29; 95% CI, 2.84-6.48; $P < .001$) and confidence in dealing with breathing problems all the time (OR, 1.74; 95% CI, 1.34-2.25; $P < .001$) but not general self-rated health (OR, 1.19; 95% CI, 0.92-1.55; $P = .19$). Specific clinician behaviors with larger associations with higher quality care included listening, caring, and attentiveness. The associations between general communication and quality care increased over time (P for interaction .03).

Conclusions.—Communication between patients and clinicians is associated with quality of care and confidence in dealing with breathing problems, and this association may change over time. Attention to specific communication strategies may lead to improvements in the care of patients with COPD.

▶ Today's patient-physician interactions are often reported by both parties to be unsatisfactory; patients complain about the 10 minutes or less they get in face time, and physicians complain about the need to rush through their patients to survive financially. The relationship is difficult to nurture and develop. But does it really matter in patient outcomes or other relevant measures if the physician takes the time to really get to know the patient and focuses on delivering patient-centered care? This study is one of the only ones I have seen that seeks to measure this. Patient-reported outcomes, such as perceived quality of care, confidence in dealing with breathing problems, perception of health, were compared with the quality of communication with the physician by scoring how well the physician used 6 general communication attributes, for example, listening to what you have to say. The best correlation was that of patient perception of high quality of care and high quality of communication; this strengthened as relationships progressed over time; however, other patient-reported health outcomes were little correlated with quality of communication. Patient-centered care is a theme of health care reform and, I think, many of us believe that a core piece of patient-centered care is more patient involvement in their care decisions. But it is not clear exactly how to do that, and this study illustrates how difficult a goal that is to achieve. A piece that is missing from this report is actual hard outcomes like rates of use of health care services. Future studies assessing improved patient-physician communications should incorporate these types of outcomes and patient perceptions.

J. R. Maurer, MD, MBA

Inhaled corticosteroid use is associated with lower mortality for subjects with COPD and hospitalised with pneumonia

Malo de Molina R, Mortensen EM, Restrepo MI, et al (Disseminations and Implementation Ctr (VERDICT)/South Texas Veterans Health Care System, San Antonio)

Eur Respir J 36:751-757, 2010

Recent studies suggest that use of inhaled corticosteroids (ICS) in chronic obstructive pulmonary disease (COPD) may be associated with a higher incidence of pneumonia. However, it is unclear whether COPD subjects on ICS who develop pneumonia have worse outcomes. Therefore, our aim was to examine the association of prior outpatient ICS therapy with mortality in hospitalised COPD subjects with pneumonia.

We included subjects ≥64 yrs of age, hospitalised with pneumonia in US Veterans Affairs hospitals, and assessed the association of ICS exposure with mortality for hospitalised COPD subjects with pneumonia in a covariate-adjusted regression model.

We identified 6,353 subjects with a diagnosis of pneumonia and prior COPD, of whom 38% were on ICS. Mortality was 9% at 30 days and 16% at 90 days. In regression analyses, outpatient ICS therapy was associated with lower mortality at both 30 days (OR 0.76, 95% CI 0.70–0.83), and 90 days (OR 0.80, 95% CI 0.75–0.86).

Outpatient therapy with ICS was associated with a significantly lower 30- and 90-day mortality in hospitalised COPD patients with pneumonia.

▶ Inhaled corticosteroids (ICS) for patients with stable, severe, and very severe chronic obstructive pulmonary disease (COPD) are widely used because of studies that showed a reduction in exacerbations when ICS are used.[1] In fact, the Global Obstructive Lung Disease guideline recommends adding ICS to bronchodilator therapy in patients with severe or worse disease. However, the finding of a reduction in exacerbations has been somewhat tempered by more recent reports that patients on ICS are more likely than those not on ICS to be hospitalized with pneumonia.[2] The piece that has been missing and is addressed by this study is a better understanding of the impact of the pneumonia in patients on ICS. This study, which is a retrospective review of a large Veteran's Administration database, found that those patients on ICS who developed pneumonia had increased, rather than decreased, survival at 30 and 90 days compared with patients without recent ICS use (Fig 2 in the original article). This is an important finding and should help clinicians feel more comfortable prescribing ICS for their patients with COPD who can benefit symptomatically and with a better quality of life. We need to keep in mind that the study, in addition to being retrospective, comprised a 98% male population with an average age of almost 75 years, making it less than representative of the usual COPD population. In addition, diagnostic codes were relied on, and pulmonary functions were not used. Thus, we would welcome a prospective study that focused more specifically on outcomes of patients with severe and very severe disease who develop pneumonia on ICS.

J. R. Maurer, MD, MBA

References

1. Nannini LJ, Cates CJ, Lasserson TJ, Poole P. Combined corticosteroid and long-acting beta-agonist in one inhaler versus placebo for chronic obstructive pulmonary disease. *Cochrane Database Syst Rev.* 2007;(4):CD003794.
2. Drummond MB, Dasenbrook EC, Pitz MW, Murphy DJ, Fan E. Inhaled corticosteroids in patients with stable chronic obstructive pulmonary disease: a systematic review and meta-analysis. *JAMA.* 2008;300:2407-2416.

Trends and Burden of Bronchiectasis-Associated Hospitalizations in the United States, 1993-2006
Seitz AE, Olivier KN, Steiner CA, et al (Natl Insts of Health, Bethesda, MD; Agency for Healthcare Res and Quality, Rockville, MD)
Chest 138:944-949, 2010

Background.—Current data on bronchiectasis prevalence, trends, and risk factors are lacking; such data are needed to estimate the burden of disease and for improved medical care and public health resource allocation. The objective of the present study was to estimate the trends and burden of bronchiectasis-associated hospitalizations in the United States.

Methods.—We extracted hospital discharge records containing International *Classification of Diseases, 9th Revision, Clinical Modification* codes for bronchiectasis (494, 494.0, and 494.1) as any discharge diagnosis from the State Inpatient Databases from the Agency for Healthcare Research and Quality. Discharge records were extracted for 12 states with complete and continuous reporting from 1993 to 2006.

Results.—The average annual age-adjusted hospitalization rate from 1993 to 2006 was 16.5 hospitalizations per 100,000 population. From 1993 to 2006, the age-adjusted rate increased significantly, with an average annual percentage increase of 2.4% among men and 3.0% among women. Women and persons aged > 60 years had the highest rate of bronchiectasis-associated hospitalizations. The median cost for inpatient care was 7,827 US dollars (USD) (range, 13-543,914 USD).

Conclusions.—The average annual age-adjusted rate of bronchiectasis-associated hospitalizations increased from 1993 to 2006. This study furthers the understanding of the impact of bronchiectasis and demonstrates the need for further research to identify risk factors and reasons for the increasing burden.

▶ Bronchiectasis is a relatively neglected pulmonary condition, although several articles in the last few years have sought to ascertain prevalence (52.3 cases/100 000 adults in the United States),[1] those most affected (women and > age 50 years),[2,3] and health care use. Bronchiectasis is not an uncommon comorbidity in other conditions such as α-1 antitrypsin deficiency emphysema, pulmonary fibrosis (traction bronchiectasis), and atypical myco-bacterial infection in older women, for example. The costs of bronchiectasis are felt to be underappreciated. In this study, the authors sought to determine bronchiectasis-associated hospitalizations and the burden of the disease using an extensive agency for health care research and quality utilization and database. These data show that bronchiectasis is an increasingly common condition among the elderly and occurs particularly in older women. More attention should be paid to the underlying causes of bronchiectasis and to approaches to preventing or mitigating them. Not only is this an increasing disease burden in the United States with an increasingly aging population, but it also has important quality of life and health care cost implications as well.

J. R. Maurer, MD, MBA

References

1. Weycker D, Edelsberg J, Oster G, Tino G. Prevalence and economic burden of bronchiectasis. *Clin Pulm Med.* 2005;12:205-209.
2. Morrissey BM, Harper RW. Bronchiectasis: sex and gender considerations. *Clin Chest Med.* 2004;25:361-372.
3. Nicotra MB, Rivera M, Dale AM, Shepherd R, Carter R. Clinical, pathophysio-logic, and microbiologic characterization of bronchiectasis in an aging cohort. *Chest.* 1995;108:955-961.

Disease Management Program for Chronic Obstructive Pulmonary Disease: A Randomized Controlled Trial
Rice KL, Dewan N, Bloomfield HE, et al (VA Med Ctr, Minneapolis, MN; VA Med Ctr, Omaha, NE; Univ of Minnesota, Minneapolis; et al)
Am J Respir Crit Care Med 182:890-896, 2010

Rationale.—The effect of disease management for chronic obstructive pulmonary disease (COPD) is not well established.

Objectives.—To determine whether a simplified disease management program reduces hospital admissions and emergency department (ED) visits due to COPD.

Methods.—We performed a randomized, adjudicator-blinded, controlled, 1-year trial at five Veterans Affairs medical centers of 743 patients with severe COPD and one or more of the following during the previous year: hospital admission or ED visit for COPD, chronic home oxygen use, or course of systemic corticosteroids for COPD. Control group patients received usual care. Intervention group patients received a single 1- to 1.5-hour education session, an action plan for self-treatment of exacerbations, and monthly follow-up calls from a case manager.

Measurements and Main Results.—We determined the combined number of COPD-related hospitalizations and ED visits per patient. Secondary outcomes included hospitalizations and ED visits for all causes, respiratory medication use, mortality, and change in Saint George's

Respiratory Questionnaire. After 1 year, the mean cumulative frequency of COPD-related hospitalizations and ED visits was 0.82 per patient in usual care and 0.48 per patient in disease management (difference, 0.34; 95% confidence interval, 0.15–0.52; $P < 0.001$). Disease management reduced hospitalizations for cardiac or pulmonary conditions other than COPD by 49%, hospitalizations for all causes by 28%, and ED visits for all causes by 27% ($P < 0.05$ for all).

Conclusions.—A relatively simple disease management program reduced hospitalizations and ED visits for COPD.

Clinical trial registered with www.clinicaltrials.gov (NCT00126776).

▶ Patients with chronic obstructive pulmonary disorder (COPD) have nearly 750 000 inpatient admissions and 500 000 emergency room visits in the United States per year, accounting for more than $20 billion per year in direct health care costs.[1] Combined with other common diseases such as asthma, diabetes, coronary disease, and heart failure, the health care cost burden of these chronic illnesses is excessive, growing, and unsustainable. Approaches to containing these costs and improving quality of life have included disease management programs like those studied here. Briefly, these are programs designed to reduce the use of health care resources by teaching people and assisting them in better caring for themselves through a better understanding of their conditions (Fig 2 in the original article). One might expect this to reduce acute care costs. Disease management programs such as the one reported here have often been hard to assess in that it often takes an extended period of time to show reductions in health care costs in patients with chronic diseases who have multiple ongoing maintenance costs, in addition to their intermittent acute care costs. In addition, many studies have not used randomized studies that apply the disease management intervention to only part of the study participants. Thus, this is a particularly welcome study because it used a robust methodology for the study, and it also used relatively easy interventions, which should be able to be replicated across other groups of patients with COPD. Because it is crucial to not only contain health care costs but also to help those with chronic conditions take more ownership of their conditions and live more fulfilling lives, we applaud this study and hope to see robust disease management programs implemented across many more chronic populations.

J. R. Maurer, MD, MBA

Reference

1. Foster TS, Miller JD, Marton JP, Caloyeras JP, Russell MW, Menzin J. Assessment of the economic burden of COPD in the U.S.: a review and synthesis of the literature. *COPD.* 2006;3:211-218.

A randomised trial of domiciliary, ambulatory oxygen in patients with COPD and dyspnoea but without resting hypoxaemia

Moore RP, Berlowitz DJ, Denehy L, et al (Austin Hosp, Heidelberg, Victoria, Australia; The Univ of Melbourne, Parkville, Victoria, Australia; et al)
Thorax 66:32-37, 2011

Background.—Patients with chronic obstructive pulmonary disease (COPD) who are not severely hypoxaemic at rest may experience significant breathlessness on exertion, and ambulatory oxygen is often prescribed in this circumstance despite a lack of conclusive evidence for benefit. This study aimed to determine whether such patients benefit from domiciliary ambulatory oxygen and, if so, which factors may be associated with benefit.

Methods.—This was a 12 week, parallel, double-blinded, randomised, placebo-controlled trial of cylinder air versus cylinder oxygen, provided at 6 l/min intranasally, for use during any activity provoking breathlessness. Patients underwent baseline measurements of arterial blood gases and lung function. Outcome measures assessed dyspnoea, health-related quality of life, mood disturbance, functional status and cylinder utilisation. Data were analysed on an intention-to-treat basis, $p \leq 0.05$.

Results.—143 subjects (44 female), mean ± SD age 71.8 ± 9.8 years, forced expiratory volume in 1 s (FEV_1) 1.16 ± 0.51 lites, PaO_2 9.5 ± 1.1 kPa (71.4 ± 8.5 mm Hg) were randomised, including 50 patients with exertional desaturation to ≤88%. No significant differences in any outcome were found between groups receiving air or oxygen. Statistically significant but clinically small improvements in dyspnoea and depression were observed in the whole study group over the 12 weeks of the study.

Conclusion.—In breathless patients with COPD who do not have severe resting hypoxaemia, domiciliary ambulatory oxygen confers no benefits in terms of dyspnoea, quality of life or function. Exertional desaturation is not predictive of outcome. Intranasal gas (either air or oxygen) may provide a placebo benefit.

Clinical Trial Number.—ACTRN12605000457640.

▶ Wow! I am surprised by these results. This is an extremely well-done study. It is hard to blind patients to oxygen use, but these investigators were able to.

We know from very old Nocturnal Oxygen Therapy Trial and MOT studies that long-term oxygen for hypoxemic chronic obstructive pulmonary disease patients improves survival. But no one has ever proven what we all believe and take for granted: that is, oxygen for exercise makes a difference in morbidity and mortality. These authors did not really have a large or long study to reach conclusions about mortality, but certainly morbidity did not change on therapy.

J. A. Barker, MD

3 Lung Cancer

Introduction

Lung cancer exacts an enormous toll globally, resulting in more than a million deaths per year worldwide. In the United States, the American Cancer Society projected that total lung cancer related deaths in 2010 would number 157,300, with mortality rates falling over the past several years in men but remaining at the same level in women. The magnitude of mortality is starkly emphasized in the recognition that lung cancer causes more deaths per year than the next four most common causes of cancer death—breast, colorectal, prostate, and pancreatic cancers—combined.

Tobacco remains the single most important epidemiologic factor associated with lung cancer risk. We have known since 1950 that cigarette smoking is causally implicated in lung cancer pathogenesis. Yet despite extensive public health educational interventions and public policy limitations on tobacco use in community settings, 20.6% of adult Americans (46.6 million individuals) continue to habitually smoke cigarettes. This glaring disconnect, as well as evidence that smoking cessation reduces not just the risk of a primary lung cancer, but renders benefit in decreasing subsequent lung cancer recurrence and mortality, as well as development of other non-lung cancers, should reinforce the goal of developing and implementing better strategies to facilitate smoking cessation.

In 2011, we await the results of the National Lung Screening Trial (NLST). Preliminary data reportedly demonstrate survival benefit with annual CT screening in patients who have smoked $\geq$30 pack-years, though these results have as yet to be formally published. Anticipating this, the report by Croswell and colleagues confirming the high false-positive rate (21%) in patients undergoing lung cancer screening with CT scanning in the context of the Prostate, Lung, Colorectal, and Ovarian Cancer Screening Trial heightens concern about how the predictable burden of false positive findings with such screening, from both physician manpower and economic perspectives, will be managed and minimized. To this end, the use of novel approaches, such as nodule volume assessment, or implementation of guidelines for managing small pulmonary nodules, both solid and subsolid, merit attention. Further, it will be important to examine the populations identified as targets for screening. The NLST participants are all smokers of 30 or more pack-years. However, we recognize that a significant minority of patients with lung cancer in the United States, and an even larger percentage of patients with lung cancer in Asia, are nonsmokers and so would not necessarily be identified for screening under the NLST criteria. Maeda and colleagues report of an 11% overall late recurrence rate after 5 years of disease-free survival following curative lung cancer resection in a large population of patients, and in particular a late recurrence rate of 8.8% in patients whose tumors were stage I, highlights the recognition that specific populations not included in the NLST may warrant screening as well, which only further study will clarify.

If CT scanning becomes more prevalent, it seems almost inevitable that the use of positron emission tomography (PET) will continue to escalate, as the use of PET imaging in the context of lung nodule evaluation has become more common. Nair and colleagues present an interesting analysis suggesting that the intensity of tumor uptake of ^{18}F-fluorodeoxyglucose (FDG) may also be a predictor of outcome in patients with non-small cell lung cancer (NSCLC). The use of PET will need to be monitored, as it is substantially more expensive than CT scanning. Cost analyses such as that presented by Barnett and colleagues will become increasingly important when considering the anticipated health care expenditures if lung cancer screening becomes a recommended intervention. Along these same lines, the prospect of lung cancer screening by CT should prompt reconsideration of the efficacy of bronchoscopic evaluation for evaluation of pulmonary nodules as well as for the evaluation of lung cancer. Gomez and Silvestri provide a comprehensive review of endobronchial ultrasound and its utility in lung cancer diagnosis and staging. Edell and Krier-Morrow review the practical aspects of navigational bronchoscopy, which has the potential to become an important tool in the evaluation of peripheral lung lesions. Development of evidence-based guidelines for the management of radiographic pulmonary abnormalities, enhancing physician adherence to guideline recommendations, and judicious use of noninvasive imaging studies as well as minimally invasive and invasive approaches will all be important in ensuring cost-effective care.

Progress continues to be made in all aspects of treatment for patients with lung cancer. Temel and colleagues present a provocative report on the benefit of early palliative care for patients with metastatic NSCLC. In their study, this intervention resulted in a magnitude of improvement in survival equivalent to that obtained with breakthroughs in pharmacologic treatments. The reasons for this benefit are not clear; though better alleviation of pain and depression associated with early palliation are likely contributing factors. This points out that the treatment of patients with lung cancer ideally should be multidisciplinary; most patients will require the input of more than one medical or surgical specialist, and clearly the role of the palliative team in this approach should be recognized.

Over the past decade, the spectrum of treatment options for lung cancer has expanded considerably, including innovations in thoracic surgical and interventional bronchoscopic approaches, refinements of adjuvant therapy for early stage patients at higher risk of postsurgical recurrence, and development of targeted biologic therapies to complement standard chemotherapy.

All of this has facilitated more flexibility in consideration of treatment for specific subpopulations of patients. We increasingly recognize that elderly persons, those with limited pulmonary reserve, patients whose cancers may elude standard staging classifications (for example those with multifocal lung cancer or multiple synchronous primaries), and patients whose tumors harbor specific genetic mutations which identify them for targeted biologic therapies all require individualized approaches, with the ultimate goal of personalized cancer treatment for all patients. At present, genetic mutations can be identified in many nonsmoking patients with NSCLC, and for these patients specific therapy directed by those molecular targets can be associated with enormous benefit, even in patients with late stage disease. For the larger majority of patients with advanced NSCLC, cytotoxic chemotherapy will remain the mainstay of treatment. For all patients, the rapidly expanding body of knowledge relating to understanding the many varied biologic aspects of cancers in general and lung cancer specifically should contribute to improve our ability to offer successful therapies for all stages of disease.

Lynn T. Tanoue, MD

Diagnostic Evaluation

Endobronchial Ultrasound for the Diagnosis and Staging of Lung Cancer

Gomez M, Silvestri GA (Med Univ of South Carolina, Charleston)
Proc Am Thorac Soc 6:180-186, 2009

The diagnosis of indeterminate mediastinal lymph nodes, masses, and peripheral pulmonary nodules constitutes a significant challenge. Options for tissue diagnoses include computed tomography–guided percutaneous biopsy, transbronchial fine-needle aspiration, mediastinoscopy, left anterior mediastinotomy, or video-assisted thoracoscopic surgery; however, these approaches have both advantages and limitations in terms of tissue yield, safety profile, and cost. Endobronchial ultrasound (EBUS) is a new minimally invasive technique that expands the view of the bronchoscopist beyond the lumen of the airway. There are two EBUS systems currently available. The radial probe EBUS allows for evaluation of central airways, accurate definition of airway invasion, and facilitates the diagnosis of peripheral lung lesions. Linear EBUS guides transbronchial needle aspiration of hilar and mediastinal lymph nodes, improving diagnostic yield. This article will review the principles and clinical applications of EBUS, and will highlight the role of this new technology in the diagnosis and staging of lung cancer (Table 2).

▶ Endobronchial ultrasound (EBUS) was introduced in the early 1990s. EBUS is minimally invasive and safe, and a growing evidence base supports its high accuracy. Though it is not a new technology, widespread availability and usage have been relatively slow, related in part to equipment cost, the need

TABLE 2.—Endobronchial Ultrasound-Guided Transbronchial Needle Aspiration Of The Mediastinum In Lung Cancer

Study/Year	Patients	Technique	Sensitivity %	Specificity %	FP %	FN %	Cancer %
Vincent/2008 (50)	152	RT-22 ga	99	100	0	1	74
Herth/2008 (42)*	100	RT-22 ga	89	100	0	1	9
Bauwens/2008 (41)†	106	RT-22 ga	95	97	0	3	55
Koh/2008 (46)	16	Rad-21 ga	83	100	0	13	63
Herth/2006 (43)	502	RT-22 ga	94	100	0	89‡	98
Herth/2006 (44)	100	RT-22 ga	94	100	0	1	17
Plat/2006 (47)	33	Rad-histo	93	100	0	25	82
Yasufuku/2005 (51)	108	RT-22 ga	95	100	0	11	69
Vilman/2005 (49)	31	RT-22 ga	85	100	0	28	65
Rintoul/2005 (48)	20	RT-22 ga	79	100	0	30	70
Kanoh/2005 (45)	54	Rad-19 ga	86	100	0	37	81
Yasufuku/2004 (52)	70	RT-22 ga	95	100	0	10	67
Summary	1292		93	100	0	9	63

Definition of abbreviations: Rad = radial probe; RT = real time.
Reprinted by permission from Reference 36.
*Nodes < 1 cm, negative mediastinal activity in PET scan.
†Increased activity in mediastinum in PET scan.
‡Excluded from calculations because NPV is less reliable with a prevalence of > 90%.

for specialized training, and uncertainties in reimbursement. This article by Gomez and Silvestri reviews the 2 types of EBUS and their clinical applications. Radial EBUS is typically used to assess tumor invasion into a bronchus and guide biopsies of peripheral nodules. Radial EBUS can be performed with 2 different types of probes: a standard probe for airway evaluation from the trachea to the level of subsegmental bronchi and an ultraminiature probe for detection of peripheral lesions. Linear (or convex probe) EBUS is most often used to sample lymph nodes in the mediastinum and typically performed in patients with known or suspected lung cancer. This function is the most common application of EBUS at the present time. The authors present a pooled analysis of 12 studies evaluating EBUS in mediastinal staging, outlined in Table 2. Overall, weighted sensitivity was 93%, specificity was 100%, and false-negative rate was 9%. Of note, 10 of the 12 studies were performed in patients with high prevalence of mediastinal cancer involvement (55%-98%), but the other 2 studies were performed in patients with no evidence on imaging studies of mediastinal adenopathy and prevalence of malignant involvement of only 9% and 17%.[1,2] EBUS performed remarkably well in these patients, with sensitivity of 89% and 94%, specificity of 99%, and false-negative rate of only 1%. It is clear that, in trained hands, EBUS is highly accurate as well as being minimally invasive and safe and offers an efficient alternative to mediastinoscopy.

L. T. Tanoue, MD

References

1. Herth FJ, Eberhardt R, Krasnik M, Ernst A. Endobronchial ultrasound-guided transbronchial needle aspiration of lymph nodes in the radiologically and positron emission tomography-normal mediastinum in patients with lung cancer. *Chest.* 2008;133:887-891.

2. Herth FJ, Ernst A, Eberhardt R, Vilmann P, Dienemann H, Krasnik M. Endobronchial ultrasound-guided transbronchial needle aspiration of lymph nodes in the radiologically normal mediastinum. *Eur Respir J.* 2006;28:910-914.

Subsolid Pulmonary Nodules and the Spectrum of Peripheral Adenocarcinomas of the Lung: Recommended Interim Guidelines for Assessment and Management
Godoy MCB, Naidich DP (New York Univ-Langone Med Ctr)
Radiology 253:606-622, 2009

Pulmonary nodule characterization is currently being redefined as new clinical, radiologic, and pathologic data are reported, necessitating a reevaluation of the clinical management, especially of subsolid nodules. These are now known to frequently, although not invariably, fall into the spectrum of peripheral adenocarcinomas of the lung. Strong correlation between the Noguchi histologic classification and computed tomographic (CT) appearances of these lesions, in particular, has been reported. Serial CT findings have further documented that stepwise progression of lesions with ground-glass opacity, manifested as an increase in size or the appearance and/or subsequent increase of solid components, does occur in a select subset of patients. As a consequence, recognition of the potential association between subsolid nodules and peripheral adenocarcinomas requires a review of current guidelines for the management of these lesions, further necessitated by a differential diagnosis that includes benign lesions such as focal inflammation, focal fibrosis, and organizing pneumonia. Specific issues that need to be addressed are the need for consensus regarding an appropriate CT classification, methods for precise measurement of subsolid nodules, including the extent of both ground-glass and solid components, as well as accurate assessment of the growth rates as means for predicting malignancy and prognosis. It is anticipated that interim guidelines may serve to standardize our current management of these lesions, pending further clarification of their natural history (Table).

▶ Technologic advances in CT scanning allow us to appreciate more detailed nuances of pulmonary anatomy. Interest in CT screening for lung cancer has heightened our awareness of the abundance and variety of small pulmonary nodules as well as the importance of density in their interpretation. Ground glass opacity (GGO) is a common feature of small nodules and appears to correlate to some extent to histopathologic features. Small malignant pulmonary nodules are more likely to be of adenocarcinoma histology, with a spectrum ranging from premalignant atypical adenomatous hyperplasia (AAH) to invasive adenocarcinoma. The original histopathologic classification for adenocarcinoma originally described by Noguchi[1]; its 2004 modification by the World Health Organization, and CT radiographic correlates are outlined in the Table. Based on their review of the available classifications and medical literature, pending further evidence relating to natural history, the authors make the

TABLE.—Correlation between the Noguchi Classification of Adenocarcinoma and World Health Organization 2004 Classifications and CT Findings

Noguchi Type	World Health Organization 2004	CT Features
...	AAH	GGO
A, Localized BAC	BAC (mucinous, nonmucinous and mixed mucinous and nonmucinous or indeterminate)	GGO
B, Localized BAC with alveolar collapse	BAC (mucinous, nonmucinous and mixed mucinous and nonmucinous or indeterminate)	GGO with possible solid component
C, Localized BAC with active fibroblastic proliferation	Adenocarcinoma, mixed subtype (with BAC component)	Part-solid nodule with increase in solid component or solid nodule
D, Poorly differentiated	Solid adenocarcinoma with mucin	Part-solid nodule with greater increase in solid component or solid nodule
E, Tubular	Acinar adenocarcinoma	Part-solid nodule with greater increase in solid component or solid nodule
F, Papillary	Papillary adenocarcinoma	Part-solid nodule with greater increase in solid component or solid nodule

Note.—Adapted, with permission, from reference 9.

following recommendations for subsolid pulmonary nodules found on CT scans: (1) Nodules with pure GGO and that are < 5 mm are likely to represent foci of AAH and do not necessarily require follow-up CT studies; (2) Nodules with pure GGO and that are between 5 and 10 mm merit further follow-up. The recommended duration of follow-up of these lesions is unclear, but the traditional 2-year monitoring for stability is likely inadequate and a 3-year minimum is suggested; (3) Nodules with pure GGO and that are > 10 mm are often bronchioloalveolar carcinoma (BAC) but may be invasive adenocarcinoma. Surgical resection should be considered if after a 3- to 6-month interval, they are demonstrated to be persistent, and in particular, if on serial imaging, there is evidence of an increasing solid component or growth; and (4) Nodules that have mixed GGO and solid components are more likely to be invasive adenocarcinoma with BAC features. Similar to pure GGO nodules, lack of resolution after a 3- to 6-month interval warrants consideration of surgical resection.

These recommendations are generalizations guided by the medical literature and based on experience and, if implemented, should be used with that understanding. They provide a useful starting point for developing a standardized approach to subsolid pulmonary nodules. Decisions regarding the management of these frequent CT findings should be made in an as organized and objective manner as possible, rather than haphazardly or an individual basis. Ultimately, guidelines for this important and challenging area of pulmonary medicine will need to be based on a larger body of evidence.

L. T. Tanoue, MD

Reference

1. Noguchi M, Morikawa A, Kawasaki M, et al. Small adenocarcinoma of the lung. Histologic characteristics and prognosis. *Cancer.* 1995;75:2844-2852.

Navigational Bronchoscopy: Overview of Technology and Practical Considerations—New Current Procedural Terminology Codes Effective 2010
Edell E, Krier-Morrow D (Mayo Clinic, Rochester, MN; Diane Krier-Morrow and Associates, Inc, Evanston, IL)
Chest 137:450-454, 2010

Navigational bronchoscopy provides a three-dimensional virtual "road-map" that enables a physician to maneuver through multiple branches of the bronchial tree to reach targeted lesions in distal regions of the lung. It is designed to be used with a standard bronchoscope to facilitate obtaining tissue samples and for placing radiosurgical or dye markers. This article overviews this technology and the Current Procedural Terminology codes that have been created for its use.

▶ Navigational bronchoscopy is a minimally invasive technique that allows the bronchoscopist-guided access to peripheral areas of the lung. This requires (1) planning software to convert CT scan images into 3-dimensional reconstruction with virtual images of the airways, (2) a steerable sensor probe able to flexibly perform the procedure, and (3) an electromagnetic navigational system consisting of an electromagnetic board and a field generator connected to a computer loaded with the planning software. This is an expensive technology, both as an initial investment and for the single-use probes. As it is new, reimbursement has been very limited, but new current procedural terminology codes were assigned this year. The role of navigational bronchoscopy is most promising in its ability to reliably guide biopsies of peripheral lung lesions, though there are no studies comparing it with conventional flexible bronchoscopy. Anticipating that routine chest CT imaging may become widespread if CT screening for lung cancer is approved, and in that setting many patients will be diagnosed with small peripheral pulmonary nodules, there may in the future be an important role for this new technology.

L. T. Tanoue, MD

PET Scan ¹⁸F-Fluorodeoxyglucose Uptake and Prognosis in Patients With Resected Clinical Stage IA Non-small Cell Lung Cancer
Nair VS, for the Veterans Affairs Solitary Nodule Accuracy Project Cooperative Studies Group (Stanford Univ School of Medicine, CA; et al)
Chest 137:1150-1156, 2010

Objective.—Our objective was to examine the association between ¹⁸F-fluorodeoxyglucose (FDG) uptake on PET scan and prognosis in patients with surgically treated, clinical stage IA non-small cell lung cancer (NSCLC).
Methods.—We reviewed data collection forms and Veterans Affairs administrative records of 75 patients with surgically treated, stage IA

NSCLC who were enrolled in a prospective study of PET imaging from 1999 to 2001. We used Cox proportional hazards analysis to examine the association between FDG uptake and survival 4 years following enrollment.

Results.—Most patients were men (97%), and the mean age was 68 ± 9 years. Almost half of the patients (44%) had adenocarcinoma, and 35% underwent a sublobar resection. The mean maximum standardized uptake value (SUV max) was 4.9 ± 2.5 in survivors and 7.1 ± 3.9 in nonsurvivors ($P = .045$). Before and after adjustment for age, tumor size, histology, and type of resection, the hazard of death was significantly higher in patients with squamous cell histology (adjusted hazard ratio [HR], 4.54; 95% CI, 1.09-18.9) and those with higher degrees of FDG uptake (adjusted HR, 1.21 per 1 unit increment; 95% CI, 1.01-1.45). At a threshold value of 5 for SUV max, 34 of 39 patients (87%) with low FDG uptake survived, compared with only 24 of 36 patients (67%) with high FDG uptake ($P = .04$). Visual assessment of FDG uptake was not associated with an increased hazard of death (HR 0.66; 95% CI, 0.19-2.29).

Conclusions.—High FDG uptake as measured by SUV max identifies individuals with clinical stage IA NSCLC who are at increased risk of death following surgery. Such high-risk patients may be good candidates for participation in future trials of adjuvant therapy.

▶ While we talk to our patients about curing early stage non–small-cell lung cancer (NSCLC), the reality is that survival after surgical resection with curative intent is imperfect even in patients with earliest stage IA disease. Based on the extensive data obtained by the International Association for the Study of Lung Cancer to inform the seventh edition of the lung cancer staging system, it is clear that 5-year survival is achieved in only 71% to 77% of patients with pathologic stage I NSCLC whose tumors are < 30 mm in diameter.[1] This recognition has triggered interest over the years in developing means by which the significant minority of stage I patients doomed to recur can be identified, with the intent of offering further intervention or treatment to increase their chances of survival. These have included examination of biomarkers, such as tumor surface protein expression, tumor gene signatures, and circulating tumor cells. This study by Nair and colleagues suggests that the intensity of tumor ^{18}F-fluorodeoxyglucose (FDG) uptake on positron emission tomography (PET) imaging might be a useful prognostic tool. This approach is appealing in that PET imaging performed on a routine basis preoperatively to look for spread of disease also yields information about the metabolic behavior of the primary site and would be information readily available without incurring further evaluation or cost. Preoperative PET images were examined in 75 patients with resected stage IA NSCLC, with specific attention to the mean maximum standardized uptake value (SUVmax), which is a semiquantitative measure of FDG uptake. As demonstrated in Fig 3 in the original article, SUVmax thresholds of both 5 and 10 discriminated survival, with tumors demonstrating higher SUVmax associated with worse outcomes.

Not all PET imaging is read quantitatively with SUV; consistent measurement can be challenging as it is affected by many variables, including the dose of the isotope, serum glucose, resolution of the scanner, time from injection to imaging, etc. However, standardization can be achieved and may be worth the required effort, as the identification of patients with resected early stage lung cancer who are destined to relapse would allow targeting for enrollment in clinical trials of adjuvant therapy and hopefully improve survival.

L. T. Tanoue, MD

Reference

1. Rami-Porta R, Ball D, Crowley J, et al. The IASLC Lung Cancer Staging Project: proposals for the revision of the T descriptors in the forthcoming (seventh) edition of the TNM classification for lung cancer. *J Thorac Oncol.* 2007;2:593-602.

Combined Endoscopic-Endobronchial Ultrasound-Guided Fine-Needle Aspiration of Mediastinal Lymph Nodes Through a Single Bronchoscope in 150 Patients With Suspected Lung Cancer

Herth FJF, Krasnik M, Kahn N, et al (Dept of Pulmonary and Critical Care Medicine, Thoraxklinik, Heidelberg, Germany; Gentofte Hosp, Copenhagen, Denmark)

Chest 138:790-794, 2010

Background.—For mediastinal lymph nodes, biopsies must often be performed to accurately stage lung cancer. Endobronchial ultrasound-guided transbronchial needle aspiration (EBUS-TBNA) allows real-time guidance in sampling paratracheal, subcarinal, and hilar lymph nodes, and endoscopic ultrasound-guided fine-needle aspiration (EUS-FNA) can sample mediastinal lymph nodes located adjacent to the esophagus. Nodes can be sampled and staged more completely by combining these procedures, but to date use of two different endoscopes has been required. We examined whether both procedures could be performed with a single endobronchial ultrasound bronchoscope.

Methods.—Consecutive patients with a presumptive diagnosis of non-small cell lung cancer (NSCLC) underwent endoscopic staging by EBUS-TBNA and EUS-FNA through a single linear ultrasound bronchoscope. Surgical confirmation and clinical follow-up was used as the reference standard.

Results.—Among 150 evaluated patients, 139 (91%; 83 men, 56 women; mean age 57.6 years) were diagnosed with NSCLC. In these 139 patients, 619 nodes were endoscopically biopsied: 229 by EUS-FNA and 390 by EBUS-TBNA. Sensitivity was 89% for EUS-FNA and 92% for EBUS-TBNA. The combined approach had a sensitivity of 96% and a negative predictive value of 95%, values higher than either approach alone. No complications occurred.

Conclusions.—The two procedures can easily be performed with a dedicated linear endobronchial ultrasound bronchoscope in one setting and by one operator. They are complementary and provide better diagnostic accuracy than either one alone. The combination may be able to replace more invasive methods as a primary staging method for patients with lung cancer.

▶ Endobronchial ultrasound (EBUS) and endoscopic ultrasound (EUS) allow minimally invasive access to mediastinal lymph nodes. Previous studies have suggested that combining the 2 procedures for the purpose of identifying lung cancer lymph node metastases results in higher sensitivity and negative predictive value than achieved by each procedure singly.[1,2] EBUS and EUS are typically performed by different operators with different equipment. This study by Herth and colleagues investigated pairing the 2 procedures using a single linear ultrasound bronchoscope. Their results demonstrate that this approach is feasible and effective. The study population had a high prevalence of lung cancer (91%) and malignant mediastinal involvement (52%). The combined approach yielded cancer diagnosis sensitivity 96%, specificity 100%, and negative predictive value 96%: performance characteristics that were superior to either procedure alone. Moreover, the combined study was very efficient, requiring only 1 anesthesia and procedural time instead of 2. Furthermore, in the hands of these highly trained operators EBUS-transbronchial needle aspiration required only 14 minutes and EUS-Fine-Needle Aspiration only 16 minutes. This emphasizes that EBUS and EUS are complementary procedures. The limitations to performing them with a single linear ultrasound bronchoscope relate to the fact that the adult bronchoscope is shorter than the adult endoscope; it is too short to reach below the diaphragm and thus cannot reach station 8 and 9 nodes accessible to endoscopy that may be important in staging. The authors note precedence for nongastroenterologists performing transesophageal procedures, citing the example of transesophageal echocardiography, and suggest that modifications to the linear ultrasound bronchoscope may facilitate such an approach combining EBUS and EUS as the primary staging procedure for lung cancer.

L. T. Tanoue, MD

References

1. Wallace MB, Pascual JM, Raimondo M, et al. Minimally invasive endoscopic staging of suspected lung cancer. *JAMA.* 2008;299:540-546.
2. Vilmann P, Krasnik M, Larsen SS, Jacobsen GK, Clementsen P. Transesophageal endoscopic ultrasound-guided fine-needle aspiration (EUS-FNA) and endobronchial ultrasound-guided transbronchial needle aspiration (EBUS-TBNA) biopsy: a combined approach in the evaluation of mediastinal lesions. *Endoscopy.* 2005; 37:833-839.

Epidemiology of Lung Cancer

Incidence of human papilloma virus in lung cancer

Klein F, Amin Kotb WFM, Petersen I (Universitätsklinikum Jena, Ziegenmühlenweg, Germany; Charité – Campus Mitte, Berlin, Germany)
Lung Cancer 65:13-18, 2009

HPV has been identified not only in gynaecological carcinomas but also in tumors of other organs, especially of the oropharynx and upper aerodigestive tract. In this study we focused on the available literature on HPV in lung carcinomas. In total, 53 publications reporting on 4508 cases were reviewed and assessed for the following parameters: continent and region of the study, number of cases, detection method, material type, HPV type, histological subtype and number of the HPV-positive cases. Overall, the mean incidence of HPV in lung cancer was 24.5%. While in Europe and America the average reported frequencies were 17% and 15%, respectively, the mean number of HPV in asian lung cancer samples was 35.7%. There was a considerable heterogeneity between certain countries and regions. Particular high frequencies of up to 80% were seen in Okinawa (Japan) and Taichung (Taiwan). However, there were also discrepant results within the same region pointing to methodological differences and the need for validation. All lung cancer subtypes were affected and especially the high risk types 16, 18, 31 and 33 as well as the low risk types 6 and 11 were found, the later mainly in association with squamous cell carcinomas. The data suggest that HPV is the second most important cause of lung cancer after cigarette smoking and strongly argues for additional research on this issue.

▶ In Western countries, cigarette smoking is clearly the most important risk factor for lung cancer, accounting for 90% of all cases.[1] However, with 15% of lung cancers in women in the United States and an even larger percentage of lung cancers in Asia occurring in nonsmokers, there is increased attention to other sources of carcinogenesis besides tobacco. Human papillomavirus (HPV) has been well established as a cause of cervical carcinoma, and evidence is increasing that it is a risk factor for squamous cell carcinoma of the head and neck.[2,3] This report by Klein and colleagues is a review of 53 studies performed across the globe analyzing HPV status in human cancers, including 4508 cases of lung cancer. The incidence of HPV in lung cancer samples from Asian studies was 35.7%, compared with 17% in European and 15% in North American studies. Oncogenic high-risk HPV subtypes include 16, 18, 31, and 33. A previous meta-analysis evaluating 2435 lung cancer cases in 37 published studies also noted geographic heterogeneity, with Asian lung cancer studies demonstrating a significantly higher HPV-16 and HPV-18 prevalence compared with studies from Europe.[4] While these analyses do not prove causation, the known oncogenic role of HPV in cervical carcinoma and its high prevalence when evaluated in patients with lung cancer support further investigation into its potential etiologic role, particularly as potential for preventive intervention would exist.

L. T. Tanoue, MD

References

1. Alberg AJ, Ford JG, Samet JM. Epidemiology of lung cancer: ACCP evidence-based clinical practice guidelines (2nd edition). *Chest.* 2007;132:29S-55S.
2. zur Hausen H. Papillomaviruses and cancer: from basic studies to clinical application. *Nat Rev Cancer.* 2002;2:342-350.
3. Ragin CC, Taioli E, Weissfeld JL, et al. 11q13 amplification status and human papillomavirus in relation to p16 expression defines two distinct etiologies of head and neck tumours. *Br J Cancer.* 2006;95:1432-1438.
4. Srinivasan M, Taioli E, Ragin CC. Human papillomavirus type 16 and 18 in primary lung cancers—a meta-analysis. *Carcinogenesis.* 2009;30:1722-1728.

Smoking as a Factor in Causing Lung Cancer
Bach PB (Memorial Sloan-Kettering Cancer Ctr, NY)
JAMA 301:539-541, 2009

Tobacco Smoking as a Possible Etiologic Factor in Bronchiogenic Carcinoma: A Study of Six Hundred and Eighty-Four Proved Cases
Ernest L. Wynder and Evarts A. Graham, MD
JAMA. 1950;143(4):329-336.
In this case-control study, the investigators compared the smoking histories of individuals with lung cancer and without lung cancer. Participants were matched for age and several dimensions of smoking history were ascertained through a standardized set of questionnaires (including age at initiation and cessation, and average amount smoked per day of cigarettes, cigars, or with a pipe). Each individual's occupational history and history of prior lung disease was captured to control for possible confounders. The investigators found that individuals with lung cancer had a more extensive smoking history than individuals without lung cancer.

▶ As part of the *JAMA* Classics series, this is a review of the classic 1950 report by Wynder and Graham linking cigarette smoking to lung cancer.[1] Any physician who has not read the original article or the analysis by Doll and Hill that same year should do so.[2] These studies elegantly and simply establish the causal link between smoking and lung cancer, though a formal acknowledgment by the US Surgeon General of the relationship would not be forthcoming until 1964.[3] A half century later, with 20% of American adults habitually smoking, we are still not successful in efforts at limiting cigarette consumption and have made minimal inroads in limiting the health consequences of smoking. This commentary by Bach outlines some highlights and failures of tobacco control policy and offers some suggestions for the future.

L. T. Tanoue, MD

References

1. Wynder EL, Graham EA. Tobacco smoking as a possible etiologic factor in bron-chiogenic carcinoma; a study of 684 proved cases. *JAMA.* 1950;143:329-336.
2. Doll R, Hill AB. Smoking and carcinoma of the lung; preliminary report. *Br Med J.* 1950;2:739-748.
3. US Public Health Service. *Smoking and health. Report of the Advisory committee to the Surgeon General of the Public Health Service.* Publication No. 1103. Washington, DC: US Department of Health, Education, and Welfare, Public Health Service; 1964.

Cancer Statistics, 2010
Jemal A, Siegel R, Xu J, et al (American Cancer Society, Atlanta, GA; Ctrs for Disease Control and Prevention, Hyattsville, MD)
CA Cancer J Clin 60:277-300, 2010

Each year, the American Cancer Society estimates the number of new cancer cases and deaths expected in the United States in the current year and compiles the most recent data regarding cancer incidence, mortality, and survival based on incidence data from the National Cancer Institute,

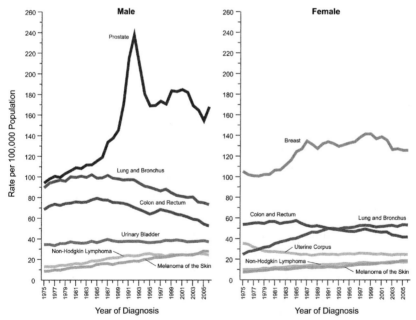

FIGURE 3.—Annual Age-Adjusted Cancer Incidence Rates* for Selected Cancers by Sex, United States, 1975 to 2006. *Rates are age adjusted to the 2000 US standard population and adjusted for delays in reporting. Source: Surveillance, Epidemiology, and End Results (SEER) program (available at: www.seer. cancer.gov). Delay-adjusted incidence database: SEER Incidence Delay-Adjusted Rates, 9 Registries, 1975-2006. Bethesda, MD: National Cancer Institute, Division of Cancer Control and Population Sciences, Surveillance Research Program, Statistical Research and Applications Branch; 2009. Released April 2009, based on the November 2008 SEER data submission. (Reprinted from Jemal A, Siegel R, Xu J, et al. Cancer statistics, 2010. *CA Cancer J Clin.* 2010;60:277-300, with permission from American Cancer Society, Inc.)

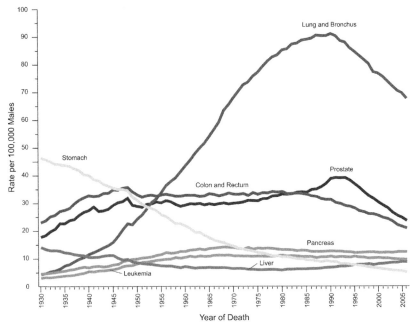

FIGURE 4.—Annual Age-Adjusted Cancer Death Rates*Among Males for Selected Cancers, United States, 1930 to 2006. *Rates are age adjusted to the 2000USstandard population. Due to changes in International Classification of Diseases (ICD) coding, numerator information has changed over time. Rates for cancers of the lung and bronchus, colon and rectum, and liver are affected by these changes. Source: US Mortality Data, 1960 to 2006, US Mortality Vol. 1930 to 1959. National Center for Health Statistics, Centers for Disease Control and Prevention. (Reprinted from Jemal A, Siegel R, Xu J, et al. Cancer statistics, 2010. CA Cancer J Clin. 2010;60:277-300, with permission from American Cancer Society, Inc.)

the Centers for Disease Control and Prevention, and the North American Association of Central Cancer Registries and mortality data from the National Center for Health Statistics. Incidence and death rates are age-standardized to the 2000 US standard million population. A total of 1,529,560 new cancer cases and 569,490 deaths from cancer are projected to occur in the United States in 2010. Overall cancer incidence rates decreased in the most recent time period in both men (1.3% per year from 2000 to 2006) and women (0.5% per year from 1998 to 2006), largely due to decreases in the 3 major cancer sites in men (lung, prostate, and colon and rectum [colorectum]) and 2 major cancer sites in women (breast and colorectum). This decrease occurred in all racial/ethnic groups in both men and women with the exception of American Indian/Alaska Native women, in whom rates were stable. Among men, death rates for all races combined decreased by 21.0% between 1990 and 2006, with decreases in lung, prostate, and colorectal cancer rates accounting for nearly 80% of the total decrease. Among women, overall cancer death rates between 1991 and 2006 decreased by 12.3%, with decreases in breast and colorectal cancer rates accounting for 60% of the total decrease. The reduction in the overall cancer death rates translates to

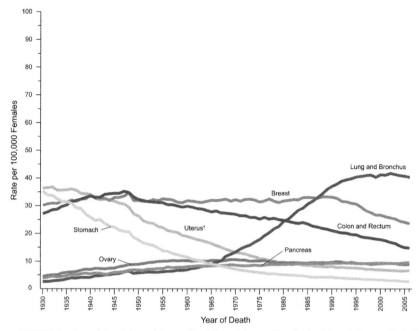

FIGURE 5.—Annual Age-Adjusted Cancer Death Rates* Among Females for Selected Cancers, United States, 1930 to 2006. *Rates are age adjusted to the 2000 US standard population. †Uterus includes uterine cervix and uterine corpus. Due to changes in International Classification of Diseases (ICD) coding, numerator information has changed over time. Rates for cancers of the uterus, ovary, lung and bronchus, and colon and rectum are affected by these changes. Source: US Mortality Data, 1960 to 2006, US Mortality Volumes 1930 to 1959. National Center for Health Statistics, Centers for Disease Control and Prevention. (Reprinted from Jemal A, Siegel R, Xu J, et al. Cancer statistics, 2010. *CA Cancer J Clin.* 2010;60:277-300, with permission from American Cancer Society, Inc.)

the avoidance of approximately 767,000 deaths from cancer over the 16-year period. This report also examines cancer incidence, mortality, and survival by site, sex, race/ethnicity, geographic area, and calendar year. Although progress has been made in reducing incidence and mortality rates and improving survival, cancer still accounts for more deaths than heart disease in persons younger than 85 years. Further progress can be accelerated by applying existing cancer control knowledge across all segments of the population and by supporting new discoveries in cancer prevention, early detection, and treatment (Figs 3, 4 and 5).

▶ Lung cancer is the leading cause of cancer death around the world, accounting for more than 1 million deaths annually.[1] In the United States, prostate cancer in men and breast cancer in women have higher incidence rates than lung cancer (Fig 3), but lung cancer has for a number of years resulted in more deaths annually than the 4 next most common causes of cancer death combined (colorectal, breast, prostate, and pancreatic cancers). This report from the American Cancer Society projected that total deaths in 2010 from lung cancer in the United States would number 157 300 (86 220 men and

71 080 women), with fewer deaths in men and more deaths in women than in 2009. Age-adjusted annual cancer death rates among men and women for selected cancers in the United States from 1930 to 2006 are demonstrated in Figs 4 and 5, which dramatically depict the lung cancer epidemic in the United States over the last 7 decades. In men, lung cancer has been the leading cause of cancer death since the 1950s, with rates steadily declining since about 1990. In women, deaths from lung cancer have exceeded deaths from breast cancer since the late 1980s, with rates appearing to reach a plateau but not declining over the past decade. These statistics remind us that lung cancer is and will remain the most prominent cause of cancer death in the United States in the foreseeable future.

L. T. Tanoue, MD

Reference

1. Parkin DM, Bray F, Ferlay J, Pisani P. Global cancer statistics, 2002. *CA Cancer J Clin.* 2005;55:74-108.

Guidelines of the European Respiratory Society and the European Society of Thoracic Surgeons for the management of malignant pleural mesothelioma

Scherpereel A, Astoul P, Baas P, et al (Hosp of the Univ (CHRU) of Lille II, France; Université de la Méditerranée, Marseille, France; The Netherlands Cancer Inst, Amsterdam; et al)
Eur Respir J 35:479-495, 2010

Malignant pleural mesothelioma (MPM) is a rare tumour but with increasing incidence and a poor prognosis. In 2008, the European Respiratory Society/European Society of Thoracic Surgeons Task Force brought together experts to propose practical and up-to-dated guidelines on the management of MPM.

To obtain an earlier and reliable diagnosis of MPM, the experts recommend performing thoracoscopy, except in cases of pre-operative contraindication or pleural symphysis. The standard staining procedures are insufficient in, ∼10% of cases. Therefore, we propose using specific immunohistochemistry markers on pleural biopsies. In the absence of a uniform, robust and validated staging system, we advise use of the most recent TNM based classification, and propose a three step pre-treatment assessment. Patient's performance status and histological subtype are currently the only prognostic factors of clinical importance in the management of MPM. Other potential parameters should be recorded at baseline and reported in clinical trials. MPM exhibits a high resistance to chemotherapy and only a few patients are candidates for radical surgery. New therapies and strategies have been reviewed.

Because of limited data on the best combination treatment, we emphasise that patients who are considered candidates for a multimodal

TABLE 6.—Prognostic Scoring Systems in Malignant Mesothelioma

First Author [ref.]	Subjects n	Parameter	Good Prognostic Group	Poor Prognostic Group
CALGB HERNDON [40]	337	Performance status	Good	Poor
		Age	<75 yrs	≥75 yrs
		Chest pain	Absent	Present
		Platelet count	$<400 \times 10^{12} \cdot L^{-1}$	$\geq 400 \times 10^{12} \cdot L^{-1}$
		LDH	$<500 \ IU \cdot L^{-1}$	$\geq 500 \ IU \cdot L^{-1}$
EORTC CURRAN [41]	204	Performance status	0	1–2
		Histological subtype	Epithelioid	Nonepithelioid
		Sex	Female	Male
		Certainty of diagnosis	Definite	Possible
		WBC count	$<8.3 \times 10^{9} \cdot L^{-1}$	$\geq 8.3 \times 10^{9} \cdot L^{-1}$
EORTC[#] VAN MEERBEECK [42]	250	Stage	I–II	III–IV
		Histology	Epithelioid	Nonepithelioid
		Interval since diagnosis	<50 days	≥50 days
		Platelet count	$<350 \times 10^{12} \cdot L^{-1}$	$\geq 350 \times 10^{12} \cdot L^{-1}$
		Haemoglobin difference[¶]	<1	>1
		Pain	Absent	Present
		Appetite loss	Absent	Present

CALGB: Cancer and Leukaemia Group B; EORTC: European Organization for Research and Treatment of Cancer; LDH: lactate dehydrogenase; WBC: white blood cell.
Editor's Note: Please refer to original journal article for full references.
[#]Performance status 0–1 was an inclusion criterion for this series.
[¶]Difference between actual value and $16 \ g \cdot dL^{-1}$ and $14 \ g \cdot dL^{-1}$ in males and females, respectively.

approach should be included in a prospective trial at a specialised centre (Table 6).

▶ Malignant mesothelioma is a rare tumor, but its incidence is unfortunately increasing around the world. Though use of asbestos, its primary etiologic agent, is prohibited in the United States, Europe, and most developed nations, asbestos is still produced and used in many countries (including China, Russia, and Canada). These guidelines are based on a systematic analysis of the literature from 1990 to 2009 and provide an extensive evidence-based review with graded recommendations relating to the epidemiology, pathology, staging, and evaluation of mesothelioma as well as a comprehensive review of the evidence relating to treatment, including palliation. Table 6 summarizes 3 prognostic scores that have been prospectively validated and may be useful tools for the practicing clinician in assessing patients with mesothelioma. Treatment options remain of limited benefit. Cure is unlikely, but palliation can be achieved, and so patients with mesothelioma should be evaluated for treatment, preferably at a center with multidisciplinary expertise in this specific area.

L. T. Tanoue, MD

Lung Cancer Screening

Management of Lung Nodules Detected by Volume CT Scanning

van Klaveren RJ, Oudkerk M, Prokop M, et al (Erasmus Med Ctr, Rotterdam, the Netherlands; Univ Med Ctr, Groningen, the Netherlands; Univ Med Ctr, Utrecht, the Netherlands; et al)
N Engl J Med 361:2221-2229, 2009

Background.—The use of multidetector computed tomography (CT) in lung-cancer screening trials involving subjects with an increased risk of lung cancer has highlighted the problem for the clinician of deciding on the best course of action when noncalcified pulmonary nodules are detected by CT.

Methods.—A total of 7557 participants underwent CT screening in years 1, 2, and 4 of a randomized trial of lung-cancer screening. We used software to evaluate a noncalcified nodule according to its volume or volume-doubling time. Growth was defined as an increase in volume of at least 25% between two scans. The first-round screening test was considered to be negative if the volume of a nodule was less than 50 mm^3, if it was 50 to 500 mm^3 but had not grown by the time of the 3-month follow-up CT, or if, in the case of those that had grown, the volume-doubling time was 400 days or more.

Results.—In the first and second rounds of screening, 2.6% and 1.8% of the participants, respectively, had a positive test result. In round one, the sensitivity of the screen was 94.6% (95% confidence interval [CI], 86.5 to 98.0) and the negative predictive value 99.9% (95% CI, 99.9 to 100.0). In the 7361 subjects with a negative screening result in round one, 20 lung cancers were detected after 2 years of follow-up.

Conclusions.—Among subjects at high risk for lung cancer who were screened in three rounds of CT scanning and in whom noncalcified pulmonary nodules were evaluated according to volume and volume-doubling time, the chances of finding lung cancer 1 and 2 years after a negative first-round test were 1 in 1000 and 3 in 1000, respectively. (Current Controlled Trials number, ISRCTN63545820.)

▶ The Dutch-Belgian randomized lung cancer screening trial (Nederlands-Leuvens Longkanker Screenings Onderzoek [NELSON]) is ongoing, having enrolled over 7000 former or current smokers (mean duration of smoking 42 pack-years) and designed to determine whether after 10 years, CT screening will have reduced lung cancer mortality by at least 25%. The NELSON study differs from other CT screening studies in its strategy of measuring nodule volume and volume-doubling time as the main criteria for determining watchful waiting or intervention, as opposed to the traditional 2-dimensional measurement of nodule diameter. The software used to perform the volume measurements is readily available. As in other CT screening studies, the incidence of lung nodules in the study population was very high; 50.5% of participants had at least one noncalcified pulmonary nodule identified on the baseline study, and an additional 21.8% had new nodules identified on the first annual screening study. The unique feature of the NELSON study is the implementation of the volume strategy to guide intervention. A positive test was defined as a noncalcified nodule with a solid component > 500 mm^3. An indeterminate test was defined as a volume of the largest solid nodule or the solid component of a partially solid nodule of 50 to 500 mm^3 or the diameter of a nonsolid nodule > 8 mm. Indeterminate tests triggered a follow-up study done approximately 3 months later to assess for growth, with a positive study defined as a volume-doubling time < 400 days and a negative study as a doubling time > 400 days. This strategy decreased the need for follow-up serial radiographic examinations without reducing the sensitivity of the screening. This approach will need to be validated but may prove beneficial if CT screening for lung cancer is ever implemented broadly.

L. T. Tanoue, MD

Cumulative Incidence of False-Positive Test Results in Lung Cancer Screening: A Randomized Trial

Croswell JM, Baker SG, Marcus PM, et al (Natl Cancer Inst, Bethesda, MD)
Ann Intern Med 152:505-512, 2010

Background.—Direct-to-consumer promotion of lung cancer screening has increased, especially low-dose computed tomography (CT). However, screening exposes healthy persons to potential harms, and cumulative false-positive rates for low-dose CT have never been formally reported.

Objective.—To quantify the cumulative risk that a person who participated in a 1- or 2-year lung cancer screening examination would receive at least 1 false-positive result, as well as rates of unnecessary diagnostic procedures.

Design.—Randomized, controlled trial of low-dose CT versus chest radiography. (ClinicalTrials.gov registration number: NCT00006382).

Setting.—Feasibility study for the ongoing National Lung Screening Trial.

Patients.—Current or former smokers, aged 55 to 74 years, with a smoking history of 30 pack-years or more and no history of lung cancer (*n* = 3190).

Intervention.—Random assignment to low-dose CT or chest radiography with baseline and 1 repeated annual screening; 1-year follow-up after the final screening. Randomization was centralized and stratified by age, sex, and study center.

Measurements.—False-positive screenings, defined as a positive screening with a completed negative work-up or 12 months or more of follow-up with no lung cancer diagnosis.

Results.—By using a Kaplan–Meier analysis, a person's cumulative probability of 1 or more false-positive low-dose CT examinations was 21% (95% CI, 19% to 23%) after 1 screening and 33% (CI, 31% to 35%) after 2. The rates for chest radiography were 9% (CI, 8% to

11%) and 15% (CI, 13% to 16%), respectively. A total of 7% of participants with a false-positive low-dose CT examination and 4% with a false-positive chest radiography had a resulting invasive procedure.

Limitations.—Screening was limited to 2 rounds. Follow-up after the second screening was limited to 12 months. The false-negative rate is probably an underestimate.

Conclusion.—Risks for false-positive results on lung cancer screening tests are substantial after only 2 annual examinations, particularly for low-dose CT. Further study of resulting economic, psychosocial, and physical burdens of these methods is warranted.

▶ From lung cancer CT screening studies done a decade ago, we know that false-positive results are an enormous issue. With the results from the National Lung Screening Trial (NLST) on the verge of release, this report from the NLST feasibility study performed within the Prostate, Lung, Colorectal, and Ovarian Cancer Screening Trial is particularly relevant. Participants had smoked > 30 pack-years, were aged 55 to 74 years, and had received either a baseline screening chest radiograph or CT scan and 1 annual screening examination with the same modality as the baseline. A false-positive result was defined as a positive (ie, abnormal) finding with a completed negative workup or follow-up of at least 12 months without a diagnosis of lung cancer. As demonstrated in Fig 2 in the original article, the cumulative probability of a false-positive finding on CT screening was 21% after the baseline screening examination, which increased to 33% after the first annual screening. In this study, positive results were communicated to participants and their physicians; follow-up was at their discretion and not directed by the study. Of the participants with false-positive findings, 9% received a minimally or moderately invasive procedure and 2% received a major surgical procedure to establish a benign diagnosis.

It is overwhelmingly likely that the NLST will present this same challenge of a high probability of false-positive findings. In the context of screening an asymptomatic (by definition) population, false-positive results have the potential to cause physical harm as well as create unnecessary emotional and economic costs. With 46.6 million Americans currently smoking[1] and more who will qualify for screening on the basis of prior cigarette use, and anticipating that CT screening for individuals at risk because of smoking appears likely to be recommended in the future, studies addressing how we will manage and/or minimize the burden of false-positive findings will be urgently required.

L. T. Tanoue, MD

Reference

1. Dube S, McClave A, James C, Caraballlo R, Kaufmann R, Pechacek T. Vital signs: current cigarette smoking among adults aged > 18 years—United States, 2009. *MMWR Morb Mortal Wkly Rep.* 2010;59:1-6.

Surgeon Specialty and Long-Term Survival After Pulmonary Resection for Lung Cancer

Farjah F, Flum DR, Varghese TK Jr, et al (Univ of Washington, Seattle)
Ann Thorac Surg 87:995-1006, 2009

Background.—Long-term outcomes and processes of care in patients undergoing pulmonary resection for lung cancer may vary by surgeon type. Associations between surgeon specialty and processes of care and long-term survival have not been described.

Methods.—A cohort study (1992 through 2002, follow-up through 2005) was conducted using Surveillance, Epidemiology, and End-Results-Medicare data. The American Board of Thoracic Surgery Diplomates list was used to differentiate board-certified thoracic surgeons from general surgeons (GS). Board-certified thoracic surgeons were designated as cardiothoracic surgeons (CTS) if they performed cardiac procedures and as general thoracic surgeons (GTS) if they did not.

Results.—Among 19,745 patients, 32% were cared for by GTS, 45% by CTS, and 24% by GS. Patient age, comorbidity index, and resection type did not vary by surgeon specialty (all $p > 0.10$). Compared with GS and CTS, GTS more frequently used positron emission tomography (36% versus 26% versus 26%, respectively; $p = 0.005$) and lymphadenectomy (33% versus 22% versus 11%, respectively; $p < 0.001$). After adjustment for patient, disease, and management characteristics, hospital teaching status, and surgeon and hospital volume, patients treated by GTS had an 11% lower hazard of death compared with those who underwent resection by GS (hazard ratio, 0.89; 99% confidence interval, 0.82 to 0.97). The risks of death did not vary significantly between CTS and GS (hazard ratio, 0.94; 99% confidence interval, 0.88 to 1.01) or GTS and CTS (hazard ratio, 0.94; 99% confidence interval, 0.87 to 1.03).

Conclusions.—Lung cancer patients treated by GTS had higher long-term survival rates than those treated by GS. General thoracic surgeons performed preoperative and intraoperative staging more often than GS or CTS.

▶ Cure for nonsmall cell lung cancer (NSCLC), as for many solid tumors, is defined as a disease-free survival after 5 years. More than 80% of NSCLC recurrences occur within the first 2 years.[1,2] There is at present no evidence basis to answer the question of whether routine re-evaluation beyond 5 years should occur or, if it were to occur, with what imaging modality and what frequency. Previous work by Okada and colleagues[3] and Martini and colleagues[4] in a large series of patients with stage I to IIIA and I to IIIB resected NSCLC respectively reported 10-year survival rates of 91% and 92.4%. Both studies concluded that age, sex, histologic condition, and stage were not predictors of late recurrence or new lung cancer. This report by Maeda evaluating late (> 5-year) recurrence of NSCLC in patients with resected stage I to III NSCLC comes to a different conclusion. In their series of 819 patients disease-free at 5 years after resection, 11% subsequently recurred, with a median recurrence-free interval of

19 months (after the first 5 years). On multivariate analysis, factors that were statistically significant predictors of late recurrence included nodal status at the time of surgery and the presence of intratumoral vascular invasion. Of note, in the group of patients with stage I NSCLC, who comprised most cases, the late recurrence rate was 8.8% compared with 19.8% in patients with stage III NSCLC. This report supports what seems intuitive: that in a disease where field cancerization is an issue for most patients, the risk of recurrence of cancer (or new malignancy) in the tissue remaining after resection remains elevated even after a number of disease-free years. The role of long-term screening for this population merits further investigation.

L. T. Tanoue, MD

References

1. Martini N, Bains MS, Burt ME, et al. Incidence of local recurrence and second primary tumors in resected stage I lung cancer. *J Thorac Cardiovasc Surg.* 1995; 109:120-129.
2. al-Kattan K, Sepsas E, Fountain SW, Townsend ER. Disease recurrence after resection for stage I lung cancer. *Eur J Cardiothorac Surg.* 1997;12:380-384.
3. Okada M, Nishio W, Sakamoto T, Harada H, Uchino K, Tsubota N. Long-term survival and prognostic factors of five-year survivors with complete resection of non-small cell lung carcinoma. *J Thorac Cardiovasc Surg.* 2003;126:558-562.
4. Martini N, Rusch VW, Bains MS, et al. Factors influencing ten-year survival in resected stages I to IIIa non-small cell lung cancer. *J Thorac Cardiovasc Surg.* 1999;117:32-36.

Cost and Outcomes of Patients With Solitary Pulmonary Nodules Managed With PET Scans

Barnett PG, for the Veterans Affairs Positron Emission Tomography Imaging in the Management of Patients with Solitary Pulmonary Nodules (VA SNAP) Cooperative Study Group (Health Economics Resource Ctr, CA; et al)
Chest 137:53-59, 2010

Background.—No prior study to our knowledge has observed the cost of managing solitary pulmonary nodules of patient groups defined by PET scan results.

Methods.—We combined study and administrative data over 2 years of follow-up.

Results.—Of 375 individuals with a definitive diagnosis, 54.4% had a malignant nodule and 62.1% had positive PET scan results. Mortality risk was 5.0 times higher (CI, 3.1-8.2) and cost was greater ($50,233 vs $22,461, $P < .0001$) among patients with malignant nodule. Mortality risk was 4.1 times higher (CI, 2.4-7.0) and cost was greater ($47,823 vs $20,744, $P < .0001$) among patients with a positive PET scan result. Among patients with a malignant nodule, 4.9% had a false-negative PET scan, but cost and survival were not different from true positives. Among patients with a benign nodule, 22.8% had a false-positive PET scan. These patients had greater cost ($33,783 vs $19,115, $P < .01$), more surgeries and biopsies, and 3.8 times the mortality risk (CI, 1.6-9.2) of true negatives. Just over one-half (54.5%) of individuals with positive PET scans received surgery. Most individuals with negative PET scans (85.2%) were managed by watchful waiting. They incurred fewer costs than patients with negative PET scans who were managed more aggressively ($19,378 vs $28,611, *P* < .01).

Conclusions.—Management of solitary pulmonary nodules is expensive, especially if the nodule is malignant or if the PET scan result is false positive. Among patients with malignant nodules, 2-year survival is poor. Compared with true-positive PET scan results, false-negative results are not associated with lower costs or better outcomes.

▶ It is very clear that the increasing use of CT scans is resulting in identification of increased numbers of solitary pulmonary nodules (SPNs). Index CT screening studies in healthy volunteers who have smoked demonstrate SPNs in 23% to 51% of subjects, most of which are small (< 10 mm), and only a very small minority is malignant.[1,2] In SPNs > 7 mm identified by means other than screening, the reported prevalence of malignancy varies widely, between 15% to 75%.[3-5] ^{18}F-fluorodeoxyglucose positron emission tomography (PET) scanning has been suggested as a cost-effective tool in managing patients with SPN, as this technology has a high negative predictive value, particularly in nodules > 10 mm. However, the cost-effectiveness of PET imaging in this approach bears evaluation, as it is an expensive technology, and the economic impact if incorporated into an algorithmic approach would potentially be quite significant. This study by Barnett and colleagues addresses this concern. The population they studied had a high prevalence of malignant SPN (54.4%). Not surprisingly, patients with positive PET scans and malignant SPN (true positives) incurred higher health care costs in the course of the diagnosis and treatment of their lung cancers. Conversely, patients with negative PET scans and benign SPN (true negatives) incurred lower costs. This is perhaps the pertinent finding that the negative PET scans facilitated a less aggressive and less costly approach of watchful waiting. However, false-positive PET scans did occur in 10% of patients; these patients incurred higher costs related to more biopsies and surgeries and also had an associated increase in mortality risk. In populations where more false positives might be anticipated (such as in regions with endemic mycoses) or where a lower prevalence of malignancy exists, these increased health care costs might be significant. With PET imaging increasingly available and being used, cost analyses such as this will be important, particularly with a heightened interest in lung cancer screening in the face of a pressing need to control escalating health care expenditure.

L. T. Tanoue, MD

References

1. Henschke CI, McCauley DI, Yankelevitz DF, et al. Early Lung Cancer Action Project: overall design and findings from baseline screening. *Lancet.* 1999;354: 99-105.

2. Swensen SJ, Jett JR, Hartman TE, et al. CT screening for lung cancer: five-year prospective experience. *Radiology.* 2005;235:259-265.
3. Swensen SJ, Morin RL, Schueler BA, et al. Solitary pulmonary nodule: CT evaluation of enhancement with iodinated contrast material–a preliminary report. *Radiology.* 1992;182:343-347.
4. Khan A, Herman PG, Vorwerk P, Stevens P, Rojas KA, Graver M. Solitary pulmonary nodules: comparison of classification with standard, thin-section, and reference phantom CT. *Radiology.* 1991;179:477-481.
5. Gould MK, Fletcher J, Iannettoni MD, et al. Evaluation of patients with pulmonary nodules: when is it lung cancer?: ACCP evidence-based clinical practice guidelines (2nd edition). *Chest.* 2007;132:108S-130S.

Lung Cancer Treatment

Stereotactic Body Radiation Therapy for Inoperable Early Stage Lung Cancer

Timmerman R, Paulus R, Galvin J, et al (Univ of Texas Southwestern Med Ctr, Dallas; Radiation Therapy Oncology Group, Philadelphia, PA; Thomas Jefferson Univ, Philadelphia, PA; et al)
JAMA 303:1070-1076, 2010

Context.—Patients with early stage but medically inoperable lung cancer have a poor rate of primary tumor control (30%-40%) and a high rate of mortality (3-year survival, 20%-35%) with current management.

Objective.—To evaluate the toxicity and efficacy of stereotactic body radiation therapy in a high-risk population of patients with early stage but medically inoperable lung cancer.

Design, Setting, and Patients.—Phase 2 North American multicenter study of patients aged 18 years or older with biopsy-proven peripheral T1-T2N0M0 non–small cell tumors (measuring <5 cm in diameter) and medical conditions precluding surgical treatment. The prescription dose was 18 Gy per fraction × 3 fractions (54 Gy total) with entire treatment lasting between $1\frac{1}{2}$ and 2 weeks. The study opened May 26, 2004, and closed October 13, 2006; data were analyzed through August 31, 2009.

Main Outcome Measures.—The primary end point was 2-year actuarial primary tumor control; secondary end points were disease-free survival (ie, primary tumor, involved lobe, regional, and disseminated recurrence), treatment-related toxicity, and overall survival.

Results.—A total of 59 patients accrued, of which 55 were evaluable (44 patients with T1 tumors and 11 patients with T2 tumors) with a median follow-up of 34.4 months (range, 4.8-49.9 months). Only 1 patient had a primary tumor failure; the estimated 3-year primary tumor control rate was 97.6% (95% confidence interval [CI], 84.3%-99.7%). Three patients had recurrence within the involved lobe; the 3-year primary tumor and involved lobe (local) control rate was 90.6% (95% CI, 76.0%-96.5%). Two patients experienced regional failure; the local-regional control rate was 87.2% (95% CI, 71.0%-94.7%). Eleven patients experienced disseminated recurrence; the 3-year rate of disseminated failure was 22.1% (95% CI, 12.3%-37.8%). The rates for disease-free survival and overall survival at 3 years were 48.3% (95% CI, 34.4%-60.8%) and 55.8% (95% CI, 41.6%-67.9%), respectively. The median overall survival was 48.1 months (95% CI, 29.6 months to not reached). Protocol-specified treatment-related grade 3 adverse events were reported in 7 patients (12.7%; 95% CI, 9.6%-15.8%); grade 4 adverse events were reported in 2 patients (3.6%; 95% CI, 2.7%-4.5%). No grade 5 adverse events were reported.

Conclusion.—Patients with inoperable non–small cell lung cancer who received stereotactic body radiation therapy had a survival rate of 55.8% at 3 years, high rates of local tumor control, and moderate treatment-related morbidity.

▶ Medically inoperable patients with early-stage non–small cell lung cancer (NSCLC) are typically treated with radiation therapy (RT). Conventional RT in this setting involves up to 30 outpatient radiation treatments spread over a number of weeks. While associated with better outcomes than supportive care alone, conventional RT is known to have relatively poor long-term control of the primary tumor and yields a 2-year survival of approximately 40% at best.[1,2] Stereotactic body RT (SBRT) is a new technology that delivers RT in high doses using small highly focused beams and is completed in a few treatments. In this report, Timmerman and colleagues report the 3-year results of the Radiation Therapy Oncology Group (RTOG) multicenter trial evaluating SBRT in medically inoperable early-stage NSCLC. All patients in the study had T1 or T2 primary tumors (< 5 cm) located more than 2 cm from the trachea, carina, and major lobar bronchi (ie, not central tumors) and were N0M0 by CT and positron emission tomography scanning. All patients underwent extensive SBRT planning, including control of tumor motion related to breathing, and received a total dose of 60 Gy divided in 3 fractions. At 3 years of follow-up, primary tumor control was 97.6%. Survival results are demonstrated in the figure in the original article. Overall 3-year survival in the entire group was 55.8%; in patients with T1 tumors, median disease-free survival was 36.1 months, and median overall survival had not been reached at the 3-year follow-up. Disseminated recurrence occurred in 22.1% of patients, suggesting that occult tumor existed at the time of SBRT that had not been detected by the noninvasive staging techniques. These results are superior to primary tumor control and survival rates achieved with conventional RT. SBRT requires meticulous planning by a multidisciplinary team of radiation oncologists and medical physicists and is not yet widely available. Side effects include fatigue, chest pain, gastrointestinal complaints, and dyspnea. Based on these results as well as other single institution reports, it appears that SBRT will have an important role in the treatment of medically inoperable patients with early-stage lung cancer. A clinical trial jointly sponsored by the American College of Surgeons Oncology Group and the RTOG comparing SBRT with sublobar surgical resection in high-risk (unable to tolerate lobectomy) patients with early-stage NSCLC is currently in progress.

L. T. Tanoue, MD

References

1. Kaskowitz L, Graham MV, Emami B, Halverson KJ, Rush C. Radiation therapy alone for stage I non-small cell lung cancer. *Int J Radiat Oncol Biol Phys.* 1993; 27:517-523.
2. Haffty BG, Goldberg NB, Gerstley J, Fischer DB, Peschel RE. Results of radical radiation therapy in clinical stage I, technically operable non-small cell lung cancer. *Int J Radiat Oncol Biol Phys.* 1988;15:69-73.

Anatomic Segmentectomy for Stage I Non-Small Cell Lung Cancer in the Elderly

Kilic A, Schuchert MJ, Pettiford BL, et al (Univ of Pittsburgh Med Ctr, PA)
Ann Thorac Surg 87:1662-1668, 2009

Background.—Anatomic segmentectomy for stage I non-small cell lung cancer (NSCLC) offers the potential of surgical cure with preservation of lung function. This may be of particular importance in elderly NSCLC patients with declining cardiopulmonary status and a limited life expectancy.

Methods.—The study compared outcomes of 78 elderly patients (aged > 75 years) with stage I NSCLC undergoing segmentectomy and 106 undergoing lobectomy for stage I NSCLC from 2002 to 2007. Primary outcome variables included perioperative morbidity and mortality, hospital course, recurrence patterns, and survival.

Results.—Age, gender, tumor histology, and surgical approach were similar between groups. Comorbidities were similar except for a higher incidence of chronic obstructive pulmonary disease and diabetes in segmentectomy patients. The tumors in the lobectomy group were significantly larger (3.5 vs 2.5 cm, $p = 0.0001$). Operative mortality was 1.3% for segmentectomy and 4.7% for lobectomy. Segmentectomy patients had fewer major complications (11.5% vs 25.5%, $p = 0.02$). There were no differences in median hospitalization (7 vs 6 days). The estimated overall survival at 2, 3, and 5 years was 76%, 69%, and 46% for segmentectomy patients and 68%, 59%, and 47% for lobectomy patients ($p = 0.28$). The 5-year disease-free survival was equivalent (segmentectomy, 49.8%; lobectomy, 45.5%; $p = 0.80$).

Conclusions.—Anatomic segmentectomy can be performed safely in elderly patients with early-stage NSCLC. This approach is associated with reduced perioperative complications and comparable oncologic efficacy compared with lobectomy in older patients with a limited life expectancy (Fig 1).

▶ More than 15 years ago, the Lung Cancer Study Group randomized trial of lobectomy versus limited sublobar resection for T1N0M0 non small cell lung cancer (NSCLC) demonstrated a significant difference in survival between the 2 approaches, leading to the current recommendation of lobectomy as the preferred treatment for stage I NSCLC patients.[1] However, lobectomy is not

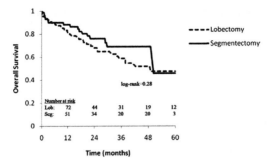

FIGURE 1.—Overall 5-year survival of elderly patients undergoing segmentectomy (solid line) or lobectomy (dashed line). (Reprinted from Kilic A, Schuchert MJ, Pettiford BL, et al. Anatomic segmentectomy for stage I non-small cell lung cancer in the elderly. *Ann Thorac Surg.* 2009;87:1662-1668, copyright The Society of Thoracic Surgeons 2009.)

always feasible because of lung function limitations, which may be of particular concern in an older population with higher frequency of comorbidities, more limited life expectancy, and age-related respiratory physiologic changes. This study is a retrospective single-center review of outcomes in patients aged > 75 years with stage I NSCLC undergoing either segmentectomy or lobectomy. Segmentectomy was performed when the patient was ineligible for a lobectomy because of medical limitations or when the surgeon believed that a complete resection could be performed with adequate margins. Of note, the definition of "adequate margins" was not strictly delineated. There were no differences in perioperative complications or 5-year survival between the 2 groups (Fig 1), a finding comparable with the early results of the American College of Surgeons Oncology Group randomized trial of sublobar resection versus lobectomy for stage I NSCLC.[2] It should be noted that the mean tumor size in the segmentectomy group was 2.5 cm as compared with 3.5 cm in the lobectomy group, and a higher percentage of patients in the segmentectomy as opposed to lobectomy group were stage IA (76% vs 49%), but the 5-year outcomes by stage (IA and IB) for the 2 groups were equivalent. While this is a relatively small study, it suggests that sublobar resection is a reasonable approach to the surgical treatment of elderly patients with stage I NSCLC.

L. T. Tanoue, MD

References

1. Ginsberg RJ, Rubinstein LV. Randomized trial of lobectomy versus limited resection for T1 N0 non-small cell lung cancer. Lung Cancer Study Group. *Ann Thorac Surg.* 1995;60:615-622.
2. Allen MS, Darling GE, Pechet TT, et al. Morbidity and mortality of major pulmonary resections in patients with early-stage lung cancer: initial results of the randomized, prospective ACOSOG Z0030 trial. *Ann Thorac Surg.* 2006;81: 1013-1019.

Surgeon Specialty and Long-Term Survival After Pulmonary Resection for Lung Cancer

Farjah F, Flum DR, Varghese TK Jr, et al (Univ of Washington, Seattle)
Ann Thorac Surg 87:995-1006, 2009

Background.—Long-term outcomes and processes of care in patients undergoing pulmonary resection for lung cancer may vary by surgeon type. Associations between surgeon specialty and processes of care and long-term survival have not been described.

Methods.—A cohort study (1992 through 2002, follow-up through 2005) was conducted using Surveillance, Epidemiology, and End-Results-Medicare data. The American Board of Thoracic Surgery Diplomates list was used to differentiate board-certified thoracic surgeons from general surgeons (GS). Board-certified thoracic surgeons were designated as cardiothoracic surgeons (CTS) if they performed cardiac procedures and as general thoracic surgeons (GTS) if they did not.

Results.—Among 19,745 patients, 32% were cared for by GTS, 45% by CTS, and 24% by GS. Patient age, comorbidity index, and resection type did not vary by surgeon specialty (all $p > 0.10$). Compared with GS and CTS, GTS more frequently used positron emission tomography (36% versus 26% versus 26%, respectively; $p = 0.005$) and lymphadenectomy (33% versus 22% versus 11%, respectively; $p < 0.001$). After adjustment for patient, disease, and management characteristics, hospital teaching status, and surgeon and hospital volume, patients treated by GTS had an 11% lower hazard of death compared with those who underwent resection by GS (hazard ratio, 0.89; 99% confidence interval, 0.82 to 0.97). The risks of death did not vary significantly between CTS and GS (hazard ratio, 0.94; 99% confidence interval, 0.88 to 1.01) or GTS and CTS (hazard ratio, 0.94; 99% confidence interval, 0.87 to 1.03).

Conclusions.—Lung cancer patients treated by GTS had higher long-term survival rates than those treated by GS. General thoracic surgeons performed preoperative and intraoperative staging more often than GS or CTS.

▶ Primary surgical resection is the recommended therapy for early-stage non-small cell lung cancer, followed by adjuvant chemotherapy for stage IB, IIA, and IIB disease. Previous studies examining surgeon specialty and operative mortality with lung resection have demonstrated that board certification is associated with lower operative mortality rates.[1,2] This provocative report by Farjah and colleagues using the Surveillance, Epidemiology, and End Results (SEER)-Medicare database demonstrated a significant difference in long-term outcomes associated with the specialty of the operating surgeon. In particular, 5-year lung cancer cause-specific survival after lung resection for early-stage (I and II) NSCLC was 70% when performed by thoracic surgeons who performed only thoracic surgery, compared with 63% when performed by general surgeons, and 67% when performed by cardiothoracic surgeons who performed both cardiac and thoracic surgery ($P < .001$). Short-term outcomes also varied by surgeon specialty; 30-day mortality after lung cancer surgery performed by general thoracic surgeons was 4.4%, compared with 6.0% when performed by general surgeons, and 5.0% when performed by cardiothoracic surgeons ($P = .005$). The reasons for these differences merit investigation. General thoracic surgeons used preoperative positron emission tomography and performed lymphadenectomy more frequently, raising the likelihood that these patients were staged more accurately, which would contribute to better-observed survival. Access to general thoracic or cardiothoracic surgeons might be limited in some regions, and the volume of cases in rural areas or smaller hospitals may limit the expertise of the rest of the medical-surgical team and hospital. Addressing these issues must take into account limitations imposed by the workforce of general thoracic surgeons, regional variations in access and volume, and the availability and cost of resources for the infrastructure requirements of multidisciplinary teams. In the SEER-Medicare patient database examined, only 24% of patients underwent surgery by general thoracic surgeons; it seems unlikely that all lung cancer surgeries in the country could be performed by this group without a substantive increase in manpower. Similarly, limiting lung cancer care to large regional centers would impose a geographic and potential economic burden on patients needing to travel distances to obtain care. Nonetheless, the differences noted in short- and long-term survival associated with surgeon specialty are significant enough to warrant further study with the goal of improving the quality of thoracic surgical care.

L. T. Tanoue, MD

References

1. Silvestri GA, Handy J, Lackland D, Corley E, Reed CE. Specialists achieve better outcomes than generalists for lung cancer surgery. *Chest.* 1998;114:675-680.
2. Goodney PP, Lucas FL, Stukel TA, Birkmeyer JD. Surgeon specialty and operative mortality with lung resection. *Ann Surg.* 2005;241:179-184.

Early Palliative Care for Patients with Metastatic Non–Small-Cell Lung Cancer

Temel JS, Greer JA, Muzikansky A, et al (Massachusetts General Hosp, Boston; et al)
N Engl J Med 363:733-742, 2010

Background.—Patients with metastatic non–small-cell lung cancer have a substantial symptom burden and may receive aggressive care at the end of life. We examined the effect of introducing palliative care early after diagnosis on patient-reported outcomes and end-of-life care among ambulatory patients with newly diagnosed disease.

Methods.—We randomly assigned patients with newly diagnosed metastatic non–small-cell lung cancer to receive either early palliative care integrated with standard oncologic care or standard oncologic care alone. Quality of life and mood were assessed at baseline and at 12 weeks with the use of the Functional Assessment of Cancer Therapy–Lung (FACT-L) scale and the Hospital Anxiety and Depression Scale, respectively. The primary outcome was the change in the quality of life at 12 weeks. Data on end-of-life care were collected from electronic medical records.

Results.—Of the 151 patients who underwent randomization, 27 died by 12 weeks and 107 (86% of the remaining patients) completed assessments. Patients assigned to early palliative care had a better quality of life than did patients assigned to standard care (mean score on the FACT-L scale [in which scores range from 0 to 136, with higher scores indicating better quality of life], 98.0 vs. 91.5; P = 0.03). In addition, fewer patients in the palliative care group than in the standard care group had depressive symptoms (16% vs. 38%, P = 0.01). Despite the fact that fewer patients in the early palliative care group than in the standard care group received aggressive end-of-life care (33% vs. 54%, P = 0.05), median survival was longer among patients receiving early palliative care (11.6 months vs. 8.9 months, P = 0.02).

Conclusions.—Among patients with metastatic non–small-cell lung cancer, early palliative care led to significant improvements in both quality of life and mood. As compared with patients receiving standard care, patients receiving early palliative care had less aggressive care at the end of life but longer survival. (Funded by an American Society of Clinical Oncology Career Development Award and philanthropic gifts; ClinicalTrials.gov number, NCT01038271.)

▶ There is broad acknowledgment that palliative care is typically delivered late, perhaps too late, in the disease process of cancer or any other illness, yet there is also general acknowledgment that good palliation improves quality of life. This provocative study by Temel and colleagues evaluated the effect of early palliative intervention integrated with standard oncologic care in patients with stage IV non–small-cell lung cancer, compared with standard oncologic care with introduction of palliative care at the discretion of the treating physician. Because the anticipated median survival of patients with metastatic lung cancer is approximately 1 year at best, these patients can be anticipated within a short time after diagnosis to develop impaired quality of life related to physical and psychological symptoms with disease progression as well as to complications of treatment. Palliative care in this study was delivered by a dedicated team of trained health care professionals. Patients in the palliative care intervention arm had better outcomes as measured by a standardized lung cancer quality of life scale, with fewer depressive symptoms. What was particularly remarkable is that median survival was longer in the intervention group by 2.7 months, as demonstrated in Fig 3 in the original article. This magnitude of benefit, while it may seem small on an absolute scale, is equivalent to the benefit obtained with intervention with standard first-line chemotherapy or with the addition of bevacizumab to chemotherapy in patients with stage IV adenocarcinoma of the lung, and so in the realm of lung cancer, care is quite significant.[1,2] The etiology of this improvement in survival is not clear, though presumably a number of factors are contributing that relate to the alleviation of suffering from physical pain and the avoidance of depression. The message is very clear that early intervention with palliative care should be part of the comprehensive care plan for patients with lung cancer.

L. T. Tanoue, MD

References

1. Schiller JH, Harrington D, Belani CP, et al. Comparison of four chemotherapy regimens for advanced non-small-cell lung cancer. *N Engl J Med.* 2002;346:92-98.
2. Sandler A, Gray R, Perry MC, et al. Paclitaxel-carboplatin alone or with bevacizumab for non-small-cell lung cancer. *N Engl J Med.* 2006;355:2542-2550.

Stage I Non-small Cell Lung Cancer (NSCLC) in Patients Aged 75 Years and Older: Does Age Determine Survival After Radical Treatment?
Palma DA, Tyldesley S, Sheehan F, et al (BC Cancer Agency, Vancouver, Canada; et al)
J Thorac Oncol 5:818-824, 2010

Introduction.—Curative treatment of stage I non-small cell lung cancer (NSCLC) in elderly patients represents a therapeutic challenge. Data examining outcomes for the elderly after radical radiotherapy (RT) or surgery in the same geographic population are limited.

Methods.—Using prospective databases from British Columbia, patients with stage I NSCLC treated curatively with either surgery or RT between 2000 and 2006 were identified. Kaplan-Meier, Cox regression, and competing risk analyses were used to assess overall survival (OS) and disease-specific survival in the elderly, and the relationship between age and survival outcomes.

Results.—Of a total of 558 patients with stage I disease, 310 (56%) received surgery and 248 (44%) received RT. Elderly patients (age ≥75 years) were less likely to undergo resection than their younger counterparts (43% versus 72%, $p < 0.0001$). Actuarial OS after surgery for elderly patients was 87% at 2 years and 69% at 5 years. On multivariate analysis, OS after surgery was dependent on tumor stage ($p = 0.034$) and performance status ($p = 0.03$), but not age ($p = 0.87$). After RT, actuarial OS for elderly patients was 53% at 2 years and 23% at 5 years. On multivariate analysis, age did not predict for OS after RT ($p = 0.43$), whereas tumor stage ($p = 0.033$), sex ($p = 0.044$), and dose ($p = 0.01$) were significant predictors.

Conclusions.—Survival after radical treatment for stage I NSCLC is dependent on factors such as tumor stage, performance status, sex, and RT dose, but not age. Elderly patients who are sufficiently fit should not be considered ineligible for radical treatment based on age alone.

▶ Lung cancer is primarily a disease of older persons. This study reports overall survival of a population of Canadian patients aged > 75 years, with stage I non–small-cell lung cancer (NSCLC). The study is particularly interesting in that it reports factors impacting outcome for patients who underwent surgery and for those who were treated primarily with radiation therapy (RT). As noted by many other studies, elderly patients were less likely to undergo curative resection when compared with younger patients (43% vs 72%), but if surgery was performed, survival was independent of age. Of the 558 patients in the study cohort, 248 (44%) were treated with curative intent RT. As was the case with surgery, overall survival after RT was independent of age (Fig 2 in the original article). These results reinforce the American College of Chest Physicians evidence-based lung cancer guidelines recommendation that healthy elderly patients with early stage NSCLC not be denied curative intent treatment.[1]

L. T. Tanoue, MD

Reference

1. Colice GL, Shafazand S, Griffin JP, Keenan R, Bolliger CT. Physiologic evaluation of the patient with lung cancer being considered for resectional surgery: ACCP evidenced-based clinical practice guidelines (2nd edition). *Chest.* 2007;132: 161S-177S.

Molecular Approach to Lung Cancer

Relationship between Tumor Size and Survival among Patients with Resection of Multiple Synchronous Lung Cancers

Tanvetyanon T, Robinson L, Sommers KE, et al (H. Lee Moffitt Cancer Ctr and Res Inst, Tampa, FL)
J Thorac Oncol 5:1018-1024, 2010

Background.—Multiple synchronous non-small cell lung cancers (NSCLCs) without extrathoracic metastasis are relatively uncommon. Some patients are treated as metastatic disease by chemotherapy alone; others are treated as multiple primary cancers by surgery. For those undergoing surgery, limited information exists on the relationship between tumor size and survival.

Methods.—We retrospectively reviewed medical records of patients with resection of at least two synchronous NSCLC located in ≥2 lobes during 1997–2008. Those with only satellite nodules in single lobe were excluded. Cox proportional hazard model was used to examine the prognostic significance of tumor size in the context of other clinical parameters including tumor stage, nodal stage, age, gender, laterality, histology, and pneumonectomy.

Results.—There were 116 patients: 57 patients had cancers distributed in one lung and 59 in both lungs. Overall, 186 thoracotomies were performed, with a 90-day mortality rate of 2.6%. The median overall survival was 65.1 months (95% confidence interval [CI]: 49.2–83.7). The median size of the largest tumor and the median sum of tumor sizes were 3.0 and 4.5 cm, respectively. Both were a significant predictor of survival: hazard ratios per centimeter increase where 1.17 (95% CI: 1.06–1.30, $p = 0.003$) and 1.15 (95% CI: 1.05–1.26, $p = 0.003$), respectively.

Multivariable regression analysis identified tumor size and lung function as independent survival predictors.

Conclusion.—Among patients with resected multiple synchronous NSCLC, tumor size is an independent predictor of survival. The size of the largest tumor performs slightly better than the sum of tumor sizes in the survival prediction; however, both are much better than the American Joint Committee on Cancer stage for this purpose.

▶ Multiple synchronous primary lung cancers are uncommon, but when they occur, they present significant challenges. The diagnostic criteria used in their identification date back to 1975, with the requirements that synchronous tumors be (1) physically separate and (2) demonstrate either (a) different histologies or (b) the same histology but in different segments, lobes, or lungs, without lymphatic spread, and without extrapulmonary metastases.[1] These tumors do not readily lend themselves to the current American Joint Committee on Cancer (AJCC) staging schema and are typically each staged separately.[2] This single-center series is a review of a large number (116) of patients who underwent resection of at least 2 synchronous nonsmall cell lung cancers. It should be noted that these were highly selected patients at a large comprehensive cancer center, all of whom were recommended for treatment with the consensus of a multidisciplinary tumor board. The notable finding is that the largest tumor size or the sum of the tumor sizes was highly predictive of survival, whereas tumor staging was not. The median overall survival was 65.1 months, which is remarkable considering the extent of the surgeries and the fact that more than 75% of patients had a cancer that was staged IIIA or higher. The authors suggest that for this particular group of patients, tumor size may be a better predictor of outcome than AJCC staging.

L. T. Tanoue, MD

References

1. Martini N, Melamed MR. Multiple primary lung cancers. *J Thorac Cardiovasc Surg.* 1975;70:606-612.
2. Goldstraw P, Crowley J, Chansky K, et al. The IASLC Lung Cancer Staging Project: proposals for the revision of the TNM stage groupings in the forthcoming (seventh) edition of the TNM Classification of malignant tumours. *J Thorac Oncol.* 2007;2:706-714.

Gefitinib or Chemotherapy for Non–Small-Cell Lung Cancer with Mutated EGFR

Maemondo M, for the North-East Japan Study Group (Miyagi Cancer Ctr, Japan; et al)
N Engl J Med 362:2380-2388, 2010

Background.—Non–small-cell lung cancer with sensitive mutations of the epidermal growth factor receptor (EGFR) is highly responsive to EGFR tyrosine kinase inhibitors such as gefitinib, but little is known about how its efficacy and safety profile compares with that of standard chemotherapy.

Methods.—We randomly assigned 230 patients with metastatic, non–small-cell lung cancer and EGFR mutations who had not previously received chemotherapy to receive gefitinib or carboplatin–paclitaxel. The primary end point was progression-free survival; secondary end points included overall survival, response rate, and toxic effects.

Results.—In the planned interim analysis of data for the first 200 patients, progression-free survival was significantly longer in the gefitinib group than in the standard-chemotherapy group (hazard ratio for death or disease progression with gefitinib, 0.36; P<0.001), resulting in early termination of the study. The gefitinib group had a significantly longer median progression-free survival (10.8 months, vs. 5.4 months in the chemotherapy group; hazard ratio, 0.30; 95% confidence interval, 0.22 to 0.41; P<0.001), as well as a higher response rate (73.7% vs. 30.7%, P<0.001). The median overall survival was 30.5 months in the gefitinib group and 23.6 months in the chemotherapy group (P = 0.31). The most common adverse events in the gefitinib group were rash (71.1%) and elevated aminotransferase levels (55.3%), and in the chemotherapy group, neutropenia (77.0%), anemia (64.6%), appetite loss (56.6%), and sensory neuropathy (54.9%). One patient receiving gefitinib died from interstitial lung disease.

Conclusions.—First-line gefitinib for patients with advanced non–small-cell lung cancer who were selected on the basis of EGFR mutations improved progression-free survival, with acceptable toxicity, as compared with standard chemotherapy. (UMIN-CTR number, C000000376.)

▶ Platinum-based combination chemotherapy is the recommended first-line treatment for advanced non–small-cell lung cancer (NSCLC), with the addition of bevacizumab in patients with adenocarcinoma. The clinical trials providing the evidence base for this approach were largely performed in North America and Europe. We now appreciate that NSCLC is a different disease in different populations. In women, nonsmokers, and individuals of Asian origin with adenocarcinoma of the lung, the incidence of somatic mutations in the region of the *EGFR* gene encoding the tyrosine kinase domain is relatively high. The Iressa Pan-Asia Study (IPASS) (First Line Iressa vs Carboplatin/Paclitaxel in Asia [IPASS]), conducted in China, Thailand, Taiwan, Japan, and Indonesia, demonstrated that in a selected population (Asian ethnicity, light or non-smokers), first-line treatment with gefitinib, an oral epidermal growth factor receptor (EGFR) tyrosine kinase inhibitor, was at least as effective, if not more effective, than standard platinum-based doublet chemotherapy.[1] The population selected for IPASS had an increased incidence of *EGFR* mutations, presumably the fundamental reason that gefitinib performed in superior fashion.

This study reported by Maemondo and colleagues from Japan was a randomized trial comparing gefitinib with platinum-based chemotherapy in a population of patients with NSCLC identified as having *EGFR* mutations sensitive to tyrosine kinase inhibition and without the T790M mutation known to confer resistance. It is a natural extension of the IPASS. The study was terminated by its data safety monitoring board after a planned interim analysis demonstrated a significant difference in progression-free survival between the 2 treatment groups in favor of gefitinib, as shown in Fig 2 in the original article. These data support the recommendation that *EGFR* mutational status should be investigated in patients with adenocarcinoma of the lung, particularly in populations identified as having a higher probability of harboring sensitive mutations, and that first-line treatment with tyrosine kinase inhibitors in patients with these mutations should be considered. These findings support the current impetus toward targeted personalized therapy, the broad application of which will depend on defining other suitable targets for therapeutic intervention.

L. T. Tanoue, MD

Reference

1. Mok TS, Wu YL, Thongprasert S, et al. Gefitinib or carboplatin-paclitaxel in pulmonary adenocarcinoma. *N Engl J Med*. 2009;361:947-957.

Clinical Features and Outcome of Patients With Non–Small-Cell Lung Cancer Who Harbor *EML4-ALK*

Shaw AT, Yeap BY, Mino-Kenudson M, et al (Massachusetts General Hosp Cancer Ctr, Boston; Beth Israel Deaconess Med Ctr, Boston, MA; et al)

J Clin Oncol 27:4247-4253, 2009

Purpose.—The *EML4-ALK* fusion oncogene represents a novel molecular target in a small subset of non–small-cell lung cancers (NSCLC). To aid in identification and treatment of these patients, we examined the clinical characteristics and treatment outcomes of patients who had NSCLC with and without *EML4-ALK*.

Patients and Methods.—Patients with NSCLC were selected for genetic screening on the basis of two or more of the following characteristics: female sex, Asian ethnicity, never/light smoking history, and adenocarcinoma histology. *EML4-ALK* was identified by using fluorescent in situ hybridization for ALK rearrangements and was confirmed by immunohistochemistry for *ALK* expression. *EGFR* and *KRAS* mutations were determined by DNA sequencing.

Results.—Of 141 tumors screened, 19 (13%) were *EML4-ALK* mutant, 31 (22%) were *EGFR* mutant, and 91 (65%) were wild type (WT/WT) for both *ALK* and *EGFR*. Compared with the *EGFR* mutant and WT/WT cohorts, patients with *EML4-ALK* mutant tumors were significantly younger $(P < .001$ and $P = .005)$ and were more likely to be men $(P = .036$ and $P = .039)$. Patients with *EML4-ALK*–positive tumors, like patients who harbored *EGFR* mutations, also were more likely to be never/light smokers compared with patients in the WT/WT cohort $(P < .001)$. Eighteen of the 19 *EML4-ALK* tumors were adenocarcinomas, predominantly the signet ring cell subtype. Among patients with metastatic disease, *EML4-ALK* positivity was associated with resistance to EGFR tyrosine kinase inhibitors (TKIs). Patients in the *EML4-ALK* cohort and the WT/WT cohort showed similar response rates to platinum-based combination chemotherapy and no difference in overall survival.

Conclusion.—*EML4-ALK* defines a molecular subset of NSCLC with distinct clinical characteristics. Patients who harbor this mutation do not benefit from EGFR TKIs and should be directed to trials of ALK-targeted agents (Table 3).

▶ There is enormous interest in genetically defining subsets of patients with non small-cell lung cancer (NSCLC). Specific mutations in the epidermal growth factor receptor (*EGFR*) gene identify patients who share clinical characteristics and demonstrate a predictable increase in response to targeted biologic therapies with tyrosine kinase inhibitors. Other genetic mutations, most notably in the *KRAS* gene, are also associated with NSCLC. An important observation has been made that *KRAS* mutations and *EGFR* mutations appear to be mutually exclusive, so the presence of a *KRAS* mutation predicts poor response to tyrosine kinase inhibition. Shaw and colleagues report on the *EML4-ALK* fusion oncogene, another mutation recently identified as associated with NSCLC. Molecular genetic typing was performed on 141 tumors, which were selected because of characteristics that would be predictive of enrichment for *EGFR* mutations (adenocarcinoma histology, female sex, Asian ethnicity, and light or never smoking history). The results of the genetic typing are shown in Table 3. Of note, *ALK* rearrangements, *EGFR* mutations, and *KRAS* mutations appear to be mutually exclusive. *EML4-ALK*–positive patients were also significantly younger and more likely to be male than patients with *EGFR* mutation and, as with *EGFR* mutation, patients were more likely to be never or light smokers. The distinction between mutations is important therapeutically. As with *KRAS* mutation, the presence of *EML4-ALK* mutation in this study was associated with clinical resistance to tyrosine kinase inhibitors. However, as opposed to *KRAS* mutations, which are more commonly found

TABLE 3.—Mutation Analysis of Screened Patients With Non–Small-Cell Lung Cancer

| | | Genotype | |
Analysis	ALK	EGFR	WT/WT
ALK rearrangement			
Positive	19	0	0
Total	19	31	91
EGFR mutation			
Positive	0	31	0
Total	19	31	74
KRAS mutation*			
Positive	0	0	6
Total	11	10	23

Abbreviation: WT, wild type.
*KRAS mutation testing was not performed on all patients because of limited amounts of tissue.

in smokers, *EML4-ALK* mutations are more commonly found in never or light smokers. If clinical factors such as smoking status were the sole basis for choosing targeted therapy in the absence of genetic testing, then patients with *EML4-ALK* mutations would probably be treated like patients with *EGFR* mutations to their clinical detriment. This argues that genetic testing should be performed whenever possible. New targeted therapies for NSCLC are being intensively developed. With specific regard to *EML4-ALK, ALK* inhibitors are now in clinical trial.

L. T. Tanoue, MD

Use of Epidermal Growth Factor Receptor/Kirsten Rat Sarcoma 2 Viral Oncogene Homolog Mutation Testing to Define Clonal Relationships Among Multiple Lung Adenocarcinomas: Comparison With Clinical Guidelines

Girard N, Deshpande C, Azzoli CG, et al (Memorial Sloan-Kettering Cancer Ctr, NY)
Chest 137:46-52, 2010

Background.—The incidence of multiple lung adenocarcinomas is rising, making it difficult to determine the stage and assign treatment in an increasing number of patients following surgery. Clinical guidelines have been developed to distinguish independent non-small cell lung cancers from metastases, that is, criteria developed by Martini and Melamed and the American College of Chest Physicians (ACCP). However, these guidelines can be difficult to apply and may give conflicting results. Here, we report on seven patients in whom epidermal growth factor receptor (*EGFR*) and Kirsten-rat sarcoma 2 viral oncogene homolog (*KRAS*) tumor mutation status was used to determine clonal relationships among multiple lung lesions.

Methods.—We identified seven patients whose paired lung adenocarcinomas were found to harbor distinct *EGFR* or *KRAS* mutations. We assessed these patients' disease status using established clinical guidelines. We also explored the use of comprehensive histologic subtyping (CHS) of tumor sections to distinguish multiple primaries.

Results.—According to the Martini-Melamed criteria, six of the seven patients had multiple primary lung tumors. By ACCP criteria, three patients had multiple primaries, and three patients had metastases. Classification of the seventh patient by ACCP criteria was indeterminate. Mutational testing suggested that all paired tumors were multiple primary adenocarcinomas, which was consistent with results from CHS.

Conclusions.—Assuming that independent tumor clones harbor distinct mutations, these seven cases highlight discrepancies between the existing clinical criteria used to distinguish independent tumor foci from metastases. *EGFR/KRAS* mutation testing of multiple lung adenocarcinomas can assist in differentiating multiple primary lung adenocarcinomas from metastatic lesions. Use of CHS in this setting should also be further explored.

▶ The diagnosis of multiple synchronous primary lung cancers is a clinical challenge. The criteria proposed by Martini and Melamed in 1975 are still widely used, with the diagnosis according to their schema requiring that synchronous tumors be (1) physically separate and (2) demonstrate either (a) different histologies or (b) the same histology but in different segments, lobes, or lungs, without lymphatic spread, and without extrapulmonary metastases.[1] The 2nd Edition of the American College of Chest Physicians Evidence-based Clinical Practice Guidelines indicated that molecular genetic characteristics should also be considered.[2] This article by Girard and colleagues involves only 7 patients but provides an interesting window on the use of molecular information to distinguish primary tumors from pulmonary metastases, an approach that will be important in advancing our ability to diagnose synchronous cancers and to more precisely characterize tumors, in general. In their report, tumors were analyzed for mutations in epidermal growth factor receptor and Kirsten rat sarcoma virus 2 genes. These mutations are found in up to 50% of lung adenocarcinomas; different mutations found in separate lung tumors presumably reflect independent clones and therefore separate primaries. Other genes whose mutations are associated with nonsmall cell lung cancer (NSCLC) include p53 and *EML4-ALK*. In future work, investigation of a broad panel of genetic mutations associated with NSCLC should further improve our ability to accurately distinguish synchronous primary tumors from a primary tumor with pulmonary metastases.

L. T. Tanoue, MD

References

1. Martini N, Melamed MR. Multiple primary lung cancers. *J Thorac Cardiovasc Surg.* 1975;70:606-612.
2. Shen KR, Meyers BF, Larner JM, Jones DR. Special treatment issues in lung cancer: ACCP evidence-based clinical practice guidelines (2nd edition). *Chest.* 2007;132:290S-305S.

Tobacco-related Issues

Impact of Smoking Cessation Before Resection of Lung Cancer: A Society of Thoracic Surgeons General Thoracic Surgery Database Study
Mason DP, Subramanian S, Nowicki ER, et al (Cleveland Clinic, OH; Duke Univ, Durham, NC)
Ann Thorac Surg 88:362-371, 2009

Background.—Smoking cessation is presumed to be beneficial before resection of lung cancer. The effect of smoking cessation on outcome was investigated.

Methods.—From January 1999 to July 2007, in-hospital outcomes for 7990 primary resections for lung cancer in adults were reported to the

Society of Thoracic Surgeons General Thoracic Surgery Database. Risk of hospital death and respiratory complications was assessed according to timing of smoking cessation, adjusted for clinical confounders.

Results.—Hospital mortality was 1.4% (n = 109), but 1.5% in patients who had smoked (105 of 6965) vs 0.39% in those who had not (4 of 1025). Compared with the latter, risk-adjusted odds ratios were 3.5 ($p = 0.03$), 4.6 ($p = 0.03$), 2.6 ($p = 0.7$), and 2.5 ($p = 0.11$) for those whose timing of smoking cessation was categorized as current smoker, quit from 14 days to 1 month, 1 to 12 months, or more than 12 months preoperatively, respectively. Prevalence of major pulmonary complications was 5.7% (456 of 7965) overall, but 6.2% in patients who had smoked (429 of 6941) vs 2.5%% in those who had not (27 of 1024). Compared with the latter, risk-adjusted odds ratios were 1.80 ($p = 0.03$), 1.62 ($p = 0.14$), 1.51 ($p = 0.20$), and 1.29 ($p = 0.3$) for those whose timing of smoking cessation was categorized as above.

Conclusions.—Risks of hospital death and pulmonary complications after lung cancer resection were increased by smoking and mitigated slowly by preoperative cessation. No optimal interval of smoking cessation was identifiable. Patients should be counseled to stop smoking irrespective of surgical timing (Fig 3, Table 4).

▶ The diagnosis of lung cancer and anticipation of a surgical resection are powerful motivators for smoking cessation. There has been discussion in the medical literature as to the optimal timing of smoking cessation, with a number of studies suggesting that cessation in the several weeks prior to cardiopulmonary surgery may actually be associated with a higher likelihood of perioperative pulmonary complications.[1,2] This report from the Society of Thoracic Surgeons registry is the largest study evaluating the effect of the timing of smoking cessation on perioperative morbidity and mortality in patients undergoing primary resection for lung cancer. Fig 3 demonstrates that mortality overall was low

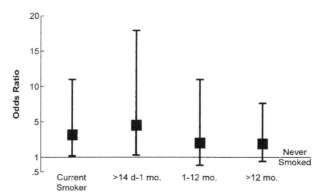

FIGURE 3.—Forest plot shows odds ratios and 95% confidence intervals for pulmonary complications according to interval of smoking cessation compared with patients who have never smoked (odds ratio of 1.0). (Reprinted from Mason DP, Subramanian S, Nowicki ER, et al. Impact of smoking cessation before resection of lung cancer: a Society of Thoracic Surgeons General Thoracic Surgery Database study. *Ann Thorac Surg.* 2009;88:362-371, with permission from The Society of Thoracic Surgeons.)

TABLE 4.—Multivariable Logistic Model of Pulmonary Complications After Resection for Lung Cancer

Variable	Coefficient ± SE	Est OR (95% CL)	p Value
Current smoker[a]	0.59 ± 0.27	1.8 (1.05, 3.1)	0.03
Pre-op smoking cessation interval			
>14 d–1 mo[a]	0.48 ± 0.33	1.6 (0.85, 3.1)	0.14
1–12 mo[a]	0.41 ± 0.32	1.5 (0.81, 2.8)	0.2
>12 mo[a]	0.26 ± 0.26	1.3 (0.77, 2.2)	0.3
Age	0.026 ± 0.0051	1.03 (1.02, 1.04)	<0.0001
Body mass index	−0.015 ± 0.0098	0.99 (0.97, 1.00)	0.13
Pack-years	0.0033 ± 0.0023	1.00 (1.00, 1.01)	0.14
FEV_1 (% of predicted)	−0.0096 ± 0.0024	0.99 (0.99, 1.00)	<0.0001
Female	−0.12 ± 0.10	0.89 (0.72, 1.09)	0.2
Zubrod score	0.14 ± 0.11	1.2 (0.92, 1.4)	0.2
ASA risk class	0.20 ± 0.090	1.2 (1.02, 1.5)	0.02
Hypertension	0.20 ± 0.095	1.2 (1.01, 1.5)	0.04
Steroids	0.61 ± 0.19	1.8 (1.3, 2.7)	0.001
Heart failure	0.58 ± 0.19	1.8 (1.2, 2.6)	0.002
Coronary artery disease	0.23 ± 0.11	1.3 (1.01, 1.6)	0.04
Peripheral arterial disease	0.16 ± 0.12	1.2 (0.92, 1.5)	0.2
Rx-treated diabetes	−0.011 ± 0.26	0.99 (0.57, 1.7)	>0.9
Renal insufficiency	0.19 ± 0.24	1.2 (0.76, 1.9)	0.4
Pre-op chemo and/or radiotherapy	0.53 ± 0.11	1.7 (1.4, 2.1)	<0.0001
Cancer stage pT	0.044 ± 0.085	1.05 (0.88, 1.2)	0.6
Cancer stage pN	0.092 ± 0.074	1.1 (0.95, 1.3)	0.2
Lobectomy	0.802 ± 0.14	2.2 (1.7, 2.9)	<0.0001
Pneumonectomy	1.3 ± 0.19	3.6 (2.5, 5.2)	<0.0001

ASA = American Society of Anesthesiologists; CL = confidence limits; FEV_1 = forced expiratory volume in 1 second; OR = odds ratio; SE = standard error.
[a]Versus never smoked.

(1.4%) and notably lowest in never smokers and lower in patients with longer intervals of smoking cessation before resection. Table 4 demonstrates that major pulmonary complications were infrequent (5.7%) but occurred more often in current or past smokers compared with never smokers, with the risk of complications steadily decreasing with duration of time between smoking cessation and surgery. No optimal time of smoking cessation was identified. This reinforces the conclusion that smoking cessation is beneficial regardless of timing of lung cancer surgery, a message that should be reinforced to patients anticipating resection.

L. T. Tanoue, MD

References

1. Warner MA, Divertie MB, Tinker JH. Preoperative cessation of smoking and pulmonary complications in coronary artery bypass patients. *Anesthesiology.* 1984;60:380-383.
2. Nakagawa M, Tanaka H, Tsukuma H, Kishi Y. Relationship between the duration of the preoperative smoke-free period and the incidence of postoperative pulmonary complications after pulmonary surgery. *Chest.* 2001;120:705-710.

Effectiveness of Extended-Duration Transdermal Nicotine Therapy: A Randomized Trial
Schnoll RA, Patterson F, Wileyto EP, et al (Univ of Pennsylvania, Philadelphia; Massachusetts General Hosp, Boston)
Ann Intern Med 152:144-151, 2010

Background.—Tobacco dependence is a chronic, relapsing condition that may require extended treatment.

Objective.—To assess whether extended-duration transdermal nicotine therapy increases abstinence from tobacco more than standard-duration therapy in adult smokers.

Design.—Parallel randomized, placebo-controlled trial from September 2004 to February 2008. Participants and all research personnel except the database manager were blinded to randomization. (ClinicalTrials.gov registration number: NCT00364156).

Setting.—Academic center.

Participants.—568 adult smokers.

Intervention.—In an unstratified small block–randomization scheme, participants were randomly assigned to standard therapy (Nicoderm CQ [GlaxoSmithKline, Research Triangle Park, North Carolina], 21 mg, for 8 weeks and placebo for 16 weeks) or extended therapy (Nicoderm CQ, 21 mg, for 24 weeks).

Measurements.—The primary outcome was biochemically confirmed point-prevalence abstinence at weeks 24 and 52. Secondary outcomes were continuous and prolonged abstinence, lapse and recovery events, cost per additional quitter, and side effects and adherence.

Results.—At week 24, extended therapy produced higher rates of point-prevalence abstinence (31.6% vs. 20.3%; odds ratio, 1.81 [95% CI, 1.23 to 2.66]; $P = 0.002$), prolonged abstinence (41.5% vs. 26.9%; odds ratio, 1.97 [CI, 1.38 to 2.82]; $P = 0.001$), and continuous abstinence (19.2% vs. 12.6%; odds ratio, 1.64 [CI, 1.04 to 2.60]; $P = 0.032$) versus standard therapy. Extended therapy reduced the risk for lapse (hazard ratio, 0.77 [CI, 0.63 to 0.95]; $P = 0.013$) and increased the chances of recovery from lapses (hazard ratio, 1.47 [CI, 1.17 to 1.84]; $P = 0.001$). Time to relapse was slower with extended versus standard therapy (hazard ratio, 0.50 [CI, 0.35 to 0.73]; $P < 0.001$). At week 52, extended therapy produced higher quit rates for prolonged abstinence only ($P = 0.027$). No differences in side effects and adverse events between groups were found at the extended-treatment assessment.

Limitation.—The generalizability of the findings may be limited because participants were smokers without medical comorbid conditions who were seeking treatment, and differences in adherence across treatment groups were detected.

Conclusion.—Transdermal nicotine for 24 weeks increased biochemically confirmed point-prevalence abstinence and continuous abstinence at week 24, reduced the risk for smoking lapses, and increased the likelihood of recovery to abstinence after a lapse compared with 8 weeks of transdermal nicotine therapy.

▶ With the appreciation that 90% of lung cancers in this country are attributable to cigarette smoking, and the fact that 46.6 million Americans are currently smoking, it is clear that we need to make even more of an effort to facilitate smoking cessation.[1,2] This study by Schnoll and colleagues confirms what seems intuitively obvious—that sustained abstinence from cigarettes is improved by extending the duration of transdermal nicotine replacement therapy. This underscores the recognition that nicotine dependence, like other addictions, is a chronic and relapsing condition. Fig 2 in the original article demonstrates that extending nicotine replacement from the standard 8 to 24 weeks doubled the likelihood of abstinence at the 24-week mark. The cost of the extended therapy was $2482 per quitter. However, at the end of 1 year, less than 40% of participants, regardless of whether they had 8 or 24 weeks of nicotine replacement, were still abstinent. Clearly, further research on optimal duration of nicotine replacement therapy and the utility of other pharmacologic or counseling interventions is warranted as well as public policy focused on tobacco taxation and limiting tobacco access and use in public areas.

L. T. Tanoue, MD

References

1. Dube S, McClave A, James C, Caraballlo R, Kaufmann R, Pechacek T. Vital signs: current cigarette smoking among adults aged >or=18 years—United States, 2009. *MMWR Morb Mortal Wkly Rep.* 2010;59:1135-1140.
2. Alberg AJ, Ford JG, Samet JM. Epidemiology of lung cancer: ACCP evidence-based clinical practice guidelines (2nd edition). *Chest.* 2007;132:29S-55S.

Vital Signs: Current Cigarette Smoking Among Adults Aged ≥18 Years — United States, 2009
Kaufmann RB, Babb S, O'Halloran A, et al (Natl Ctr for Chronic Disease Prevention and Health Promotion, Atlanta, GA; et al)
MMWR Morb Mortal Wkly Rep 59:1135-1140, 2010

Background.—Cigarette smoking continues to be the leading cause of preventable morbidity and mortality in the United States, causing approximately 443,000 premature deaths annually.

Methods.—The 2009 National Health Interview Survey and the 2009 Behavioral Risk Factor Surveillance System were used to estimate national and state adult smoking prevalence, respectively. Cigarette smokers were defined as adults aged ≥18 years who reported having smoked ≥100 cigarettes in their lifetime and now smoke every day or some days.

Results.—In 2009, 20.6% of U.S. adults aged ≥18 years were current cigarette smokers. Men (23.5%) were more likely than women (17.9%) to be current smokers. The prevalence of smoking was 31.1% among persons below the federal poverty level. For adults aged ≥25 years, the prevalence of smoking was 28.5% among persons with less than a high school diploma, compared with 5.6% among those with a graduate degree. Regional differences were observed, with the West having the lowest prevalence (16.4%) and higher prevalences being observed in the South (21.8%) and Midwest (23.1%). From 2005 to 2009, the proportion of U.S. adults who were current cigarette smokers did not change (20.9% in 2005 and 20.6% in 2009).

Conclusions.—Previous declines in smoking prevalence in the United States have stalled during the past 5 years; the burden of cigarette smoking continues to be high, especially in persons living below the federal poverty level and with low educational attainment. Sustained, adequately funded, comprehensive tobacco control programs could reduce adult smoking.

Implications for Public Health Practice.—To further reduce disease and death from cigarette smoking, declines in cigarette smoking among adults must accelerate. The Patient Protection and Affordable Care Act is expected to expand access to evidence-based smoking-cessation services and treatments; this likely will result in additional use of these services and reductions of current smoking and its adverse effects among U.S. adults. Population-based prevention strategies such as tobacco taxes, media campaigns, and smoke-free policies, in concert with clinical cessation interventions, can help adults quit and prevent the uptake of tobacco use, furthering the reduction in the current prevalence of tobacco use in the United States across age groups.

▶ Cigarette smoking is the leading cause of preventable morbidity and mortality in the United States. An estimated 443 000 premature deaths, including 30% of all cancer deaths, are attributable to cigarettes. Despite extensive efforts at heightening public knowledge of the health consequences of smoking, 20.6% of Americans (46.6 million individuals) currently smoke, a prevalence that has been unfortunately stable over the past 5 years. The objective of Healthy People 2010 (US Department of Health and Human Services, Office of Disease Prevention and Health Promotion) with regard to tobacco use was to achieve nationally a < 12% prevalence of cigarette smoking, a goal that was clearly not met. Among adult Americans, smoking is more common in persons with less education (28.5% among persons with less than a high school diploma compared with 5.6% among persons with a graduate degree) and economic status below the federal poverty level (31.1%). Identification of more effective strategies targeting high-risk populations, including tobacco taxation, incentives, and opportunities for smoking cessation, and public policy to extend the reach of enforced nonsmoking, will be necessary to achieve success in reducing tobacco consumption.

L. T. Tanoue, MD

Influence of smoking cessation after diagnosis of early stage lung cancer on prognosis: systematic review of observational studies with meta-analysis
Parsons A, Daley A, Begh R, et al (Univ of Birmingham, Edgbaston)
BMJ 340:b5569, 2010

Objective.—To systematically review the evidence that smoking cessation after diagnosis of a primary lung tumour affects prognosis.

Design.—Systematic review with meta-analysis.

Data Sources.—CINAHL (from 1981), Embase (from 1980), Medline (from 1966), Web of Science (from 1966), CENTRAL (from 1977) to December 2008, and reference lists of included studies.

Study Selection.—Randomised controlled trials or observational longitudinal studies that measured the effect of quitting smoking after diagnosis of lung cancer on prognostic outcomes, regardless of stage at presentation or tumour histology, were included.

Data Extraction.—Two researchers independently identified studies for inclusion and extracted data. Estimates were combined by using a random effects model, and the I^2 statistic was used to examine heterogeneity. Life tables were used to model five year survival for early stage nonsmall cell lung cancer and limited stage small cell lung cancer, using death rates for continuing smokers and quitters obtained from this review.

Results.—In 9/10 included studies, most patients studied were diagnosed as having an early stage lung tumour. Continued smoking was associated with a significantly increased risk of all cause mortality (hazard ratio 2.94, 95% confidence interval 1.15 to 7.54) and recurrence (1.86, 1.01 to 3.41) in early stage non-small cell lung cancer and of all cause mortality (1.86, 1.33 to 2.59), development of a second primary tumour (4.31, 1.09 to 16.98), and recurrence (1.26, 1.06 to 1.50) in limited stage small cell lung cancer. No study contained data on the effect of quitting smoking on cancer specific mortality or on development of a second primary tumour in nonsmall cell lung cancer. Life table modelling on the basis of these data estimated 33% five year survival in 65 year old patients with early stage non-small cell lung cancer who continued to smoke compared with 70% in those who quit smoking. In limited stage small cell lung cancer, an estimated 29% of continuing smokers would survive for five years compared with 63% of quitters on the basis of the data from this review.

Conclusions.—This review provides preliminary evidence that smoking cessation after diagnosis of early stage lung cancer improves prognostic outcomes. From life table modelling, the estimated number of deaths prevented is larger than would be expected from reduction of cardiorespiratory deaths after smoking cessation, so most of the mortality gain is likely to be due to reduced cancer progression. These findings indicate that offering smoking cessation treatment to patients presenting with early stage lung cancer may be beneficial (Figs 2 and 3).

▶ Ninety percent of lung cancer cases are attributable to cigarette smoking in countries where cigarette smoking is common.[1] Lifelong smokers incur on average a 20-fold increase in lung cancer risk compared with people who have never smoked, and by the age of 75 years, a cumulative risk of approximately 16% is observed.[2,3] It is well recognized that smoking cessation at any age reduces the risk of lung cancer.[3] It is perhaps less appreciated that smoking cessation after lung cancer diagnosis and treatment may be associated with better outcomes. A remarkable percentage of individuals, as many as 60%, continue to smoke after treatment of lung cancer.[4] In this systematic review with meta-analysis, 10 longitudinal observational studies measuring the effect of smoking cessation after lung cancer diagnosis on clinical outcomes were identified and combined. Most patients in these studies had early-stage cancer. The results of the meta-analysis are shown in Figs 2 and 3. The risk of all primary outcomes measures—all-cause mortality and cancer recurrence in early-stage non–small cell lung cancer and all-cause mortality, cancer recurrence, and development of a second primary tumor in limited-stage small cell lung cancer—were increased in patients who continued to smoke after

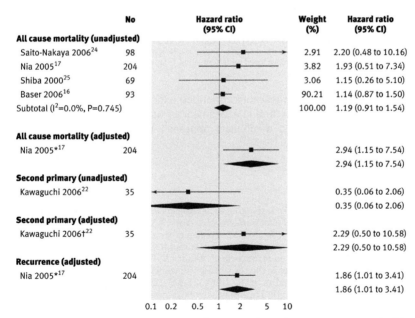

FIGURE 2.—Effect of continued smoking on all cause mortality and recurrence in non-small cell lung cancer. Weights are from random effects analysis. *Adjusted for age, sex, type of operation, histology, postoperative radiotherapy, N status, T status, and previous malignancies. †Adjusted for sex, histology, and cumulative smoking. (Reprinted from Parsons A, Daley A, Begh R, et al. Influence of smoking cessation after diagnosis of early stage lung cancer on prognosis: systematic review of observational studies with meta-analysis. *BMJ.* 2010;340:b5569, reproduced with permission from the BMJ Publishing Group Ltd.)

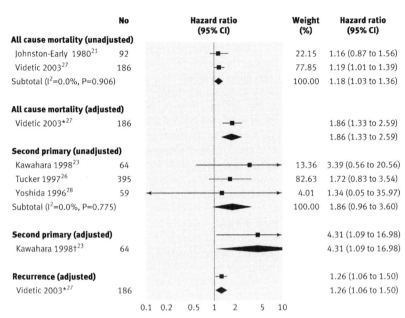

FIGURE 3.—Effect of continued smoking on all cause mortality, development of a second primary, or recurrence in small cell lung cancer. Weights are from random effects analysis. *Adjusted for sex, age, and volume of limited disease. †Adjusted for sex, age, performance status, etoposide, radiotherapy, and cumulative smoking. (Reprinted from Parsons A, Daley A, Begh R, et al. Influence of smoking cessation after diagnosis of early stage lung cancer on prognosis: systematic review of observational studies with meta-analysis. *BMJ.* 2010;340:b5569, reproduced with permission from the BMJ Publishing Group Ltd.)

treatment. These data suggest that continued exposure to tobacco smoke has a significant effect on the biologic behavior of early-stage lung cancers and also clearly argue against a nihilistic approach to smoking cessation after lung cancer diagnosis.

L. T. Tanoue, MD

References

1. Peto R. *Mortality from smoking in developed countries 1950–2000: indirect estimates from national vital statistics.* New York, NY: Oxford University Press; 1994.
2. Alberg AJ, Ford JG, Samet JM. Epidemiology of lung cancer: ACCP evidence-based clinical practice guidelines (2nd edition). *Chest.* 2007;132:29S-55S.
3. Peto R, Darby S, Deo H, Silcocks P, Whitley E, Doll R. Smoking, smoking cessation, and lung cancer in the UK since 1950: combination of national statistics with two case-control studies. *BMJ.* 2000;321:323-329.
4. Pinto BM, Trunzo JJ. Health behaviors during and after a cancer diagnosis. *Cancer.* 2005;104:2614-2623.

4 Pleural, Interstitial Lung, and Pulmonary Vascular Disease

Interstitial Lung Disease

Cryptogenic Organizing Pneumonia: Serial High-Resolution CT Findings in 22 Patients

Lee JW, Lee KS, Lee HY, et al (Sungkyunkwan Univ School of Medicine, Seoul, Republic of Korea)

AJR Am J Roentgenol 195:916-922, 2010

Objective.—We conducted a review of serial high-resolution CT (HRCT) findings of cryptogenic organizing pneumonia (COP).

Materials and Methods.—Over the course of 14 years, we saw 32 patients with biopsy-confirmed COP. Serial HRCT scans were available for only 22 patients (seven men and 15 women; mean age, 52 years; median follow-up period, 8 months; range, 5–135 months). Serial CT scans were evaluated by two chest radiologists who reached a conclusion by consensus. Overall changes in disease extent were classified as cured, improved (i.e., ≥10% decrease in extent), not changed, or progressed (i.e., ≥10% increase in extent). When there were remaining abnormalities, the final follow-up CT images were analyzed to express observers' ideas regarding what type of interstitial lung disease the images most likely suggested.

Results.—The two most common patterns of lung abnormality on initial scans were ground-glass opacification (86% of patients [19/22]) and consolidation (77% of patients [17/22]), distributed along the bronchovascular bundles or subpleural lungs in 13 patients (59%). In six patients (27%), the disease disappeared completely; in 15 patients (68%), the disease was decreased in extent; and in one patient (5%), no change in extent was detected on follow-up CT. When lesions remained, the final follow-up CT findings were reminiscent of fibrotic nonspecific interstitial pneumonia in 10 of 16 patients (63%).

Conclusion.—Although COP is a disease with a generally good prognosis, most patients (73%) with COP have some remaining disease seen on follow-up CT scans, and, in such cases, the lesions generally resemble a fibrotic nonspecific interstitial pneumonia pattern.

▶ I included this retrospective study with its limitations of being small sample size to press on the following points:

1. Long-term follow-up shows complete resolution of the cryptogenic organizing pneumonia in only 27%, a lower number than that previously described.
2. The patients who are going to resolve versus who will not get complete resolution have more restrictive disease (forced vital capacity 93 ± 7.2% vs 58 ± 16.2% predicted) and lower single-breath carbon monoxide diffusing capacity of the lung (86 ± 15.8% vs 65 ± 14.2% predicted).
3. There is no evidence of any crucial decline in pulmonary function tests after initial assessment in any of the patients with the right treatment.
4. If reticulation is the initial picture on high-resolution CT, then the patients are less likely to respond to therapy.
5. The relapse rate is about 10%.[1,2]

M. Ali Raza, MD

References

1. Cordier JF, Loire R, Brune J. Idiopathic bronchiolitis obliterans organizing pneumonia: definition of characteristic clinical profiles in a series of 16 patients. *Chest.* 1989;96:999-1004.
2. Epler GR, Colby TV, McLoud TC, Carrington CB, Gaensler EA. Bronchiolitis obliterans organizing pneumonia. *N Engl J Med.* 1985;312:152-158.

Bosentan Improves Skin Perfusion of Hands in Patients with Systemic Sclerosis with Pulmonary Arterial Hypertension
Rosato E, Molinaro I, Borghese F, et al (Sapienza Univ of Rome, Italy)
J Rheumatol 37:2531-2539, 2010

Objective.—Our aim was to investigate effects of bosentan on hand perfusion in patients with systemic sclerosis (SSc) with pulmonary arterial hypertension (PAH), using laser Doppler perfusion imaging (LDPI).

Methods.—We enrolled 30 SSc patients with PAH, 30 SSc patients without PAH, and 30 healthy controls. In SSc patients and healthy controls at baseline, skin blood flow of the dorsum of the hands was determined with a Lisca laser Doppler perfusion imager. The dorsal surface of the hands was divided into 3 regions of interest (ROI). ROI 1 included 3 fingers of the hand from the second to the fourth distally to the proximal interphalangeal finger joint. ROI 2 included the area between the proximal interphalangeal and the metacarpophalangeal joint. ROI 3 included only the dorsal surface of the hand without the fingers. LDPI was repeated in SSc patients and controls after 4, 8, and 16 weeks of treatment. In SSc patients, nailfold videocapillaroscopy and Raynaud Condition Score (RCS) were performed at baseline and at 4, 8, and 16 weeks.

Results.—SSc patients with PAH enrolled in the study received treatment with bosentan as standard care for PAH. In these patients with PAH, after 8 and 16 weeks of treatment, bosentan improved minimum, mean, and maximum perfusion and the perfusion proximal-distal gradient. Bosentan seems to be most effective in patients with the early and active capillaroscopic pattern than in patients with the late pattern. Bosentan improved skin blood flow principally in the ROI 1 compared to the ROI 2 and ROI 3. Bosentan restored the perfusion proximal-distal gradient in 57% of SSc patients with the early capillaroscopic pattern. No significant differences from baseline were observed in the RCS in SSc patients with PAH.

Conclusion.—Bosentan improved skin perfusion in SSc patients with PAH, although it did not ameliorate symptoms of Raynaud's phenomenon. Skin blood perfusion increased in SSc patients with PAH, particularly in the skin region distal to the proximal interphalangeal joint, and in patients with the early/active capillaroscopic pattern. Double-blind randomized clinical trials are needed to evaluate the effects of bosentan on skin perfusion of SSc patients without PAH and with active digital ulcers.

▶ Bosentan has significant therapeutic advantage in pulmonary arterial hypertension (PAH) and more so in the connective tissue diseases. The above study shows the effect of 62.5 mg and 125 mg doses of bosentan on digital perfusion. These changes were more evident in patients with the early/active capillaroscopic pattern than in patients with the late pattern. Because activation of the endothelin-I system also plays a role in determining endothelial dysfunction in systemic sclerosis, we can suppose that bosentan ameliorates endothelial dysfunction and consequently microcirculatory flow. The study is restricted by its limitations namely, correction for temperature, the open-label approach, the lack of a run-in treatment-free period, the lack of a crossover design, including the diagnosis of PAH in these patients without right heart catheter. I personally believe that endothelin receptor blockers have significant added advantages pertaining to the microvascular remodelling and prevention of microthrombi formation, which is the ultimate cause of end-organ damage and ischemia.

M. Ali Raza, MD

Impaired Heart Rate Recovery Index in Patients With Sarcoidosis

Ardic I, Kaya MG, Yarlioglues M, et al (Erciyes Univ School of Medicine, Kayseri, Turkey)
Chest 139:60-68, 2011

Background.—Sarcoidosis, an inflammatory granulomatous disease, is associated with various cardiac disorders, including threatening ventricular arrhythmias and sudden cardiac death. Heart rate recovery (HRR) after exercise is a function of vagal reactivation, and its impairment is an independent prognostic indicator for cardiovascular and all-cause mortality. The aim of our study was to evaluate HRR in patients with sarcoidosis.

Methods.—The study population included 56 patients with sarcoidosis (23 men, mean age = 47.3 ± 13.0 years, and mean disease duration = 38.4 ± 9.7 months) and 54 healthy control subjects (20 men, mean age = 46.5 ± 12.9 years). Basal ECG, echocardiography, and treadmill exercise testing were performed on all patients and control participants. The HRR index was defined as the reduction in the heart rate at peak exercise to the first-minute rate (HRR_1), second-minute (HRR_2), third-minute (HRR_3), and fifth-minute (HRR_5) after the cessation of exercise stress testing.

Results.—There are significant differences in HRR_1 and HRR_2 indices between patients with sarcoidosis and the control group (25 ± 6 vs 34 ± 11; $P < 001$ and 45 ± 10 vs 53 ± 12; $P < .001$, respectively). Similarly, HRR_3 and HRR_5 indices of the recovery period were lower in patients with sarcoidosis when compared with indices in the control group (53 ± 12 vs 61 ± 13; $P < .001$ and 60 ± 13 vs 68 ± 13; $P < .001$, respectively). Exercise capacity was notably lower (9.2 ± 2.1 vs 11.6 ± 2.8 METs; $P = .001$, respectively) and systolic pulmonary arterial pressure at rest was significantly higher in patients with sarcoidosis compared with the control group (29.7 ± 5.5 mm Hg vs 25.6 ± 5.7 mm Hg, $P = .001$, respectively). Furthermore, HRR indices were found to be different among radiographic stage groups.

Conclusions.—The HRR index was impaired in patients with sarcoidosis as compared with control subjects. When the prognostic significance of the HRR index is considered, these results may partially explain the increased occurrence of arrhythmias and sudden cardiac death in patients with sarcoidosis. Our findings suggest that the HRR index may be clinically helpful in identifying high-risk patients with sarcoidosis.

▶ It is interesting to note that heart rate recovery index can be applied to patients with sarcoidosis, shows increased incidence of arrhythmias, and identifies patients with pulmonary arterial hypertension and morbidity. This is also different in radiologic stages.

M. Ali Raza, MD

Pleural Disease

Management of pleural infection in adults: British Thoracic Society pleural disease guideline 2010

Davies HE, on behalf of the BTS Pleural Disease Guideline Group (Oxford Radcliffe Hosp, UK; et al)
Thorax 65:ii41-ii53, 2010

Background.—Prompt evaluation and therapeutic intervention for pleural infection can reduce morbidity, mortality, and healthcare costs for this common clinical problem. Guidelines were developed from a peer-reviewed systematic literature review and expert opinion of the preferred management.

Considerations.—The care of all patients who require chest tube drainage for a pleural infection should be directed by a chest physician or thoracic surgeon. The clinician should ensure that patients with pleural infection are adequately nourished. These patients are at high risk for developing venous thromboembolism, so adequate thrombosis prophylaxis with heparin is advisable unless contraindicated. If patients with pneumonia progress to ongoing sepsis and elevated C reactive protein levels within 3 days, pleural infection is a possibility and blood cultures for aerobic and anaerobic bacteria are recommended. If pleural effusion accompanies sepsis or pneumonic illness, diagnostic pleural fluid sampling is needed. The pH of pleural fluid is measured in all nonpurulent effusions when pleural infection is suspected. If such data cannot be obtained, the pleural fluid glucose level should be assessed.

Management.—Patients with purulent or turbid/cloudy pleural fluid should be managed with prompt pleural space chest tube drainage. Samples are tested using Gram stain and/or culture to determine if the infection is established. Chest tube drainage is indicated for patients whose samples contain pathogenic organisms and those whose pleural fluid pH exceeds 7.2. Antibiotics alone may be sufficient for patients whose parapneumonic effusions do not meet these criteria. Patient review, repeat pleural fluid sampling, and chest tube drainage are advised for patients whose clinical progress is poor. Early chest tube drainage aids patients with a loculated pleural collection. To relieve symptoms, large nonpurulent effusions are drained by aspiration or chest tube.

If chest tube drainage is chosen, usually a small-bore catheter (10 to 14 F) is used, but no specific size is considered optimal. Small-bore flexible catheters require regular flushing to avoid catheter blockage. Chest tubes placement is guided by imaging.

Antibiotics include agents targeted to treat the bacterial profile of modern pleural infection and consider local antibiotic policies and resistance patterns. All patients except those with culture-proven pneumococcal infection need antibiotics directed at anaerobic infection. Unless objective evidence reveals a high clinical index of suspicion for atypical pathogens, macrolide antibiotics are not indicated. Bacterial culture results and advice

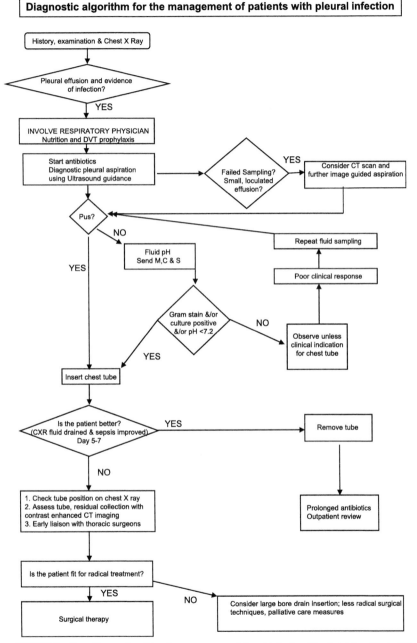

Diagnostic algorithm for the management of patients with pleural infection

History, examination & Chest X Ray

Pleural effusion and evidence of infection?

YES

INVOLVE RESPIRATORY PHYSICIAN
Nutrition and DVT prophylaxis

Start antibiotics
Diagnostic pleural aspiration
using Ultrasound guidance

Failed Sampling?
Small, loculated effusion?

YES

Consider CT scan and further image guided aspiration

Pus?

NO

Fluid pH
Send M,C & S

Repeat fluid sampling

Poor clinical response

YES

Gram stain &/or culture positive &/or pH <7.2

NO

Observe unless clinical indication for chest tube

YES

Insert chest tube

Is the patient better?
(CXR fluid drained & sepsis improved)
Day 5-7

YES

Remove tube

NO

1. Check tube position on chest X ray
2. Assess tube, residual collection with contrast enhanced CT imaging
3. Early liaison with thoracic surgeons

Prolonged antibiotics
Outpatient review

Is the patient fit for radical treatment?

YES

Surgical therapy

NO

Consider large bore drain insertion; less radical surgical techniques, palliative care measures

FIGURE 1.—Flow diagram describing the management of pleural infection. (Reprinted from Davies HE, on behalf of the BTS Pleural Disease Guideline Group, Management of pleural infection in adults: British Thoracic Society pleural disease guideline 2010. *Thorax*. 2010;65:ii41-ii53, and reproduced/amended with permission from the BMJ Publishing Group.)

from a microbiologist should guide antibiotic choice. Pleural space penetration is quite adequate with penicillins, pencillins plus β-lactamase inhibitors, metronidazole, and cephalosporins. Aminoglycosides are avoided. With negative bacterial cultures, antibiotics must cover both common community-acquired bacterial pathogens and anaerobic organisms. Empirical antibiotic therapy for hospital-acquired empyema includes coverage for anaerobic organisms and methicillin-resistant *Staphylococcus aureus* (MRSA). Once sepsis improves both clinically and objectively, oral therapy can be substituted for intravenous antibiotics. There is no indication for intrapleural antibiotics, and intrapleural fibrinolytics are not routinely needed. Antibiotics can be given for an extended time on an outpatient basis.

Chest drains are removed once radiographs show successful pleural drainage. If sepsis or a residual pleural collection persists, additional radiographic imaging is needed, along with a thoracic surgical consultation.

Surgery is needed for patients with persistent sepsis and pleural collection despite chest tube drainage and antibiotic therapy. A thoracic surgical consultation is also helpful, allowing better assessment of the suitability for anesthesia. Among the less radical approaches are rib resection and placement of a large-bore drain, particularly useful in frail patients. Sometimes these less invasive procedures are accomplished under local or epidural anesthesia. If effusion drainage is ineffective and sepsis persists in patients who cannot tolerate general anesthesia, reimaging of the thorax, and placement of a small-bore catheter under image guidance, the thoracic surgeon may choose to use a larger-bore chest tube or an intrapleural fibrinolytic. Some patients may benefit from palliative treatment and active symptom control measures. Bronchoscopy is needed only when there is a high index of suspicion of bronchial obstruction.

Conclusions.—Outpatient follow-up is needed for all patients who develop empyema and pleural infection. With prompt treatment, the long-term survival of patients with pleural infection is good. However, long-term sequelae associated with pleural empyema include residual pleural thickening. Patients with pyothorax present for over 20 years may rarely develop pleural lymphoma (Fig 1).

▶ These are new guidelines for treating pleural infection. I suggest every pulmonologist go over the Web site since access is free. There is always a debate on how big a catheter to place and when to place it for infected pleural effusions. According to British Thoracic Society, the catheter size could be as small as 10 to 14 F and needs frequent flushing. The other point is to put a chest tube in if only the Gram stain is positive even if the effusion does not look complicated.

M. Ali Raza, MD

Rapid Pleurodesis for Malignant Pleural Effusions: A Pilot Study

Reddy C, Ernst A, Lamb C, et al (Univ of Utah Health Sciences Ctr, Salt Lake City; Beth Israel Deaconess Med Ctr, Boston, MA; Lahey Clinic, Burlington MA; et al)
Chest 2010 [Epub ahead of print]

Background.—Malignant pleural effusions affect more than 150,000 people each year in the United States. Current palliative options include pleurodesis and placement of an indwelling catheter, each with their own associated benefits. This study was conducted to determine the safety, efficacy and feasibility of a rapid pleurodesis protocol by combining medical thoracoscopy with talc pleurodesis and simultaneous placement of a tunneled pleural catheter (TPC) in patients with symptomatic malignant pleural effusions (MPE).

Methods.—Patients with recurrent, symptomatic MPEs underwent medical thoracoscopy with placement of a TPC and talc poudrage. The TPC was drained per protocol until the output was less than 150 mL/day on two consecutive drainage attempts and then removed. Patients were followed for up to 6 months.

Results.—Between October of 2005 and September of 2009, thirty patients underwent the procedure. The median duration of hospitalization following the procedure was 1.79 days. All patients had an improvement in dyspnea and quality of life. Pleurodesis was successful in 92% of patients, and the TPC was removed at a median of 7.54 days. Complications included fever in two patients, the need for replacement of tunneled pleural catheter in one patient and empyema in one patient.

Conclusion.—Rapid pleurodesis can be safely achieved by combining medical thoracoscopy and talc poudrage with simultaneous TPC placement. Both hospital length of stay and duration of the tunneled pleural catheter can be significantly reduced as compared to historical controls of either procedure alone. Future randomized trials are needed to confirm these results.

▶ I selected this article because it shows how patients with malignant pleural effusion can get the best quality of life with their limited time. Usually, these patients are in the hospital for a few days to sometimes weeks to be treated for their recurrent large effusions. This protocol of early pleurodesis with a placement of tunneled pleural catheter makes it possible for them to stay at home. This palliative approach makes all the sense.

M. Ali Raza, MD

Bedside Transthoracic Sonography in Suspected Pulmonary Embolism: A New Tool for Emergency Physicians
Hoffmann B, Gullett JP (Johns Hopkins Univ, Baltimore, MD; Johns Hopkins Bayview Med Ctr, Baltimore, MD)
Acad Emerg Med 17:e88-e93, 2010

Background.—The signs and symptoms of pulmonary embolism (PE) are nonspecific, making it difficult to diagnose without a high index of suspicion. Technical advances including D-dimer and multidetector-row computed tomography (MDCT) scan have increased detection rates, especially for segmental and subsegmental PE, but with lower specificity. MDCT drawbacks include not being widely available; not being feasible for all patients who require a PE workup, particularly unstable patients; exposing patients to radiation; and requiring more time than bedside ultrasound (US). Bedside pulmonary US has successfully diagnosed pneumothorax, pleural effusion, pneumonia, lung edema, and PE. Little information exists on the use of bedside US in emergency department (ED) settings. Three patients were diagnosed provisionally using chest/pulmonary US and confirmed using MDCT.

Case Reports.—*Case 1*: Woman, 21, came to the ED complaining of several days of severe and worsening chest pain that disturbed her sleep. Symptoms began about 24 hours after an elective surgical abortion at gestational age 8 2/7 weeks. She smoked but had no other known risk factors for PE. The pain was located inferior to the right breast and was accompanied by palpitations, periodic shortness of breath, and cough with minor hemoptysis the day she came for treatment. Her vital signs were blood pressure 127/81 mm Hg, heart rate 109 beats/min, respirations 18 breaths/min, oxygen saturation 100% on room air, and temperature 38.2°C. Respirations increased and pain worsened when she spoke. Heart tones were normal with coarse rhonchi over the right lung and diminished breath sounds over the right lung base. Chest pain was reproducible on chest wall palpation of the right lower chest. Focused bedside US showed the right lower lung had multiple wedge-shaped hypodense parenchymal defects at the lung periphery with localized and basal effusion. Doppler US showed no perfusion of the edematous lung tissue. PE with lung infarction was diagnosed.

Case 2: Woman, 65, had a past history of hypertension and stroke and came for treatment of sudden-onset sharp chest pain worsening with deep breathing. Her blood pressure was 168/69 mm Hg, heart rate 69 beats/min, respirations 18 breaths/min, and oxygen saturation 99% on 2 L of oxygen by nasal cannula. Her lungs were clear and she had a regular heart rate and rhythm with no murmurs or rubs. Chest x-ray was negative, but sonography showed several subtle wedge-shaped or rounded hypodense

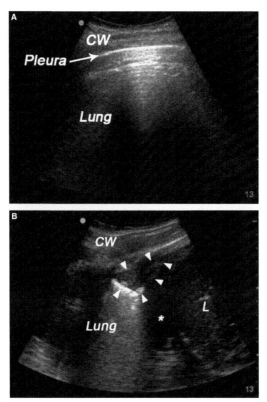

FIGURE 1.—(A) TUS showing normal left lung. The transducer is placed at the left mid-axillary line above the diaphragm parallel to the fourth intercostal space. The pleura is identified as a bright hyperechoic line. (B) The transducer is placed in the right coronal plane at the level of the diaphragm. The lung parenchyma is seen with a pleural-based, wedge-shaped, parenchymal hypodense area (white arrowheads) marking the visible area of lung infarction. There is strong posterior enhancement and parenchymal consolidation (white hyperdense area central to the peripheral defect). *Pleural effusion between liver (L) and right lung. CW = chest wall; TUS = transthoracic ultrasound. (Reprinted from Hoffmann B, Gullett JP. Bedside transthoracic sonography in suspected pulmonary embolism: a new tool for emergency physicians. *Acad Emerg Med.* 2010;17:e88-e93, with permission from the Society for Academic Emergency Medicine.)

parenchymal areas adjacent to the pleural space, suggesting PE. Transthoracic US found large areas of normal lung. A contrast-enhanced MDCT with PE protocol revealed bilateral PE.

Case 3: Man, 52, came to the ED with chest pain and shortness of breath while walking to work. He felt diaphoretic and febrile. His blood pressure was 153/87 mm Hg, heart rate 132 beats/min (tachycardic), and respirations 20 breaths/min (mildly tachypneic). Initial oxygen saturation on room air was 83%, but this improved to 96% on 3 L of oxygen by nasal cannula. On auscultation he had a regular heart rate with no murmurs, coarse breath sounds bilaterally, and chest pain on deep breathing. Focused bedside sonography found no pneumothorax but multiple small wedge-shaped parenchymal defects at the lung periphery with localized pleural effusion, suggesting multiple PE.

Conclusions.—Using bedside US of the thorax and heart may improve the assessment of patients with suspected PE. This approach may be especially useful for patients in an intermediate risk group or when D-dimer and chest CT are not available or feasible. The effectiveness of US for adults and children and the possible inclusion of this modality into clinical decision-making algorithms will need to be assessed through large multicenter studies. Transthoracic US for the diagnosis of PE in the ED should be considered, especially for patients who have contraindications for CT radiation exposure or contrast application (Fig 1).

▶ Ultrasound used at bedside in the critical care areas and emergency room is becoming a norm now. It has a great advantage in timely and accurate assessment of the clinical condition. Ultrasound of the lung has not been catching fame, but I believe in the right clinical context, it has a great role to play, and this study is a great example of that. I am sure that this scenario has happened to all of us as described in the cases, and at least in few instances, we have overlooked the possibility of pulmonary embolism because the patient is pregnant and infiltrates are shown with fever and high white blood cell count. I am including this article so that all of us know about the future application of bedside ultrasound when it is at its prime in the coming years.

M. Ali Raza, MD

Investigation of a unilateral pleural effusion in adults: British Thoracic Society pleural disease guideline 2010
Hooper C, on behalf of the BTS Pleural Guideline Group (Southmead Hosp, Bristol, UK; et al)
Thorax 65:ii4-ii17, 2010

Pleural effusions are a common medical problem with more than 50 recognised causes including disease local to the pleura or underlying lung, systemic conditions, organ dysfunction and drugs.

Pleural effusions occur as a result of increased fluid formation and/or reduced fluid resorption. The precise pathophysiology of fluid accumulation varies according to underlying aetiologies. As the differential diagnosis for a unilateral pleural effusion is wide, a systematic approach to investigation is necessary. The aim is to establish a diagnosis swiftly while minimising unnecessary invasive investigations and facilitating treatment, avoiding the need for repeated therapeutic aspirations when possible.

Since the 2003 guideline, several clinically relevant studies have been published, allowing new recommendations regarding image guidance of

TABLE 1.—Pleural Fluid Tests and Sample Collection Guidance

Test	Notes
Recommended tests for all sampled pleural effusions	
Biochemistry: LDH and protein	2–5 ml in plain container or serum blood collection tube depending on local policy. Blood should be sent simultaneously to biochemistry for total protein and LDH so that Light's criteria can be applied
Microscopy and culture (MC and S)	5 ml in plain container. If pleural infection is particularly suspected, a further 5 ml in both anaerobic and aerobic blood culture bottles should be sent
Cytological examination and differential cell count	Maximum volume from remaining available sample in a plain universal container. Refrigerate if delay in processing anticipated (eg, out of hours)
Other tests sent only in selected cases as described in the text	
pH	In non-purulent effusions when pleural infection is suspected. 0.5–1 ml drawn up into a heparinised blood gas syringe immediately after aspiration. The syringe should be capped to avoid exposure to air. Processed using a ward arterial blood gas machine
Glucose	Occasionally useful in diagnosis of rheumatoid effusion. 1–2 ml in fluoride oxalate tube sent to biochemistry
Acid-fast bacilli and TB culture	When there is clinical suspicion of TB pleuritis. Request with MC and S. 5 ml sample in plain container
Triglycerides and cholesterol	To distinguish chylothorax from pseudochylothorax in milky effusions. Can usually be requested with routine biochemistry (LDH, protein) using the same sample
Amylase	Occasionally useful in suspected pancreatitis-related effusion. Can usually be requested with routine biochemistry
Haematocrit	Diagnosis of haemothorax. 1–2 ml sample in EDTA container sent to haematology

LDH, lactate dehydrogenase; PH, pulmonary hypertension; TB, tuberculosis.

pleural procedures with clear benefits to patient comfort and safety, optimum pleural fluid sampling and processing and the particular value of thoracoscopic pleural biopsies. This guideline also includes a review of recent evidence for the use of new biomarkers including N-terminal pro-brain natriuretic peptide (NT-proBNP), mesothelin and surrogate markers of tuberculous pleuritis (Table 1).

▶ British Thoracic Society guidelines are a must read. The updates for unilateral pleural effusion are:

1. Aspiration should not be performed for bilateral effusions in a clinical setting strongly suggestive of a transudate unless there are atypical features or they fail to respond to therapy.
2. An accurate drug history should be taken during clinical assessment.
3. Ultrasound detects pleural fluid septations with greater sensitivity than CT.
4. The appearance of the pleural fluid and any odor should be recorded.
5. *N*-terminal probrain natriuretic peptide levels in blood and pleural fluid correlate closely, and the measurement of both has been shown in several series to be effective in discriminating transudates associated with congestive heart failure from other transudative or exudative causes. The cutoff value of these studies varies from 600 to 4000 pg/mL (with 1500 pg/mL being most commonly used).
6. There is no significant increase in cytology yield after 2 samples.

M. Ali Raza, MD

Management of a malignant pleural effusion: British Thoracic Society pleural disease guideline 2010
Roberts ME, on behalf of the BTS Pleural Disease Guideline Group (Sherwood Forest Hosps NHS Foundation Trust, UK; et al)
Thorax 65:ii32-ii40, 2010

Background.—Finding malignant cells in pleural fluid and/or parietal pleura indicates a disseminated or advanced disease and reduced life expectancy in patients who have cancer. The management of malignant pleural effusion was outlined.

Clinical Presentation.—Most malignant effusions produce symptoms. If the pleural effusions are massive, with complete or almost complete opacification of a hemithorax on the chest x-ray, malignancy is the most common cause.

Management.—Asymptomatic patients who have a known tumor type can be observed. Symptomatic malignant effusions prompt consultation with the respiratory team and/or respiratory multidisciplinary team. If pleural effusions are treated by aspiration alone, recurrence of effusion within 1 month is likely. If the patient's life expectancy exceeds 1 month, aspiration is not recommended. Caution is needed if more than 1.5 L is removed in a single episode. Except in patients with short life expectancies, small-bore chest tubes and pleurodesis are preferred to repeat aspiration. Pleurodesis after intercostal drainage prevents recurrence except with significant trapped lung.

For effusion drainage plus pleurodesis, small-bore (10 to 14 F) intercostal catheters are chosen initially. For large pleural effusions, controlled drainage will reduce the risk of re-expansion pulmonary edema. If only partial pleural apposition can be done, chemical pleurodesis may provide relief of symptoms. If pleural apposition is not possible in a patient with symptoms, an indwelling pleural catheter is more efficacious than repeat aspiration. Radiographic confirmation of effusion drainage and lung re-expansion should be immediately followed by pleurodesis. Usually suction to help pleural drainage is unnecessary, but if used, a high-volume low-pressure system is needed.

Because intrapleural administration of sclerosing agents can be painful, 3 mg/kg of lidocaine (maximum 250 mg) is given intrapleurally just before the sclerosant is given. The use of premedication can alleviate both anxiety and pain associated with pleurodesis. The most effective sclerosant available is talc. Graded talc is preferred to ungraded talc because of the lower risk of arterial hypoxemia. Either a slurry or insufflation can be used. An alternative to talc is bleomycin, which has modest efficacy. Sclerosant administration can be complicated by pleuritic chest pain and fever. After intrapleural instillation of sclerosant, it is not necessary to rotate the patient. The intercostal tube is clamped for 1 hour after administering the sclerosant. The tube is removed within 24 to 48 hours if fluid drainage is not excessive (less than 250 mg/day).

In patients with proven or suspected mesothelioma, prophylactic radiotherapy may be used at the site of thoracoscopy, surgery, or insertion of a large-bore chest tube. However, for pleural aspiration or biopsy, such prophylaxis is not needed. For the relief of distressing dyspnea caused by multiloculated malignant effusion resistant to simple drainage, fibrinolytic drugs can be instilled intrapleurally.

Thoracoscopy is recommended to diagnose suspected malignant pleural effusion and for drainage and pleurodesis of known malignant pleural effusion in patients with good performance status. To control recurrent malignant pleural effusion, thoracoscopic talc poudrage may be helpful. Thorascopy is safe and has low complication rates. To control recurrent and symptomatic malignant effusions, ambulatory indwelling pleural catheters may be useful. Pleurectomy cannot be recommended as an alternative to pleurodesis or an indwelling pleural catheter in patients with recurrent effusions or trapped lung.

Conclusions.—Lung cancer is the most common metastatic tumor (50% to 65% of cases) to the pleura in men and breast tissue in women, followed by lymphomas and tumors of the genitourinary tract and gastrointestinal tract (25% of cases). The primary is unknown in 7% to 15% of malignant pleural effusions. The clinical characteristics of pleural fluid have not yet

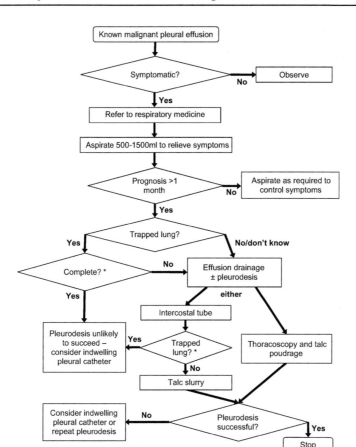

* There is no evidence as to what proportion of unapposed
pleura prevents pleurodesis. We suggest that <50% pleural
apposition is unlikely to lead to successful pleurodesis

FIGURE 1.—Management algorithm for malignant pleural effusion. (Reprinted from Roberts ME, on behalf of the BTS Pleural Disease Guideline Group. Management of a malignant pleural effusion: British Thoracic Society pleural disease guideline 2010. *Thorax.* 2010;65:ii32-ii40, and reproduced/amended with permission from the BMJ Publishing Group.)

been shown to correlate with survival. Guidelines for the management of malignant pleural effusions were offered (Fig 1, Table 1).

▶ I would encourage all pulmonologists to review the guidelines. New information is summarized as follows:

1. No need to only aspirate pleural effusion in patients with life expectancy of > 1 month. Better to drain it with chest tube.
2. Size 10 to 14 F catheters are good enough as an initial choice for drainage and pleurodesis.
3. In cases of trapped lung, indwelling pleural catheters have a role.
4. Suction to aid pleurodesis is not necessary.

TABLE 1.—Primary Tumour Site in Patients with Malignant Pleural Effusion

Primary Tumour Site	Salyer[14] (n=95)	Chernow[1] (n=96)	Johnston[13] (n=472)	Sears[4] (n=592)	Hsu[12] (n=785)	Total (%)
Lung	42	32	168	112	410	764 (37.5)
Breast	11	20	70	141	101	343 (16.8)
Lymphoma	11	–	75	92	56	234 (11.5)
Gastrointestinal	–	13	28	32	68	141 (6.9)
Genitourinary	–	13	57	51	70	191 (9.4)
Other	14	5	26	88	15	148 (7.8)
Unknown primary	17	13	48	76	65	219 (10.7)

Editor's Note: Please refer to original journal article for full references.

5. Graded talc is the sclerosing agent of choice.
6. For suspected mesothelioma, biopsy or drainage of effusion is not proven to be associated with seeding of chest wall but should be radiated before any other major intervention.
7. Chest tube can be removed if drainage is < 250 mL/d.
8. Recurrent pleural effusion with good performance status should be treated with thoracoscopy. Please review Fig 1.

M. Ali Raza, MD

Pulmonary Vascular Disease

Pulmonary embolism risk stratification: Pulse oximetry and pulmonary embolism severity index

Nordenholz K, Ryan J, Atwood B, et al (Univ of Colorado, Aurora; Univ of Texas Med School at Houston)
J Emerg Med 40:95-102, 2011

Background.—Risk stratification of pulmonary embolism (PE) patients is important to determine appropriate management.

Objectives.—We evaluated two published risk-stratification tools in emergency department (ED) PE patients: a pulse oximetry cutoff below 92.5% oxygen (at 5280 feet elevation) and the Pulmonary Embolism Severity Index (PESI).

Methods.—Electronic medical records of all patients diagnosed with PE were abstracted to identify their triage vital signs, co-morbidities, and adverse short-term outcomes (AO) either requiring interventions (defined as respiratory failure, hypotension requiring pressors, and hemodynamic impairment requiring thrombolytics) or resulting in death. We applied these models to our ED PE patients and assessed their performance.

Results.—There were 168 PE patients identified, with an overall AO rate of 7.1% (12/168), including a 3.0% mortality rate. A room-air pulse oximetry cutoff of 92.5%, for values measured at 5280 feet, classified 89/136 patients as low risk, 1.1% of which had an AO, and 47/136 patients as high risk, of which 10.6% had AO. This pulse oximetry cutoff had a sensitivity of 83% (95% confidence interval [CI] 36–99%), specificity of 68% (95% CI 58–76%), and a negative predictive value (NPV) of 99% (95% CI 93–100%). PESI classified 91/168 patients as low risk (class I or II): 2.2% had AO but none died, and 77/168 were classified as high risk (class III, IV, or V), with an AO rate of 13.0%. A PESI cutoff score of II had a sensitivity of 83% (95% CI 52–98%), specificity of 57% (95% CI 49–65%), and NPV of 98% (95% CI 92–100%).

Conclusion.—Both PESI and pulse oximetry measurements are moderately accurate identifiers of low-risk patients with PE.

▶ I wanted you to think about a combined approach of risk assessment and treatment strategy for patients with submassive pulmonary embolism (PE) and stable hemodynamics. A number of parameters, including vital signs, blood markers, CT assessment, and echocardiographic assessments of right heart failure, have been proposed and evaluated in the literature. I believe that it is still open to interpretation. I would also strongly suggest paying close attention to the clinical scenario since not every patient is the same. In general, the use of saturation < 92.5%, probrain natriuretic peptide (proBNP) > 300 pmol/mL, troponin-T (Tn-T) > 0.027, CT evaluation of right ventricular (RV)/left ventricular > 0.9 and signs of RV dysfunction (RVD) on echo is substantially increasing the odds of death up to 26.5 times in the above study. The mortality is 60% in patients with Tn-T ≥0.027 ng/mL and echocardiographic evidence of RVD. A *N*-terminal proBNP (NT-proBNP) of < 90 pmol/mL confers a negative predictive value of 98% all-cause and 100% PE-related mortality. So the echo may not be needed in these cases. Three previous studies[1-3] show that the negative predictive value of low-level NT-proBNP for mortality ranges from 97% to 100%. I would suggest aggressive treatment in these patients with high risk even though they have normal hemodynamics.

M. Ali Raza, MD

References

1. British Thoracic Society Standards of Care Committee Pulmonary Embolism Guideline Development Group. British Thoracic Society guidelines for the management of suspected acute pulmonary embolism. *Thorax.* 2003;58:470-483.
2. Wells PS, Ginsberg JS, Anderson DR, et al. Use of a clinical model for safe management of patients with suspected pulmonary embolism. *Ann Intern Med.* 1998;129: 997-1005.
3. Torbicki A, Perrier A, Konstantinides S, et al. Guidelines on the diagnosis and management of acute pulmonary embolism. the Task Force for the Diagnosis and Management of Acute Pulmonary Embolism of the European Society of Cardiology (ESC). *Eur Heart J.* 2008;29:2276-2315.

Central thromboembolism is a possible predictor of right heart dysfunction in normotensive patients with acute pulmonary embolism

Berghaus TM, Haeckel T, Behr W, et al (Intensive Care and Endocrinology, Klinikum Augsburg, Germany; Dept of Diagnostic Radiology and Neuroradiology, Klinikum Augsburg, Germany; Inst of Laboratory Medicine, Klinikum Augsburg, Germany; et al)
Thromb Res 126:e201-e205, 2010

Background.—Right heart dysfunction is a crucial factor in risk stratification of normotensive patients with pulmonary embolism. Apart from biomarkers, determinants of right heart dysfunction in this group of patients are not yet well established.

Aim and Method.—In order to identify such determinants, we analysed data of 252 patients with acute pulmonary embolism admitted to our hospital in 2008.

Results.—69 out of 140 patients showed right heart dysfunction by echocardiography within 24 hours after diagnosis, 71 did not. Right ventricular dysfunction was significantly more frequent in patients with central clots on computed tomography (p = 0.004), a history of syncope (p < 0.001) and among women on oral contraceptives (p = 0.003). In multiple regression analysis, only central thromboembolism (p < 0.001) was identified as individual predictor of right ventricular dysfunction. Age, gender, body mass index, idiopathic or recurrent thromboembolism, duration of symptoms, preceding surgery, room air oxygen saturation, carcinoma, hypertension, diabetes, renal disease, congestive left heart failure and concomitant lung disease were equally distributed. In comparison with NT-pro brain natriuretic peptide (PPV 67%, NPV 75%, p = 0.782) and troponin I (PPV 76%, NPV 62%, p = 0.336), central thromboembolism has shown to have a greater statistical power in predicting right heart dysfunction in normotensive patients with pulmonary embolism (PPV 78%, NPV 88%, p < 0.001).

Conclusion.—Among normotensive patients with acute pulmonary embolism, those with central clots seem to be at greater risk for echocardiographically evaluated right ventricular dysfunction (Table 4).

▶ The patients with acute pulmonary embolism (PE) are divided into 2 main groups. One with massive PE (hemodynamically instable patients with large clot burden) and others with submassive PE (hemodynamically stable patients with small to moderate clot burden). The choice of urgent treatment like medical thrombolysis and surgical thromboendartectomy is easier and straightforward in massive PE, but treatment of submassive PE with hemodynamic stability is always met with controversy. One way to divide these patients into a high-risk group is to see if they have evidence of significant right heart dysfunction (RHD). This study evaluates the surrogate markers of RHD. Central thromboembolism is seen in this series as an independent predictor of RHD. The other markers like troponin, probrain natriuretic peptide (proBNP) and history of syncope were not significant when plotted in multiple regression

TABLE 4.—Ability to Predict Right Heart Dysfunction (RHD) on Echocardiography

	Sensitivity	Specificity	NPV	PPV
NT-proBNP >125 pg/ml	94%	28%	75%	67%
Troponin I >0.09 ng/ml	56%	80%	62%	76%
Central thrombus on CT scan	89%	75%	88%	78%

NPV: negative predictive value PPV: positive predictive value.

analysis. The authors postulate that central PE is presenting more acutely with less time of the right ventricle for pressure adaptation, although central thromboembolism probably cannot be proclaimed as a single surrogate marker for right ventricular dysfunction. The limitations of the study were that the troponin was done very early at presentation, may not have given enough time to elevate significantly, and proBNP cutoff was chosen low. It shows us another interesting point that a low *N*-terminal proBNP <125 pg/mL excludes the possibility of RHD in these patients with good specificity.

M. Ali Raza, MD

Combined risk stratification with computerized tomography /echocardiography and biomarkers in patients with normotensive pulmonary embolism
Ozsu S, Karaman K, Mentese A, et al (Karadeniz Technical Univ, Trabzon, Turkey)
Thromb Res 126:486-492, 2010

Background.—Right ventricular dysfunction (RVD) detected by computerized tomography (CT)/echocardiography or elevated biomarkers is associated with a poor prognosis for pulmonary embolism (PE). However, these prognostic factors have not previously been concomitantly elucidated in the same patient group.

Methods.—This prospective study included 108 consecutive patients with normotensive PE confirmed by CT pulmonary angiography (CTPA). On admission, patient serum NT-proBNP and troponin T (Tn-T) levels were measured, and echocardiography was performed within 24 hours after diagnosis of PE. Receiver operating characteristic (ROC) analysis was performed to determine the optimal echocardiographic end-diastolic diameters of the right ventricle, the ratio of the right ventricle to left ventricle (RV/LV ratio) on CTPA, and NT-proBNP and Tn-T cut-off levels with regard to prognosis.

Results.—All-cause 30-day mortality was 13% and PE-related mortality was 5.6%. RVD was defined as a right/left ventricular dimension ratio ≥1.1 on CTPA and RV >30 mm on echocardiography by ROC analysis. A cut-off level of NT-proBNP ≤90 pmol/ml had a high positive predictive value of 98% for survival, whereas NT-proBNP >300 and Tn-T ≥0.027

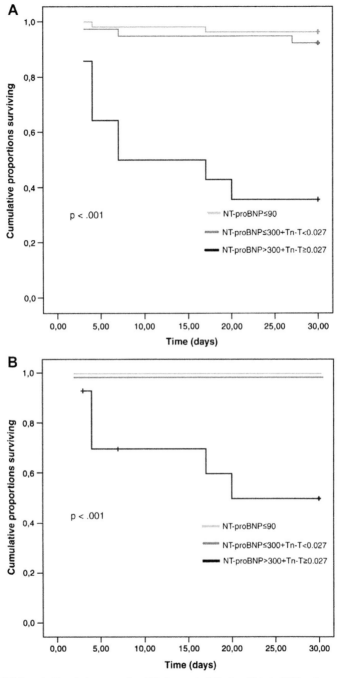

FIGURE 3.—a-b. Cumulative proportional 30-day survival (Kaplan–Meier) of 108 patients with APE, grouped according to the cut-off values: NT-proBNP >300 and TnT ≥0.027 (A) All-cause mortality and (B) PE-related mortality. (Reprinted from Ozsu S, Karaman K, Mentese A, et al. Combined risk stratification with computerized tomography /echocardiography and biomarkers in patients with normotensive pulmonary embolism. *Thromb Res*. 2010;126:486-492, with permission from Elsevier.)

had a negative predictive value, for all-cause deaths, of 95% and 96%, respectively. PE mortality in patients with NT-proBNP >300 and Tn-T ≥0.027 reached 64%. In univariable analysis, the combination of Tn-T ≥0.027 ng/ml with a echocardiographic RVD were the most significant predictors of overall mortality and PE-related death [HR: 14 (95% CI: 4.6–42,) and HR: 37.6 (95% CI: 4.4–324)], respectively. In multivariable Cox's regression analysis, NT-proBNP >300 and Tn-T ≥0.027 HR: 26.5 (95% CI: 4.1-169.9, p < 0.001) were the best combination to predict all-cause of mortality.

Conclusions.—The combination of NT-proBNP and Tn-T clearly appears to be a better risk stratification predictor than biomarkers plus RVD on CT/ echocardiography in patients with normotensive PE (Fig 3).

▶ I wanted to get you to think about a combined approach of risk assessment and treatment strategy for patients with submassive pulmonary embolism (PE) and stable hemodynamics. A number of parameters, including vital signs, blood markers, CT assessment, and echocardiographic assessments of right heart failure, have been proposed and evaluated in the literature. I believe that it is still open to interpretation. I would also strongly suggest paying close attention to the clinical scenario because not every patient is the same. In general, the use of saturation of < 92.5%, probrain natriuretic peptide (proBNP) of > 300pmol/mL, troponin-T (Tn-T) of > 0.027, CT evaluation of right ventricle/left ventricle of > 0.9, and signs of right ventricular dysfunction (RVD) on echo are substantially increasing the odds of death up to 26.5 times in the above study. The mortality is 60% in patients with Tn-T of ≥0.027 ng/mL and echocardiographic evidence of RVD. A *N*-terminal-proBNP (NT-proBNP) of < 90 pmol/mL confers a negative predictive value of 98% all-cause and 100% PE-related mortality. So the echo may not be needed in these cases. Three previous studies[1–3] show that the negative predictive value of low-level NT-proBNP for mortality range from 97% to 100%. I would suggest aggressive treatment in these patients with high risk even when they have normal hemodynamics.

M. Ali Raza, MD

References

1. British Thoracic Society Standards of Care Committee Pulmonary Embolism Guideline Development Group. British Thoracic Society guidelines for the management of suspected acute pulmonary embolism. *Thorax.* 2003;58:470-484.
2. Wells PS, Ginsberg JS, Anderson DR, et al. Use of a clinical model for safe management of patients with suspected pulmonary embolism. *Ann Intern Med.* 1998;129: 997-1005.
3. Torbicki A, Perrier A, Konstantinides S, et al. Guidelines on the diagnosis and management of acute pulmonary embolism. the Task Force for the Diagnosis and Management of Acute Pulmonary Embolism of the European Society of Cardiology (ESC). *Eur Heart J.* 2008;29:2276-2315.

Combinations of prognostic tools for identification of high-risk normotensive patients with acute symptomatic pulmonary embolism

Jiménez D, Aujesky D, Moores L, et al (Ramón y Cajal Hosp, Madrid, Spain; Univ of Lausanne, Switzerland; Uniformed Services Univ, Bethesda, MD; et al)
Thorax 66:75-81, 2011

Background.—In haemodynamically stable patients with acute symptomatic pulmonary embolism (PE), studies have not evaluated the usefulness of combining the measurement of cardiac troponin, transthoracic echocardiogram (TTE), and lower extremity complete compression ultrasound (CCUS) testing for predicting the risk of PE-related death.

Methods.—The study assessed the ability of three diagnostic tests (cardiac troponin I (cTnI), echocardiogram, and CCUS) to prognosticate the primary outcome of PE-related mortality during 30 days of follow-up after a diagnosis of PE by objective testing.

Results.—Of 591 normotensive patients diagnosed with PE, the primary outcome occurred in 37 patients (6.3%; 95% CI 4.3% to 8.2%). Patients with right ventricular dysfunction (RVD) by TTE and concomitant deep vein thrombosis (DVT) by CCUS had a PE-related mortality of 19.6%, compared with 17.1% of patients with elevated cTnI and concomitant DVT and 15.2% of patients with elevated cTnI and RVD. The use of any two-test strategy had a higher specificity and positive predictive value compared with the use of any test by itself. A combined three-test strategy did not further improve prognostication. For a subgroup analysis of high-risk patients, according to the pulmonary embolism severity index (classes IV and V), positive predictive values of the two-test strategies for PE-related mortality were 25.0%, 24.4% and 20.7%, respectively.

Conclusions.—In haemodynamically stable patients with acute symptomatic PE, a combination of echocardiography (or troponin testing) and CCUS improved prognostication compared with the use of any test by itself for the identification of those at high risk of PE-related death.

▶ I wanted you to think about a combined approach of risk assessment and treatment strategy for patients with submassive pulmonary embolism (PE) and stable hemodynamics. A number of parameters, including vital signs, blood markers, CT assessment, and echocardiographic assessments of right heart failure, have been proposed and evaluated in the literature. I believe that it is still open to interpretation. I would also strongly suggest paying close attention to the clinical scenario since not every patient is the same. In general, the use of saturation < 92.5%, pro-brain natriuretic peptide (proBNP) > 300 pmol/mL, troponin-T (Tn-T) > 0.027, CT evaluation of right ventricular (RV)/left ventricular > 0.9, and signs of RV dysfunction (RVD) on echo is substantially increasing the odds of death up to 26.5 times in the above study. The mortality is 60% in patients with Tn-T ≥0.027 ng/mL and echocardiographic evidence of RVD. A *N*-terminal proBNP (NT-proBNP) of < 90 pmol/mL confers a negative predictive value of 98% all-cause and 100% PE-related mortality. So the echo may not be needed in these cases. Three previous studies[1-3] show that the negative predictive value of low-level NT-proBNP for mortality ranges from 97% to 100%. I would suggest aggressive treatment in these patients with high risk even though they have normal hemodynamics.

M. Ali Raza, MD

References

1. British Thoracic Society Standards of Care Committee Pulmonary Embolism Guideline Development Group. British Thoracic Society guidelines for the management of suspected acute pulmonary embolism. *Thorax.* 2003;58:470-483.
2. Wells PS, Ginsberg JS, Anderson DR, et al. Use of a clinical model for safe management of patients with suspected pulmonary embolism. *Ann Intern Med.* 1998;129: 997-1005.
3. Torbicki A, Perrier A, Konstantinides S, et al. Guidelines on the diagnosis and management of acute pulmonary embolism. the Task Force for the Diagnosis and Management of Acute Pulmonary Embolism of the European Society of Cardiology (ESC). *Eur Heart J.* 2008;29:2276-2315.

Elevated Levels of Inflammatory Cytokines Predict Survival in Idiopathic and Familial Pulmonary Arterial Hypertension

Soon E, Holmes AM, Treacy CM, et al (Univ of Cambridge, UK; Novartis Insts for Biomedical Res, West Sussex, UK; Papworth Hosp, Cambridge, UK; et al)
Circulation 122:920-927, 2010

Background.—Inflammation is a feature of pulmonary arterial hypertension (PAH), and increased circulating levels of cytokines are reported in patients with PAH. However, to date, no information exists on the significance of elevated cytokines or their potential as biomarkers. We sought to determine the levels of a range of cytokines in PAH and to examine their impact on survival and relationship to hemodynamic indexes.

Methods and Results.—We measured levels of serum cytokines (tumor necrosis factor-α, interferon-γ and interleukin-1β, -2, -4, -5, -6, -8, -10, -12p70, and -13) using ELISAs in idiopathic and heritable PAH patients (n=60). Concurrent clinical data included hemodynamics, 6-minute walk distance, and survival time from sampling to death or transplantation. Healthy volunteers served as control subjects (n=21). PAH patients had significantly higher levels of interleukin-1β, -2, -4, -6, -8, -10, and -12p70 and tumor necrosis factor-α compared with healthy control subjects. Kaplan-Meier analysis showed that levels of interleukin-6, 8, 10, and 12p70 predicted survival in patients. For example, 5-year survival with interleukin-6 levels of >9 pg/mL was 30% compared with 63% for patients with levels $\leq$9 pg/mL (P=0.008). In this PAH cohort, cytokine levels were superior to traditional markers of prognosis such as 6-minute walk distance and hemodynamics.

Conclusions.—This study illustrates dysregulation of a broad range of inflammatory mediators in idiopathic and familial PAH and demonstrates that cytokine levels have a previously unrecognized impact on patient survival. They may prove to be useful biomarkers and provide insight into the contribution of inflammation in PAH.

▶ This study highlights the broad range of dysfunction in the inflammatory mediators in the idiopathic pulmonary arterial hypertension (PAH) and familial PAH. The strength of the study is the long 6 years follow-up, which showed, for example that interleukin-6 level of > 9 pg/mL was associated with significantly decreased 5-year survival of 30%. This is better than the 6-minute walk distance in predicting 5-year survival. There was a lack of correlation between levels of cytokines and hemodynamic parameters as measured by right heart catheterization. This may mean that cytokines are potentially involved in the pathogenesis of PAH and are not just due to right ventricular dysfunction.

M. Ali Raza, MD

Comparison of Brain Natriuretic Peptide (BNP) and NT-proBNP in Screening for Pulmonary Arterial Hypertension in Patients with Systemic Sclerosis
Cavagna L, Caporali R, Klersy C, et al (University and IRCCS Foundation Policlinico S. Matteo, Pavia, Italy)
J Rheumatol 37:2064-2070, 2010

Objective.—To compare the performance of brain natriuretic peptide (BNP) and N-terminal pro-brain natriuretic peptide (NT-proBNP) in screening for pulmonary arterial hypertension (PAH) in systemic sclerosis (SSc).

Methods.—Between January 2008 and March 2009, outpatients referred to our unit and satisfying LeRoy criteria for SSc were assessed for PAH. Doppler echocardiography, BNP measurement, and NT-proBNP measurement were done concomitantly for a complete clinical, instrumental, and biochemical evaluation. Right-heart catheterization was carried out in cases of suspected PAH [estimated pulmonary arterial pressure (PAP) ≥ 36 mm Hg; diffusion capacity for carbon monoxide (DLCO) ≤ 50% of predicted value; 1-year DLCO decline ≥ 20% in absence of pulmonary fibrosis; unexplained dyspnea].

Results.—One hundred thirty-five patients were enrolled (124 women, 11 men; 96 limited SSc, 39 diffuse SSc); precapillary PAH was found in 20 patients (15 limited SSc, 5 diffuse SSc). The estimated PAP correlated with both BNP (R = 0.3; 95% CI 0.14–0.44) and NT-proBNP (R = 0.3, 95% CI 0.14-0.45). BNP [area under the curve (AUC) 0.74, 95% CI 0.59–0.89] was slightly superior to NT-proBNP (AUC 0.63, 95% CI 0.46–0.80) in identification of PAH, with diagnosis cutoff values of 64 pg/ml (sensitivity 60%, specificity 87%) and 239.4 pg/ml (sensitivity 45%, specificity 90%), respectively. BNP (log-transformed, p = 0.032) and creatinine (p = 0.049) were independent predictors of PAH, while NT-proBNP was not (p = 0.50).

Conclusion.—In our single-center study, the performance of BNP was slightly superior to that of NT-proBNP in PAH screening of patients with SSc, although normal levels of these markers do not exclude diagnosis. We observed that impaired renal function is associated with an increased risk of PAH in SSc. Further multicenter studies are needed to confirm our results (ClinicalTrials.gov ID NCT00617487).

▶ Circulating natriuretic peptides (CNPs) have been found effective for the evaluation of patients with suspected pulmonary arterial hypertension (PAH); among CNPs, plasma *N*-terminal pro-brain natriuretic peptide (NT-proBNP) and BNP are the most commonly used markers, although in systemic sclerosis (SSc) only NT-proBNP has been tested. These 2 markers are also used in the evaluation of left heart failure, and in a recent meta-analysis, testing for BNP was found to be superior to NT-proBNP in this setting. This study is meant to compare the performance of BNP and NT-proBNP in the screening of PAH in a cohort of out-patients with SSc. The results showed that both BNP and NT-proBNP correlated linearly with estimated pulmonary arterial pressure.

Accounting for univariable results, a closer association between BNP levels and PAH was observed, while NT-proBNP values were not statistically associated with the final diagnosis of PAH, although a trend toward the association was found. The receiver-operating characteristic curve also confirmed that the performance of BNP is better than that of NT-proBNP in the diagnosis of PAH in this setting. Moreover, in multivariable analysis, only BNP could be regarded as an independent predictor of PAH. Almost all of the studies that I come across in patients with SSc are done with NT-proBNP. I wonder whether the BNP has better accuracy when chosen.

M. Ali Raza, MD

Incidence and risk factors for fatal pulmonary embolism after major trauma: a nested cohort study
Ho KM, Burrell M, Rao S, et al (Univ of Western Australia, Australia; Royal Perth Hosp, Australia; et al)
Br J Anaesth 105:596-602, 2010

Background.—Venous thromboembolism is common after major trauma. Strategies to prevent fatal pulmonary embolism (PE) are widely utilized, but the incidence and risk factors for fatal PE are poorly understood.

Methods.—Using linked data from the intensive care unit, trauma registry, Western Australian Death Registry, and post-mortem reports, the incidence and risk factors for fatal PE in a consecutive cohort of major trauma patients, admitted between 1994 and 2002, were assessed. Non-linear relationships between continuous predictors and risk of fatal PE were modelled by logistic regression.

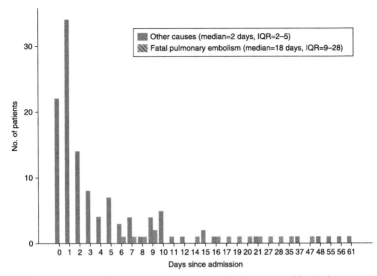

FIGURE 2.—The timing of fatal pulmonary embolism and other causes of death after major trauma. IQR, inter-quartile range. (Reprinted from Ho KM, Burrell M, Rao S, et al. Incidence and risk factors for fatal pulmonary embolism after major trauma: a nested cohort study. Br J Anaesth. 2010;105:596-602, by permission of The Board of Management and Trustees of the British Journal of Anaesthesia, Oxford University Press.)

Results.—Of the 971 consecutive trauma patients considered in the study, 134 (13.8%) died after their injuries. Fatal PE accounted for 11.9% of all deaths despite unfractionated heparin prophylaxis being used in 44% of these patients. Fatal PE occurred in those who were older (mean age 51- *vs* 37-yr-old, $P = 0.01$), with more co-morbidities (Charlson's co-morbidity index 1.1 *vs* 0.2, $P = 0.01$), had a larger BMI (31.8 vs 24.5, $P = 0.01$), and less severe head and systemic injuries when compared with those who died of other causes. Sites of injuries were not significantly related to the risk of fatal PE. Fatal PE occurred much later than deaths from other causes (median 18 *vs* 2 days, $P = 0.01$), and the estimated attributable mortality of PE was 49% (95% confidence interval 36-62%).

Conclusions.—Fatal PE appeared to be a potential preventable cause of late mortality after major trauma. Severity of injuries, co-morbidity, and BMI were important risk factors for fatal PE after major trauma (Fig 2).

▶ I included this study to press the fact that most patients with major trauma are faced with a dilemma for when to start anticoagulation and/or to think of inferior vena cava (IVC) filter. The new trauma guidelines suggest the early use of IVC in certain patients, but the interesting point made in this study is that a pulmonary embolism is usually seen late in the course (18 days); it has occurred even in patients with heparin prophylaxis. Obesity and age are significant risk factors. High mortality of up to 45% is associated with it. I personally would be extra cautious toward all patients with major trauma and would begin doing prophylaxis, scanning their legs more frequently, and placing IVC filters in older patients who are obese.

M. Ali Raza, MD

Clinical Outcomes of Pulmonary Arterial Hypertension in Patients Carrying an *ACVRL1* (*ALK1*) Mutation
Girerd B, Montani D, Coulet F, et al (Université Paris-Sud, Kremlin Bicêtre, Clamart, France; Université Pierre et Marie Curie-Paris 6, France; et al)
Am J Respir Crit Care Med 181:851-861, 2010

Rationale.—Activin A receptor type II-like kinase-1 (*ACVRL1*, also known as *ALK1*) mutation is a cause of hereditary hemorrhagic telangiectasia (HHT) and/or heritable pulmonary arterial hypertension (PAH).

Objectives.—To describe the characteristics of patients with PAH carrying an *ACVRL1* mutation.

Methods.—We reviewed clinical, functional, and hemodynamic characteristics of 32 patients with PAH carrying an *ACVRL1* mutation, corresponding to 9 patients from the French PAH Network and 23 from literature analysis. These cases were compared with 370 patients from the French PAH Network (93 with a bone morphogenetic protein receptor type 2 [*BMPR2*] mutation and 277 considered as idiopathic cases without identified mutation). Distribution of mutations in the *ACVRL1* gene in patients with PAH was compared with the HHT Mutation Database.

Measurements and Main Results.—At diagnosis, *ACVRL1* mutation carriers were significantly younger (21.8 ± 16.7 yr) than *BMPR2* mutation carriers and noncarriers (35.7 ± 14.9 and 47.6 ± 16.3 yr, respectively; $P < 0.0001$). In seven of the nine patients from the French PAH Network, PAH diagnosis preceded manifestations of HHT. *ACVRL1* mutation carriers had better hemodynamic status at diagnosis, but none responded to acute vasodilator challenge and they had shorter survival when compared with other patients with PAH despite similar use of specific therapies. *ACVRL1* mutations in exon 10 were more frequently observed in patients with PAH, as compared with what was observed in the HHT Mutation Database (33.3 vs. 5%; $P < 0.0001$).

Conclusions.—*ACVRL1* mutation carriers were characterized by a younger age at PAH diagnosis. Despite less severe initial hemodynamics and similar management, these patients had worse prognosis compared with other patients with PAH, suggesting more rapid disease progression.

▶ Several genes have been implicated in the pathogenesis of hereditary hemorrhagic telangiectasia (HHT), including activin receptor-like kinase-1 (*ACVRL1* or *ALK1*) located on chromosome 12. *ACVRL1* has been implicated in producing pulmonary arterial hypertension (PAH). In this series, it is shown that *ACVRL1* mutation carriers may develop severe PAH without any clinical evidence of HHT. The distribution and frequency of mutations in the *ACVRL1* gene is different in PAH than in HHT. The important point to highlight this subgroup is the high mortality in this cohort much closer to connective tissue disease-PAH than familial PAH. This may be another variable to keep in mind when treating severely progressive PAH patients.

M. Ali Raza, MD

Adrenergic Receptor Blockade Reverses Right Heart Remodeling and Dysfunction in Pulmonary Hypertensive Rats

Bogaard HJ, Natarajan R, Mizuno S, et al (Virginia Commonwealth Univ, Richmond; et al)
Am J Respir Crit Care Med 182:652-660, 2010

Rationale.—Most patients with pulmonary arterial hypertension (PAH) die from right heart failure. β-Adrenergic receptor blockade reduces mortality by about 30% in patients with left-sided systolic heart failure, but is not used in PAH.

Objectives.—To assess the effect of the adrenergic receptor blocker carvedilol on the pulmonary circulation and right heart in experimental pulmonary hypertension in rats.

Methods.—Angioproliferative pulmonary hypertension was induced in rats by combined exposure to the vascular endothelial growth factor–receptor antagonist SU5416 and hypoxia. Carvedilol treatment was started after establishment of pulmonary hypertension and right heart dysfunction.

Measurements and Main Results.—Compared with vehicle-treated animals, treatment with carvedilol resulted in increased exercise endurance; improved right ventricular (RV) function (increased tricuspid annular plane systolic excursion and decreased RV dilatation); and an increased cardiac output. The morphology of the pulmonary vessels and the RV afterload were not affected by carvedilol. Carvedilol treatment was associated with enhancement of RV fetal gene reactivation, increased protein kinase G (PKG) activity, and a reduction in capillary rarefaction and fibrosis. Metoprolol had similar but less pronounced effects in the SU5416 and hypoxia model. Cardioprotective effects were noted of both carvedilol and metoprolol in the monocrotaline model. In the case of carvedilol, but not metoprolol, part of these effects resulted from a prevention of monocrotaline-induced lung remodeling.

Conclusions.—Adrenergic receptor blockade reverses RV remodeling and improves RV function in experimental pulmonary hypertension. β-Adrenergic receptor blockers are not recommended in humans with PAH before their safety and efficacy are assessed in well-designed clinical trials (Fig 1).

▶ This is an interesting study showing significant benefit of carvedilol and not metoprolol in improving right ventricular (RV) function and reducing RV hypertrophy

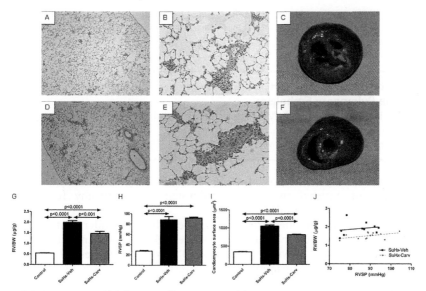

FIGURE 1.—Carvedilol does not affect SU5416 and hypoxia (SuHx)–induced angioproliferative pulmonary vascular remodeling. (A) Vehicle treated, SuHx-Veh and (D) carvedilol treated, SuHx-Carv are lower (25×) magnifications of SuHx lungs, whereas (B) SuHx-Veh and (E) SuHx-Carv show closeups (100× magnifications) of vasoobliterative lesions, which are not found in normal lungs. (H) Right ventricular systolic pressure (RVSP) is not different between SuHx-Veh and SuHx-Carv animals. However, carvedilol treatment is associated with less RV hypertrophy: macroscopically (compare [C], SuHx-Veh with [F], SuHx-Carv) expressed as (G) RV weight per body weight and expressed as (I) cardiomyocyte surface area on hematoxylin-eosin stains. (Reprinted from Bogaard HJ, Natarajan R, Mizuno S, et al. Adrenergic receptor blockade reverses right heart remodeling and dysfunction in pulmonary hypertensive rats. *Am J Respir Crit Care Med*. 2010;182:652-660, Official Journal of the American Thoracic Society © American Thoracic Society.)

despite the persistence of a high RV afterload in experimental rat model. Carvedilol treatment also prevents myocardial cell death, fibrosis, and capillary rarefaction. The general consensus formed in the pulmonary arterial hypertension–treating community[1,2] is to not use β-blockers for their detrimental effects on decreasing cardiac output by mainly decreasing heart rate. This notion comes from studies performed on patients treated with metoprolol as the main β-blocker and some with propranolol. It will be interesting to see how the use of carvedilol pans out in humans since the medication will decrease heart rate a lot more than it does in mice and may lose its other anti-inflammatory benefits to decreased cardiac output.

M. Ali Raza, MD

References

1. McLaughlin VV, Archer SL, Badesch DB, et al. ACCF/AHA 2009 expert consensus document on pulmonary hypertension a report of the American College of Cardiology Foundation Task Force on Expert Consensus Documents and the American Heart Association developed in collaboration with the American College of Chest Physicians; American Thoracic Society, Inc.; and the Pulmonary Hypertension Association. *J Am Coll Cardiol*. 2009;53:1573-1619.

2. Velez-Roa S, Ciarka A, Najem B, Vachiery JL, Naeije R, van de Borne P. Increased sympathetic nerve activity in pulmonary artery hypertension. *Circulation*. 2004; 110:1308-1312.

Early and Late Clinical Outcomes of Pulmonary Embolectomy for Acute Massive Pulmonary Embolism

Vohra HA, Whistance RN, Mattam K, et al (Southampton Univ Hosps NHS Trust, UK)
Ann Thorac Surg 90:1747-1752, 2010

Background.—The aim of this study was to investigate the early and late outcomes of patients undergoing pulmonary embolectomy for acute massive pulmonary embolus.

Methods.—Twenty-one patients (15 male, 6 female) underwent pulmonary embolectomy at our institution between March 2001 and July 2010. The median age was 55 years (range, 24 to 70 years). Of these, 9 patients presented with out-of-hospital cardiac arrest and 8 presented with New York Heart Association class III or IV. Sixteen patients underwent preoperative transthoracic echocardiography, which showed evidence of right ventricular dilatation in all, whereas in 14 patients (66.6%) pulmonary artery pressures were significantly elevated with moderate to severe tricuspid regurgitation. The median preoperative Euroscore was 9 (range, 3 to 16), and 11 patients (52.1%) received systemic thrombolysis preoperatively. There were 6 salvage (28.5%), 10 emergency (47.6%), and 5 urgent (23.8%) procedures. Concomitant procedures were performed in 3 patients (14.2%), and surgery was performed without the use of cardiopulmonary bypass in 3 patients (14.2%). The median follow-up was 38 months (range, 0 to 114 months).

Results.—The in-hospital mortality was 19% (n = 4). Postoperative complications included stroke (n = 3, 14.2%), lower respiratory tract infection (n = 6, 28.5%), wound infection (n = 3, 14.2%), acute renal failure requiring hemofiltration (n = 4, 19%), and supraventricular tachyarrhythmias (n = 4, 19%). At discharge, transthoracic echocardiography showed mild to moderate right ventricular dysfunction and dilatation in 11 survivors (64.7%). Two patients died during follow-up, and actuarial survival at 5 years was 76.9% ± 10.1% and at 8 years was 51.2% ± 22.0%. At final follow-up, 11 of the 15 survivors (73.3%) were New York Heart Association class I, and no patients required further intervention.

Conclusions.—Patients who undergo surgery for massive pulmonary embolism have an acceptable outcome despite being high-risk.

▶ I am including this article to show that except for 1 or 2 large centers, who have exceptionally low rates of morbidity and mortality associated with thromboendarterectomy, there is at least 20% mortality associated with this procedure in major centers. This may also be related to low number of cases done and only taking cases who are in impending arrest. This treatment is still much better than thrombolytics used for patients with unstable pulmonary embolism, which is close to 40%. There is another approach that minimizes the mortality to even lower 6%, showed by Leacche et al,[1,2] where they take all patients with large central clot burden and impending right ventricular failure for operation.

M. Ali Raza, MD

References

1. Leacche M, Unic D, Goldhabe SZ, et al. Modern surgical treatment of massive pulmonary embolism: results of 47 consecutive patients after rapid diagnosis and aggressive surgical approach. *J Thorac Cardiovasc Surg.* 2005;129: 1018-1023.
2. Kadner A, Schmidli J, Schönhoff F, et al. Excellent outcome after surgical treatment of massive pulmonary embolism in critically ill patients. *J Thorac Cardiovasc Surg.* 2008;136:448-451.

Characterization of Connective Tissue Disease-Associated Pulmonary Arterial Hypertension From REVEAL: Identifying Systemic Sclerosis as a Unique Phenotype
Chung L, Liu J, Parsons L, et al (Stanford Univ, CA; ICON Clinical Res, San Francisco, CA; et al)
Chest 138:1383-1394, 2010

Background.—REVEAL (the Registry to Evaluate Early and Long-term Pulmonary Arterial Hypertension Disease Management) is the largest US cohort of patients with pulmonary arterial hypertension (PAH) confirmed by right-sided heart catheterization (RHC), providing a more comprehensive subgroup characterization than previously possible. We used REVEAL to analyze the clinical features of patients with connective tissue disease-associated PAH (CTD-APAH).

Methods.—All newly and previously diagnosed patients with World Health Organization (WHO) group 1 PAH meeting RHC criteria at 54 US centers were consecutively enrolled. Cross-sectional and 1-year mortality and hospitalization analyses from time of enrollment compared CTD-APAH to idiopathic disease and systemic sclerosis (SSc) to systemic lupus erythematosus (SLE), mixed connective tissue disease (MCTD), and rheumatoid arthritis (RA).

Results.—Compared with patients with idiopathic disease (n = 1,251), patients with CTD-APAH (n = 641) had better hemodynamics and favorable right ventricular echocardiographic findings but a higher prevalence of pericardial effusions, lower 6-min walk distance (300.5 ± 118.0 vs 329.4 ± 134.7 m, $P = .01$), higher B-type natriuretic peptide (BNP) levels (432.8 ± 789.1 vs 245.6 ± 427.2 pg/mL, $P < .0001$), and lower diffusing capacity of carbon monoxide (D_{LCO}) (44.9% ± 18.0% vs 63.6% ± 22.1% predicted, $P < .0001$). One-year survival and freedom from hospitalization were lower in the CTD-APAH group (86% vs 93%, $P < .0001$;

67% vs 73%, $P = .03$). Compared with patients with SSc-APAH (n = 399), those with other CTDs (SLE, n = 110; MCTD, n = 52; RA, n = 28) had similar hemodynamics; however, patients with SSc-APAH had the highest BNP levels (552.2 ± 977.8 pg/mL), lowest D_{LCO} (41.2% ± 16.3% predicted), and poorest 1-year survival (82% vs 94% in SLE-APAH, 88% in MCTD-APAH, and 96% in RA-APAH).

Conclusions.—Patients with SSc-APAH demonstrate a unique phenotype with the highest BNP levels, lowest D_{LCO}, and poorest survival of all CTD-APAH subgroups.

Trial Registry.—ClinicalTrials.gov; No.: NCT00370214; URL: clinicaltrials.gov.

▶ The Registry to Evaluate Early and Long-term PAH Disease Management is a multicenter (54 centers), observational, US-based registry that includes information about current demographics and treatment practices for patients with pulmonary arterial hypertension (PAH). Historically, patients with connective tissue disease–associated PAH (CTD-APAH) have been characterized as having the most severe disease with the highest mortality rates of all PAH subgroups. It is proven in the aforementioned study, which found that patients with systemic sclerosis (SSc)-APAH have a unique phenotype characterized by markedly elevated B-type natriuretic peptide (BNP) levels, reduced diffusing capacity of carbon monoxide (D_{LCO}), and poor short-term survival rates. The CTD-PAH have better hemodynamics but with poor 6-minute walk and prognosis. There are many hypotheses why this discrepancy is present. Langleben et al[1] have shown that patients with CTD-APAH have significantly reduced endothelial metabolic function. Moreover, for a given cardiac index, patients with CTD-APAH have a lower functional capillary surface area than an idiopathic PAH (IPAH) cohort, which is directly correlated with the degree of D_{LCO} reduction. The low D_{LCO} in patients with CTD-APAH reflects diminishing vascular area with reduced metabolic activity. The other possibility is the use of less aggressive therapy since the chance of adverse effects are perceived more in these patients than IPAH—such as diminished fine motor dexterity, prohibiting them from injecting themselves with the drugs and less proper handling of them. This trend is not surely seen in the registry data by the way. The inconsistent use of the best immunosupression may also be a possibility. The reason for higher BNP in patients with scleroderma may be related to the fact that they have been shown to have myocardial fibrosis[2] and inflammation. Short-term survival was significantly worse in patients with SSc-APAH than those with systemic lupus erythematosus-APAH and rheumatoid arthritis-APAH, with 1-year survival rates of 82% versus 94% and 96%, respectively.

M. Ali Raza, MD

References

1. Langleben D, Orfanos SE, Giovinazzo M, et al. Pulmonary capillary endothelial metabolic dysfunction: severity in pulmonary arterial hypertension related to connective tissue disease versus idiopathic pulmonary arterial hypertension. *Arthritis Rheum.* 2008;58:1156-1164.

2. Tzelepis GE, Kelekis NL, Plastiras SC, et al. Pattern and distribution of myocardial fibrosis in systemic sclerosis: a delayed enhanced magnetic resonance imaging study. *Arthritis Rheum.* 2007;56:3827-3836.

Exercise-Induced Pulmonary Hypertension Associated With Systemic Sclerosis: Four Distinct Entities

Saggar R, Khanna D, Furst DE, et al (David Geffen School of Medicine at Univ of California, Los Angeles; et al)
Arthritis Rheum 62:3741-3750, 2010

Objective.—Exercise-induced pulmonary hypertension (PH) may represent an early but clinically relevant phase in the spectrum of pulmonary vascular disease. There are limited data on the prevalence of exercise-induced PH determined by right heart catheterization in scleroderma spectrum disorders. We undertook this study to describe the hemodynamic response to exercise in a homogeneous population of patients with scleroderma spectrum disorders at risk of developing pulmonary vascular disease.

Methods.—Patients with normal resting hemodynamics underwent supine lower extremity exercise testing. A classification and regression tree (CART) analysis was used to assess combinations of variables collected during resting right heart catheterization that best predicted abnormal exercise physiology, applicable to each individual subject.

Results.—Fifty-seven patients who had normal resting hemodynamics underwent subsequent exercise right heart catheterization. Four distinct hemodynamic groups were identified during exercise: a normal group, an exercise-induced pulmonary venous hypertension (ePVH) group, an exercise out of proportion PH (eoPH) group, and an exercise-induced PH (ePH) group. The eoPH and ePVH groups had higher pulmonary capillary wedge pressure (PCWP) than the ePH group ($P < 0.05$). The normal and ePH groups had exercise PCWP ≤ 18 mm Hg, which was lower than that in the ePVH and eoPH groups ($P < 0.05$). During submaximal exercise, the transpulmonary gradient and pulmonary vascular resistance (PVR) were elevated in the ePH and eoPH groups as compared with the normal and ePVH groups ($P < 0.05$). CART analysis suggested that resting mean pulmonary artery pressure (mPAP) ≥ 14 mm Hg and PVR ≥ 160 dynes/seconds/cm^{-5} were associated with eoPH and ePH (positive predictive value 89% for mPAP 14-20 mm Hg and 100% for mPAP >20 mm Hg).

Conclusion.—We characterized the exercise hemodynamic response in at-risk patients with scleroderma spectrum disorders who did not have resting PH. Four distinct hemodynamic groups were identified during exercise. These groups may have potentially different prognoses and treatment options (Fig 2).

▶ This study is pushing the normal assessment tools and treatment strategies for at-risk patients because we know that we have to eradicate more than 70% of

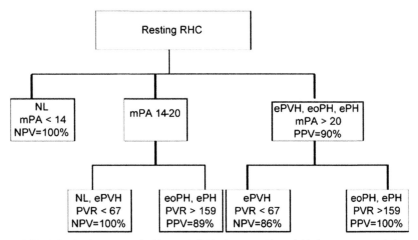

FIGURE 2.—Decision tree applicable to an individual patient with available data on resting right heart catheterization (RHC) hemodynamics. The baseline mean pulmonary artery pressure (mPA; in mm Hg) is the primary mode. PVR values are in dynes/seconds/cm^{-5}. NPV = negative predictive value; PPV = positive predictive value (see Figure 1 for other definitions). (Reprinted from Saggar R, Khanna D, Furst DE, et al. Exercise-induced pulmonary hypertension associated with systemic sclerosis: four distinct entities. *Arthritis Rheum.* 2010;62:3741-3750, with permission from American College of Rheumatology.)

the pulmonary vasculature to start treatment and appropriate life-prolonging therapy.

The authors' hypothesis is that patients with normal exercise physiology and exercise-induced pulmonary venous hypertension (ePVH) have a different pathophysiology from those with exercise-induced pulmonary hypertension (ePH) and exercise out of proportion pulmonary hypertension (eoPH). They have a decision model that shows that a resting mean pulmonary artery pressure (mPAP) of 14 mm Hg excludes ePH and eoPH (negative predictive value [NPV], 100%). While a resting mPAP > 20 mm Hg had a positive predictive value (PPV) of 90% for abnormal physiology (ePH, eoPH, or ePVH), a concurrent pulmonary vascular resistance (PVR) ≥160 dynes/seconds/cm^{-5} had a PPV of 100%. Similarly, for patients with mPAP 14-20 mm Hg (inclusive), PVR < 67 dynes/seconds/cm^{-5} had an NPV of 100% and PVR ≥160 dynes/seconds/cm^{-5} had a PPV of 89% for predicting ePH and eoPH.

Collectively, these studies suggest an abnormal phenotype in at-risk populations after assessing the response of the pulmonary vasculature to exercise. Limitations aside from being a single-center study with a low number of subjects, this gives us a tool to predict and treat at-risk patients aggressively since their natural history is very strongly predicting the pulmonary arterial hypertension.

M. Ali Raza, MD

Venous Thromboembolism with Chronic Liver Disease

Saleh T, Matta F, Alali F, et al (St Joseph Mercy Oakland Hosp, Pontiac, MI; Michigan State Univ, East Lansing)
Am J Med 124:64-68, 2011

Background.—Patients with chronic liver disease have both antithrombotic and prothrombotic coagulation abnormalities. Published data conflict on whether patients with chronic liver disease have a high or low prevalence of venous thromboembolism.

Methods.—The number of patients discharged from hospitals throughout the US with a diagnostic code for chronic alcoholic and chronic nonalcoholic liver disease from 1979 through 2006 was obtained from the National Hospital Discharge Survey. We compared prevalences of venous thromboembolism among patients with chronic alcoholic liver disease and chronic nonalcoholic liver disease.

Results.—Among 4,927,000 hospitalized patients with chronic alcoholic liver disease from 1979-2006, the prevalence of venous thromboembolism was 0.6%, compared with 0.9% among 4,565,000 hospitalized patients with chronic nonalcoholic liver disease.

Conclusion.—The prevalence of venous thromboembolism in hospitalized patients with chronic liver disease, both alcoholic and nonalcoholic, was low. The prevalence of venous thromboembolism was higher in those with chronic non-alcoholic liver disease, but the difference was small and of no clinical consequence. Based on the literature, both showed a lower prevalence of venous thromboembolism than in hospitalized patients with most other medical diseases. It may be that both chronic alcoholic liver disease and chronic nonalcoholic liver disease have protective antithrombotic mechanisms, although the mechanisms differ (Table 3).

▶ It is always a question of whether to do venous thromboembolism (VTE) prophylaxis for patients with chronic liver disease or not because they are mostly autoanticoagulated.[1] The above study is a big step in alleviating the concern because it agrees with the previous work done on the incidence of pulmonary embolism (PE)/deep venous thrombosis (DVT) in liver cirrhosis. The risk of PE is 0.1% to 0.3% and DVT is 0.5% to 0.6% in the cohort of all patients with chronic liver disease. In our center, we consider it simply by looking at the prothrombin time and international normalized ratio (INR) of the patients with chronic liver disease, and if the INR is more than 2, then we don't give DVT prophylaxis. Prophylaxis is recommended for an INR less than 1.5, and an INR between 1.5 and 2.0 is even more tricky. To date, I don't see a study approving this approach but it makes sense and we have not had a major problem so far. Please remember that it is anecdotal rather than evidence.

The strength of the investigation is the large number of patients identified with alcoholic liver disease and VTE (30 000 patients) and nonalcoholic liver disease[2] with VTE (42 000 patients).

TABLE 3.—Prevalence of Deep Venous Thrombosis and Venous Thromboembolism in Selected Medical Illnesses

Medical Illness	Prevalence of DVT (%)	Prevalence of VTE (%)	Age Group	Reference (First Author)
Non-alcoholic liver disease	0.6	0.9	≥18 years	Present study
Alcoholic liver disease	0.5	0.6	≥18 years	Present study
Cancer of pancreas	3.9	5.1	All ages	Stein[20]
Cancer of brain	3.7	4.9	All ages	Stein[20]
Myeloproliferative, lymphatic/ hematopoietic	3.0	3.4	All ages	Stein[20]
Cancer of stomach	2.2	2.6	All ages	Stein[20]
Obesity	2.0	–	All ages	Stein[21]
Cancer of prostate	1.7	2.2	All ages	Stein[20]
Rheumatoid arthritis	1.6	2.3	All ages	Matta[22]
Cancer of colon	1.5	2.1	All ages	Stein[20]
Ulcerative colitis	1.5	1.9	All ages	Saleh[23]
Nephrotic syndrome	1.5	–	>1 month	Kayali[24]
Hemorrhagic stroke	1.4	1.9	All ages	Skaf[25]
Hypothyroidism	1.4	1.8	All ages	Danescu[26]
Human immunodeficiency virus	1.4	1.7	≥18 years	Matta[27]
Heart failure	1.0	1.6	All ages	Beemath[28]
Crohn disease	1.1	1.2	All ages	Saleh[23]
COPD	1.1	1.6	>20 years	Stein[29]
Diabetes mellitus	1.0	1.4	All ages	Stein[30]
Ischemic stroke	0.7	1.2	All ages	Skaf[25]
Sickle cell disease	0.6	–	All ages	Stein[31]

COPD = chronic obstructive pulmonary disease; DVT = deep venous thrombosis; VTE = venous thromboembolism. *Editor's Note*: Please refer to original journal article for full references.

Diversity of the population ranges in terms of age, race, sex, and geographic regions (all 50 states and the District of Columbia), and the extensive duration of observation (28 years).

Limitations include lack of data on the severity of the liver disease, the proportion with ascites, hepatic decompensation, reason for hospitalization, proportion of patients hospitalized more than once, and the basis for the diagnosis of liver disease.

M. Ali Raza, MD

References

1. Northup PG, McMahon MM, Ruhl AP, et al. Coagulopathy does not fully protect hospitalized cirrhosis patients from peripheral venous thromboembolism. *Am J Gastroenterol.* 2006;101:1524-1528.
2. García-Fuster MJ, Abdilla N, Fabiá MJ, Fernández C, Oliver V, Forner MJ. [Venous thromboembolism and liver cirrhosis]. *Rev Esp Enferm Dig.* 2008;100: 259-262.

Effect of Balloon Inflation Volume on Pulmonary Artery Occlusion Pressure in Patients With and Without Pulmonary Hypertension

Tonelli AR, Mubarak KK, Li N, et al (Univ of Florida, Gainesville)
Chest 139:115-121, 2011

Background.—Pulmonary artery occlusion pressure (PAOP) is used to differentiate patients with pulmonary hypertension (PH) associated with left-sided heart disease from other etiologies. Technical errors in the measurement of PAOP are common and lead to incorrect classification of the etiology of PH. We investigated the agreement among PAOP measurements obtained from both pulmonary arteries with balloon full (1.5 mL) and half (0.75 mL) inflation in patients undergoing right-sided heart catheterization for suspected PH.

Methods.—Thirty-seven patients suspected or known to have PH who underwent right-sided heart catheterization were included. Seventy-six percent had PH (mean pulmonary arterial pressure >25 mm Hg). The validity of the measurements was assessed by using five preestablished criteria based on hemodynamic, fluoroscopic, and gasometric data. For each patient, the measurement that most likely represented the left atrial pressure was labeled "best PAOP."

Results.—Seventy percent of all the PAOP measurements met at least four of the five preestablished criteria for validity. In patients with PH (n = 28), the mean ± SE PAOP was 23.1 ± 2 and 19.1 ± 2 mm Hg for balloon full and half inflation, respectively, in the right pulmonary artery and 23.54 ± 2 and 19.07 ± 2 mm Hg for balloon full and half inflation, respectively, in the left pulmonary artery ($P = .05$). Bland-Altman analysis revealed lower bias and narrower limits of agreement with balloon half inflation. Wedge angiography showed that some balloon inflations failed to occlude upstream flow, whereas others had collateral vessels draining after the occlusion.

Conclusions.—PAOP can be falsely elevated in patients with PH according to the balloon inflation volume. Balloon half inflation was safe and correlated with higher precision and lower bias in the PAOP measurements.

▶ This study hypothesized that the difficulty in the measurement of pulmonary artery occlusion pressure (PAOP) in the patients with pulmonary arterial hypertension (PAH) is because of the distortion of the proximal pulmonary vasculature, which prevents complete occlusion of the vessels by the pulmonary artery catheter (PAC) balloon. In certain cases,[1] therefore, it might be possible to overcome this anatomic difficulty by reducing the volume of air injected in the PAC balloon, allowing an occlusion of a more distal and less-distorted vessel.

The finding itself is not new because Swan et al[2] has showed in his study that lower balloon volumes 0.8 mL is shown to increase the likelihood of measuring PAOP up to 72%. The important point is that in PAH, the occlusion pressure calculation is harder by many folds and the reliability matters the most.

The authors have also identified that less volume also meets with some problems like no flow from the distal end of the catheter and some times low saturation from the distal port. So no method is 100% accurate in all instances but using the following helped.

First, obtain a PAOP measurement in the right pulmonary artery (PA) with balloon inflation of 1.5 mL and, if not reliable, use an inflation of 0.75 mL. If the PAOP measurement does not meet at least 4 of the 5 criteria, advance the PAC to the left PA using a balloon inflation of 1.5 mL and, if necessary, 0.75 mL. In their hands, this sequential approach improved the yield of obtaining a reliable PAOP measurement from 73% to 84% and 95% to 100%, respectively. In patients without PAH, there were no major discrepancies and the normal method was working.[3]

M. Ali Raza, MD

References

1. Leatherman JW, Shapiro RS. Overestimation of pulmonary artery occlusion pressure in pulmonary hypertension due to partial occlusion. *Crit Care Med.* 2003;31: 93-97.
2. Swan HJ, Ganz W, Forrester J, Marcus H, Diamond G, Chonette D. Catheterization of the heart in man with use of a flow-directed balloon-tipped catheter. *N Engl J Med.* 1970;283:447-451.
3. Morris AH, Chapman RH, Gardner RM. Frequency of wedge pressure errors in the ICU. *Crit Care Med.* 1985;13:705-708.

Miscellaneous

Efficacy of Prophylactic Placement of Inferior *Vena Cava* Filter in Patients Undergoing Spinal Surgery

Ozturk C, Ganiyusufoglu K, Alanay A, et al (Florence Nightingale Hosp, Istanbul, Turkey)
Spine 35:1893-1896, 2010

Study Design.—Retrospective case series.

Objective.—To evaluate the safety and efficacy of prophylactic inferior *vena cava* filter (IVCF) to prevent pulmonary embolism (PE) in high risk patients undergoing major complex spinal surgery.

Summary of Background Data.—PE has been reported to be the major cause of death after spinal reconstructive surgery. Mechanical prophylaxis alone is often not sufficient whereas anticoagulation therapy carries a significant risk of bleeding complications. Prophylactic IVCF placement is advocated in high-risk patients.

Methods.—A total of 129 high-risk patients undergoing complex spine surgery, having prophylactic IVCF were compared to a matched cohort of age, diagnosis, and risk factors of 193 patients for whom only mechanical prophylaxis was used. Patients were observed for potential complications related to the IVCF and also for clinical signs and symptoms of PE.

Results.—Eight cases (4.2%) of symptomatic PE were detected in the matched cohort control group (5 cases having combined anterior + posterior surgery and 3 patients having only posterior surgery). One of them died due to massive PE (0.5%). Symptomatic PE was detected in only 2 patients (1.5%), having combined anterior + posterior surgery due to lumbar spinal stenosis in IVCF group who responded well to medical treatment (*P* < 0.05). No complications were associated with filter insertion.

Conclusion.—Prophylactic IVCF is effective and safe in prevention of pulmonary embolism in patients with risk factors for PE.

▶ As the inferior vena cava filters are evolving to be safer and easily retrievable, it makes sense to use them in patients with high risk of deep vein thrombosis and pulmonary embolism (PE) to limit the morbidity and mortality. In this study, the authors show a small but significant decline in death and symptomatic PE by using retrievable filter in patients who underwent spine surgery.

M. Ali Raza, MD

Improving Inferior Vena Cava Filter Retrieval Rates: Impact of a Dedicated Inferior Vena Cava Filter Clinic

Minocha J, Idakoji I, Riaz A, et al (Northwestern Univ, Chicago, IL)
J Vasc Interv Radiol 21:1847-1851, 2010

Purpose.—To test the hypothesis that an inferior vena cava (IVC) filter clinic increases the retrieval rate of optional IVC filters.

Materials and Methods.—Patients who had optional IVC filters placed at the authors' institution between January 2000 and December 2008 were identified and retrospectively studied. A dedicated IVC filter clinic was established at this institution in January 2009, and there is a comprehensive database of prospectively acquired data for patients seen in the IVC filter clinic. Patients were chronologically classified into preclinic and postclinic groups. The number of optional filters retrieved and failed retrieval attempts were recorded.

Results.—In the preclinic and postclinic periods, 369 and 100 optional IVC filters were placed. Median (interquartile range) number of optional filters placed per month for preclinic and postclinic periods was 3 (range 2–5) and 10 (range 6.5–10.5) (*P* < .001). Retrieval rates in preclinic and postclinic periods were 108 of 369 (29%) and 60 of 100 (60%) (*P* < .001). The median time to filter retrieval in the postclinic group was 1.5 months (95% confidence interval 1.2–1.8). The number of failed retrieval attempts in preclinic and postclinic periods was 23 of 369 (6%) and 5 of 100 (5%) (*P* = .823).

Conclusions.—The retrieval rate of optional IVC filters at this institution was significantly increased by the establishment of a dedicated IVC filter clinic. This retrieval increase is not related to a decrease in technical failures but more likely relates to more meticulous patient management and clinical follow-up.

▶ Inferior vena cava filter placement is indicated by trauma guidelines for patients with increased risk of deep venous thrombosis (DVT) during ineligibility for anticoagulation. It is also a rising trend in our medical patients who have significantly high potential of bleeding if anticoagulated or have a DVT with massive pulmonary embolism in acute setting. More important than putting these filters in is their removal when the underlying problem is resolved because it increases the chance of chronic edema, persistent DVT, and morbidity. Historically, the retrieval rate of these so-called retrievable filters is very low. The largest study so far by the American Association for the Surgery of Trauma multicenter trial[1] reported that only 22% of these filters were removed. In medical patients, the rates are even lower. The above study is important because it shows that with formal follow-up and protocol, we can increase the retrieval rate by > 50%.[2]

M. Ali Raza, MD

References

1. Karmy-Jones R, Jurkovich GJ, Velmahos GC, et al. Practice patterns and outcomes of retrievable vena cava filters in trauma patients: an AAST multicenter study. *J Trauma.* 2007;62:17-24.
2. Ray CE Jr, Mitchell E, Zipser S, Kao EY, Brown CF, Moneta GL. Outcomes with retrievable inferior vena cava filters: a multicenter study. *J Vasc Interv Radiol.* 2006;17:1595-1604.

A Policy of Dedicated Follow-Up Improves the Rate of Removal of Retrievable Inferior Vena Cava Filters in Trauma Patients

O'Keeffe T, Thekkumel JJ, Friese S, et al (Univ of Arizona College of Medicine, Tucson; et al)
Am Surg 77:103-108, 2011

Retrievable Inferior Vena Cava Filters (IVCF) for prophylaxis against pulmonary embolus have been associated with low rates of removal. Strategies for improving the rates of retrieval have not been described. We hypothesized that a policy of dedicated follow-up would achieve a higher rate of filter removal. Trauma and Nontrauma patients who had a retrievable IVCF placed during 2006 were identified. A protocol existed for trauma patients with chart stickers, arm bracelets, and dedicated follow-up by nurse practitioners from three trauma teams. No protocol existed for nontrauma patients. Statistical analysis was performed using χ^2 analysis or analysis of variance. One hundred sixty-seven retrievable IVCFs were placed over 12 months; 91 in trauma patients and 76 in nontrauma patients. Trauma patients were more likely to have their IVCF removed than nontrauma patients, 55 per cent *versus* 19 per cent, $P < 0.001$. There were differences between the three trauma teams, with removal rates of 44 per cent, 42 per cent, and 86 per cent respectively ($P < 0.05$). On multivariate analysis young age and trauma patient status were independent predictors of filter removal. A policy of dedicated follow-up of patients with IVCFs can achieve significantly higher rates of filter removal than have been previously reported. Similar policies should be adopted by all centers placing retrievable IVCFs to maximize retrieval rates.

▶ Inferior vena cava filter placement is indicated by trauma guidelines for patients with increased risk of deep venous thrombosis (DVT) while not eligible for anticoagulation. It is also a rising trend in our medical patients who have significantly high potential of bleeding if anticoagulated or have a DVT with massive pulmonary embolism in acute setting. More important than putting these filters in is the removal of these filters when the underlying problem resolves because it increases the chance of chronic edema, persistent DVT, and morbidity. Historically, the retrieval rate of these so-called retrievable filters is very low. The largest study so far by the American Association for the Surgery of Trauma multicenter trial[1] reported that only 22% of these filters were removed. In medical patients, the rates are even lower. The above study is important because it shows that with formal follow-up and protocol, we can increase the retrieval rate > 50%.[2]

M. Ali Raza, MD

References

1. Karmy-Jones R, Jurkovich GJ, Velmahos GC, et al. Practice patterns and outcomes of retrievable vena cava filters in trauma patients: an AAST multicenter study. *J Trauma.* 2007;62:17-24.
2. Ray CE Jr, Mitchell E, Zipser S, Kao EY, Brown CF, Moneta GL. Outcomes with retrievable inferior vena cava filters: a multicenter study. *J Vasc Interv Radiol.* 2006;17:1595-1604.

5 Community-Acquired Pneumonia

Introduction

Community-acquired pneumonia (CAP) continues to be a major cause of morbidity and mortality in the United States. The most recent final National Vital Statistics Report (2007) shows that influenza and pneumonia have been listed as the eighth most common cause of death, accounting for 52,717 of the 2,423,712 deaths that year.[1] The morbidity rate is far greater, with the number of cases per year estimated at up to 20 times the death rate.[2] This year's selections about CAP address prevention, diagnosis, identification of risk factors for the development of pneumonia, approaches to determining risk of poor outcome, and treatment.

In an article by Maruyama et al, the authors were able to evaluate pneumococcal polysaccharide vaccine against placebo in a Japanese population that is relatively vaccination-naïve. The same population typically has a high rate of pneumococcal disease, making it relatively easy to evaluate the impact of the vaccine.

Two articles address the role of specific diagnosis in managing CAP. A prospective randomized trial by Falguera et al using urine antigen studies to try to better target therapy to specific organisms concludes by questioning the value of this approach. A second article, by Chandra et al, looked at the hospital discharge diagnoses of patients who were given an emergency department diagnosis of CAP and found the discharge diagnoses were often different.

Risk-factor assessment has been a favorite topic of researchers in the last few years. This chapter contains articles looking at risk factors associated with the development of pneumonia and, once one has pneumonia, risk for a poor outcome. In terms of risk factors for pneumonia developing in the elderly, Trifiro et al investigate the role of antipsychotics that are often given to elderly patients in the development of pneumonia and the mortality associated with those pneumonia episodes. Neupane et al investigate a completely different type of risk factor for CAP in elderly patients, the impact of long-term exposure to ambient air pollution. At the other end of the age spectrum, O'Grady et al observed in an Australian population of infants receiving both conjugate pneumococcal vaccine boostered by polysaccharide vaccine that there are increased rates of respiratory-related hospitalizations. The cause is unclear. Teepe and colleagues studied the population between those extremes, children and young adults. This is somewhat of a neglected population in terms of CAP studies because the mortality rate is low. Interestingly, in this Dutch population, the authors found risk factors for pneumonia can be identified in this typically healthy population.

Risk factors identified as potential predictors of poor outcomes include a comorbidity of diabetes mellitus (Yende et al), the hospital in which a person is hospitalized (Ross et al), uncertain factors other than bacteremia in health care–associated pneumonia (Rello et al), culture positivity in health care–associated pneumonia (LaBelle et al), the level of specific biomarkers (Kruger et al), and platelet abnormalities at the time of hospitalization (Mirsaeidi et al). Though intriguing, many of these require larger, better designed studies for confirmation. A final article in this section (Chalmers et al) is a meta-analysis comparing the performance of 3 different severity predictors—PSI, CURB65, and CRB65—in predicting 30-day mortality from CAP.

Janet R. Maurer, MD, MBA

References

1. http://www.cdc.gov/NCHS/data/nvsr/nvsr58/nvsr58_19.pdf
2. Mandell LA, Wunderink RG, Anzueto A, et al. Infectious Diseases Society of America/American Thoracic Society consensus guidelines on the management of community-acquired pneumonia in adults. *Clin Infect Dis.* 2007;44:S27-S72.

Long-Term Exposure to Ambient Air Pollution and Risk of Hospitalization with Community-acquired Pneumonia in Older Adults
Neupane B, Jerrett M, Burnett RT, et al (McMaster Univ, Hamilton, Ontario, Canada; Univ of California, Berkeley; Health Canada, Ottawa, Ontario; et al)
Am J Respir Crit Care Med 181:47-53, 2010

Rationale.—Little is known about the long-term effects of air pollution on pneumonia hospitalization in the elderly.

Objectives.—To assess the effect of long-term exposure to ambient nitrogen dioxide, sulfur dioxide, and fine particulate matter with diameter equal to or smaller than 2.5 μm ($PM_{2.5}$) on hospitalization for community-acquired pneumonia in older adults.

Methods.—We used a population-based case–control study in Hamilton, Ontario, Canada. We enrolled 345 hospitalized patients aged 65 years or more for community-acquired pneumonia and 494 control participants, aged 65 years and more, randomly selected from the same community as cases from July 2003 to April 2005. Health data were collected by personal interview. Annual average levels of nitrogen dioxide, sulfur dioxide, and $PM_{2.5}$ before the study period were estimated at the residential addresses of participants by inverse distance weighting, bicubic splined and land use regression methods and merged with participants' health data.

Measurements and Main Results.—Long-term exposure to higher levels of nitrogen dioxide and $PM_{2.5}$ was significantly associated with hospitalization for community-acquired pneumonia (odds ratio [OR], 2.30; 95% confidence interval [CI], 1.25 to 4.21; $P = 0.007$ and OR, 2.26; 95% CI, 1.20 to 4.24; $P = 0.012$, respectively, over the 5th–95th percentile range increase of exposure). Sulfur dioxide did not appear to have any association (OR, 0.97; 95% CI, 0.59 to 1.61; $P = 0.918$). Results were somewhat sensitive to the choice of methods used to estimate air pollutant levels at residential addresses, although all risks from nitrogen dioxide and $PM_{2.5}$ exposure were positive and generally significant.

Conclusions.—In older adults, exposure to ambient nitrogen dioxide and $PM_{2.5}$ was associated with hospitalization for community-acquired pneumonia.

▶ It is known that as patients age and particularly as patients above the age of 65 get older, the rate of pneumonia increases and mortality from pneumonia also increases. Not only does increasing age correlate with increased risk of pneumonia, there is evidence that there are increasing hospitalization rates in these older age groups for the diagnosis of pneumonia.[1] Age-related risk factors include relative immunosuppression, comorbidities, especially cardiopulmonary disease and cognitive issues, and use of drugs that impair mental clarity. However, the fact that rates of hospitalization are increasing suggests there may be other environmental factors that create additional risk. The authors hypothesized that long-term exposures to certain types of air pollutants might create part of this additional risk. They also note that most previous studies on the impact of air pollution have focused on short-term exposures and have used administrative databases. This study uses the residential addresses of actual cases and controls, the average annual amount of air pollutants and an inverse distance weighting approach to determine the approximate exposures of cases and controls to particulate matter (2.5 micrometers), NO_2, and SO_2. Also patients were carefully assessed to identify covariates that might impact their risk for pneumonia independent of exposures to air pollution. Higher levels of NO_2 and particulate matter correlated with higher rates of hospitalization for pneumonia. SO_2 did not, a finding consistent with other studies of short-term exposures. However, NO_2 has been shown in animal models to impair alveolar macrophage function and epithelial cell function.[2] In an elderly population with an already impaired immune response, that kind of impact would certainly increase pneumonia risk. Risk modification is difficult but could include situating assisted living and other living facilities for the elderly in areas of less traffic density and away from industrial areas as well as informing the appropriate population of this risk.

J. R. Maurer, MD, MBA

References

1. Fry A, Shay DK, Holman RC, Curns AT, Anderson IJ. Trends in hospitalizations for pneumonia among persons aged 65 years or older in the United States, 1988-2002. *JAMA*. 2005;294:2712-2719.
2. Frampton MW, Smeglin AM, Roberts NJ Jr, Finkelstein JN, Morrow PE, Utell MJ. Nitrogen dioxide exposure in vivo and human alveolar macrophage inactivation of influenza virus in vitro. *Environ Res.* 1989;48:179-192.

Prospective, randomised study to compare empirical treatment versus targeted treatment on the basis of the urine antigen results in hospitalised patients with community-acquired pneumonia
Falguera M, Ruiz-González A, Schoenenberger JA, et al (Universitat de Lleida, Spain)
Thorax 65:101-106, 2010

Background.—Recommendations for diagnostic testing in hospitalised patients with community-acquired pneumonia remain controversial. The aim of the present study was to evaluate the impact of a therapeutic strategy based on the microbiological results provided by urinary antigen tests for *Streptococcus pneumoniae* and *Legionella pneumophila*.

Methods.—For a 2-year period, hospitalised patients with community-acquired pneumonia were randomly assigned to receive either empirical treatment, according to international guidelines, or targeted treatment, on the basis of the results from antigen tests. Outcome parameters, monetary costs and antibiotic exposure levels were compared.

Results.—Out of 194 enrolled patients, 177 were available for randomisation; 89 were assigned to empirical treatment and 88 were assigned to targeted treatment. Targeted treatment was associated with a slightly higher overall cost (€1657.00 vs €1617.20, p=0.28), reduction in the incidence of adverse events (9% vs 18%, p=0.12) and lower exposure to broad-spectrum antimicrobials (154.4 vs 183.3 defined daily doses per 100 patient days). No statistically significant differences in other outcome parameters were observed. Oral antibiotic treatment was started according to the results of antigen tests in 25 patients assigned to targeted treatment; these patients showed a statistically significant higher risk of clinical relapse as compared with the remaining population (12% vs 3%, p=0.04).

Conclusions.—The routine implementation of urine antigen detection tests does not carry substantial outcome-related or economic benefits to hospitalised patients with community-acquired pneumonia. Narrowing the antibiotic treatment according to the urine antigen results may in fact be associated with a higher risk of clinical relapse.

▶ Following a series of articles several years ago that reported little contribution of sputum or blood cultures to the eventual outcome in patients with community-acquired pneumonia,[1,2] many frontline practitioners began treating these patients empirically following accepted guidelines.[3] However, physicians still felt a bit uncomfortable not knowing what they were treating, so when specific urine antigen tests became widely available, they became widely adopted by many practitioners. The same sort of careful study of antigen tests in terms of their impact on outcomes has not been previously reported. The purposes of this study were to prospectively evaluate clinical and economic consequences of routine use of urine antigen tests in hospitalized patients. This is a well-designed, prospective, randomized trial, but it is quite small in that less than 200 patients overall were randomized. There was no outcome benefit from targeting therapy based on urine antigen studies. The authors note that this might have been predicted based on previous studies of other diagnostic modalities and rate of successful outcomes generally seen when the guideline recommendations are followed. One of the more interesting findings was that in the group randomized to have targeted treatment, the 25 patients with urine antigen positivity who had therapy narrowed to specifically address pneumococcal disease had a higher failure rate than patients receiving empirical treatment. There were slightly more adverse advents, primarily gastrointestinal distress, in patients with empirical treatment. In general, the results of this trial are similar to another small similar trial[4] and both fail to support the routine use of urine antigen tests in community-acquired pneumonia, except possibly in very unusual situations.

J. R. Maurer, MD, MBA

References

1. Theerthakari R, El-Halees W, Ismail M, Solis RA, Khan MA. Nonvalue of the initial microbiological studies in the management of nonsevere community-acquired pneumonia. *Chest.* 2001;119:181-184.
2. Sanyal S, Smith PR, Saha AC, Gupta S, Berkowitz L, Homel P. Initial microbiologic studies did not affect outcome in adults hospitalized with community-acquired pneumonia. *Am J Respir Crit Care Med.* 1999;160:346-348.
3. Mandell LA, Wunderink RG, Anzueto A, et al. Infectious Diseases Society of America/American Thoracic Society consensus guidelines on the management of community-acquired pneumonia in adults. *Clin Infect Dis.* 2007;44:S27-S72.
4. van der Eerden MM, Vlaspolder F, de Graaff CS, et al. Comparison between pathogen directed antibiotic treatment and empirical broad spectrum antibiotic treatment in patients with community acquired pneumonia: a prospective, randomized study. *Thorax.* 2005;60:672-678.

Thrombocytopenia and Thrombocytosis at Time of Hospitalization Predict Mortality in Patients With Community-Acquired Pneumonia

Mirsaeidi M, Peyrani P, Aliberti S, et al (Univ of Louisville, KY; Univ of Milan, Italy; et al)

Chest 137:416-420, 2010

Background.—Platelets are inflammatory cells with an important role in antimicrobial host defenses. We speculate that an abnormal platelet count may be a marker of severity in patients with community-acquired

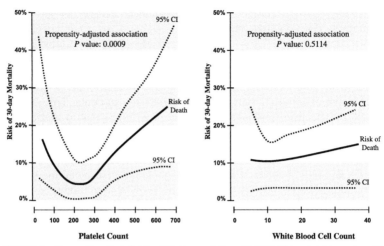

FIGURE 1.—Propensity-adjusted risk of 30-day mortality with 95% CI by platelet count and WBC count at time of hospitalization for patients with community-acquired pneumonia. (Reprinted from Mirsaeidi M, Peyrani P, Aliberti S, et al. Thrombocytopenia and thrombocytosis at time of hospitalization predict mortality in patients with community-acquired pneumonia. *Chest.* 2010;137:416-420, with permission from American College of Chest Physicians.)

pneumonia (CAP). The objectives of this study were to evaluate if abnormal platelet count in hospitalized patients with CAP was associated with 30-day mortality and to compare platelet count and leukocyte count as predictors of 30-day mortality.

Methods.—We performed a retrospective cohort study of 500 consecutive patients hospitalized with CAP at the Veterans Hospital of Louisville, Kentucky, between June 2001 and March 2006 to investigate the association of platelet count and leukocyte count with 30-day mortality. Predictor variables were platelet count and leukocyte count. Abnormal platelet count was < 100,000/L (thrombocytopenia) and > 400,000/L (thrombocytosis). The outcome variable was 30-day mortality. To control for potential confounding, a propensity score that incorporated 33 variables was used.

Results.—Platelet count was strongly associated ($P = .0009$) with 30-day mortality, whereas no association was observed for leukocyte count ($P = .5114$). High platelet counts resulted in a significantly increased risk of mortality.

Conclusions.—Thrombocytopenia and thrombocytosis are associated with mortality in patients hospitalized with CAP. When evaluating an initial CBC test in patients with CAP, an abnormal platelet count is a better predictor of outcome than an abnormal leukocyte count (Fig 1).

▶ Platelet abnormalities have been associated with outcomes in children with pneumonia[1] but are rarely mentioned in studies of adults. In this Veterans Administration population study of 500 consecutively admitted adults with a diagnosis of community-acquired pneumonia, thrombocytosis in particular was a very useful predictor of death. There are several theoretical reasons why platelet counts may be useful indicators. They are immunologically active cells that undergo chemotaxis and release proinflammatory molecules.[2] The authors suggest that the finding of thrombocytosis may be a marker for an exaggerated inflammatory response. Potentially more important is the possibility of enhanced thrombus formation, which could have a multiorgan systemic impact on outcomes. Interestingly, the authors found that thrombocytosis was a much better predictor of outcomes than white blood cell counts, a popular clinical indicator. It would be interesting to add the platelet counts to some of the commonly used predictors of severity to determine if that element provides any added value. However, probably the most important next step is to do a prospective study in a larger population that is more diverse at least in age and sex to determine the generalizability of the findings of this study.

J. R. Maurer, MD, MBA

References

1. Wolach B, Morag H, Drucker M, Sadan N. Thrombocytosis after pneumonia with empyema and other bacterial infections in children. *Pediatr Infect Dis J.* 1990;9: 718-721.
2. Elzey BD, Sprague DL, Ratliff TL. The emerging role of platelets in adaptive immunity. *Cell Immunol.* 2005;238:1-9.

Increased Risk of Hospitalization for Acute Lower Respiratory Tract Infection among Australian Indigenous Infants 5–23 Months of Age Following Pneumococcal Vaccination: A Cohort Study

O'Grady K-AF, Lee KJ, Carlin JB, et al (Charles Darwin Univ, Tiwi, London, England; Royal Children's Hosp, Melbourne, Australia; et al)

Clin Infect Dis 50:970-978, 2010

Background.—Australian Indigenous children are the only population worldwide to receive the 7-valent pneumococcal conjugate vaccine (7vPCV) at 2, 4, and 6 months of age and the 23-valent pneumococcal polysaccharide vaccine (23vPPV) at 18 months of age. We evaluated this program's effectiveness in reducing the risk of hospitalization for acute lower respiratory tract infection (ALRI) in Northern Territory (NT) Indigenous children aged 5–23 months.

Methods.—We conducted a retrospective cohort study involving all NT Indigenous children born from 1 April 2000 through 31 October 2004. Person-time at-risk after 0, 1, 2, and 3 doses of 7vPCV and after 0 and 1 dose of 23vPPV and the number of ALRI following each dose were used to calculate dose-specific rates of ALRI for children 5–23 months of age. Rates were compared using Cox proportional hazards models, with the number of doses of each vaccine serving as time-dependent covariates.

Results.—There were 5482 children and 8315 child-years at risk, with 2174 episodes of ALRI requiring hospitalization (overall incidence, 261 episodes per 1000 child-years at risk). Elevated risk of ALRI requiring hospitalization was observed after each dose of the 7vPCV vaccine, compared with that for children who received no doses, and an even greater elevation in risk was observed after each dose of the 23vPPV (adjusted hazard ratio [HR] vs no dose, 1.39; 95% confidence interval [CI], 1.12–1.71; $P = .002$). Risk was highest among children vaccinated with the 23vPPV who had received <3 doses of the 7vPCV (adjusted HR, 1.81; 95% CI, 1.32–2.48).

Conclusions.—Our results suggest an increased risk of ALRI requiring hospitalization after pneumococcal vaccination, particularly after receipt of the 23vPPV booster. The use of the 23vPPV booster should be reevaluated.

▶ When 7-valent pneumococcal vaccine became available in 2000-2001 for young children, it was administered in different ways in different settings. In the United States, it was administered widely and subsequent reports of its impact documented a decrease in pneumococcal disease both in the children given the vaccine as well as in adults who might otherwise have developed disease because of their proximity to infected children.[1,2] In other countries such as Spain, where it was not as widely administered across the population, the results were less impressive. In this study of administration to Australian indigenous infants, the 7-valent conjugate vaccine was administered in conjunction with a 23-valent polysaccharide vaccine at 18 months as a sort of booster shot. This resulted in an unexpected increase in lower respiratory tract infections that had been previously reported only sporadically in vaccinated infants. The authors speculate that this phenomenon may be caused by rapid emergence of noncovered serotypes or other organisms. Another potential explanation noted is the development of immune hyporesponsiveness after the use of meningococcal vaccine,[3] though this is considered unlikely. Most of the increased lower respiratory tract infections occurred after the polysaccharide vaccine booster, leading the authors to suggest caution in using this approach. Lower respiratory tract infections in these infants is not without long-term consequences as repeated infections not uncommonly result in bronchiectasis, which can be a cause of lifelong morbidity. The message here, I think, is that any intervention, no matter how beneficial in most, can have adverse and unintended side effects in select populations.

J. R. Maurer, MD, MBA

References

1. Grijalva CG, Nuorti JP, Arbogast PG, Martin SW, Edwards KM, Griffin MR. Decline in pneumonia admissions after routine childhood immunisation with pneumococcal conjugate vaccine in the USA: a time series analysis. *Lancet.* 2007;369:1179-1186.
2. Nelson JC, Jackson M, Yu O, et al. Impact of the introduction of pneumococcal conjugate vaccine on rates of community acquired pneumonia in children and adults. *Vaccine.* 2008;26:4947-4954.
3. O'Brien KL, Hochman M, Goldblatt D. Combined schedules of pneumococcal conjugate and polysaccharide vaccines: is hyporesponsiveness an issue? *Lancet Infect Dis.* 2007;7:597-606.

Efficacy of 23-valent pneumococcal vaccine in preventing pneumonia and improving survival in nursing home residents: double blind, randomised and placebo controlled trial

Maruyama T, Taguchi O, Niederman MS, et al (Mie Univ Graduate School of Medicine, Japan; Winthrop Univ Hosp, Mineola, NY; et al)
BMJ 340:c1004, 2010

Objective.—To determine the efficacy of a 23-valent pneumococcal polysaccharide vaccine in people at high risk of pneumococcal pneumonia.

Design.—Prospective, randomised, placebo controlled double blind study.

Setting.—Nursing homes in Japan.

Participants.—1006 nursing home residents.

Interventions.—Participants were randomly allocated to either 23-valent pneumococcal polysaccharide vaccine (n=502) or placebo (n=504).

Main Outcome Measures.—The primary end points were the incidence of all cause pneumonia and pneumococcal pneumonia. Secondary end points were deaths from pneumococcal pneumonia, all cause pneumonia, and other causes.

Results.—Pneumonia occurred in 63 (12.5%) participants in the vaccine group and 104 (20.6%) in the placebo group. Pneumococcal pneumonia was diagnosed in 14 (2.8%) participants in the vaccine group and 37 (7.3%) in the placebo group (P<0.001). All cause pneumonia and pneumococcal pneumonia were significantly more frequent in the placebo group than in the vaccine group: incidence per 1000 person years 55 *v* 91 (P<0.0006) and 12 *v* 32 (P<0.001), respectively. Death from pneumococcal pneumonia was significantly higher in the placebo group than in the vaccine group (35.1% (13/37) *v* 0% (0/14), P<0.01). The death rate from all cause pneumonia (vaccine group 20.6% (13/63) *v* placebo group 25.0% (26/104), P=0.5) and from other causes (vaccine group 17.7% (89/502) *v* placebo group (80/504) 15.9%, P=0.4) did not differ between the two study groups.

Conclusion.—The 23-valent pneumococcal polysaccharide vaccine prevented pneumococcal pneumonia and reduced mortality from pneumococcal pneumonia in nursing home residents.

Trial registration.—Japan Medical Association Center for Clinical Trials JMA-IIA00024 (Fig 3).

▶ Most data reported on the value of pneumococcal polysaccharide vaccine are equivocal in terms of its efficacy in nursing home residents, and this has probably resulted in a relatively low rate of vaccination of these patients.[1] In addition, as the authors of this study note, it is difficult to do a prospective randomized controlled trial in areas (such as the United States) where rates of pneumococcal pneumonia are relatively low, as the numbers required to power such a study would be extremely large. This is not the situation, however, in Japan. Only 3% of the population older than 65 years has been vaccinated with pneumococcal vaccine, and the rate of disease is very high in nursing

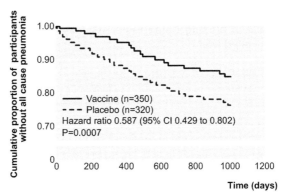

FIGURE 3.—Kaplan-Meier survival curves of participants without all cause pneumonia in vaccine and placebo groups. (Reprinted from Maruyama T, Taguchi O, Niederman MS, et al. Efficacy of 23-valent pneumococcal vaccine in preventing pneumonia and improving survival in nursing home residents: double blind, randomised and placebo controlled trial. *BMJ*. 2010;340:c1004, reproduced with permission from the BMJ Publishing Group Ltd.)

home patients in rural areas. This made an ideal milieu in which to conduct a prospective placebo controlled trial, especially because there is no national recommendation to provide pneumococcal vaccine to this population, thus minimizing potential ethical issues. Pneumococcal disease was suspected by a new infiltrate. Cultures of blood and sputum were done as was urine antigen analysis. Thus, this study gives some of the most methodologically pure results to date of the impact of pneumococcal vaccine in a highly susceptible population. It supports the current US recommendation to vaccinate all patients entering chronic care facilities,[1] especially because the rates of pneumococcal disease are several times higher than those of the community-dwelling population.

J. R. Maurer, MD, MBA

Reference

1. Centers for Disease Control and Prevention. Prevention of pneumococcal disease: recommendation of the Advisory Committee on Immunization Practices (ACIP). *MMWR Morb Mortal Wkly Rep.* 1997;46:1-24.

Pro-atrial natriuretic peptide and pro-vasopressin for predicting short-term and long-term survival in community-acquired pneumonia: results from the German Competence Network CAPNETZ

Krüger S, the CAPNETZ Study Group (RWTH Univ, Aachen, Germany; et al)
Thorax 65:208-214, 2010

Background.—Community-acquired pneumonia (CAP) is the most important clinical infection with a high long-term mortality rate. The aim of this study was to evaluate the value of biomarkers for the prediction of short-term and long-term mortality in CAP.

Methods.—A total of 1740 patients of mean ± SD age 60 ± 18 years (45% female) with proven CAP were enrolled in the study. Mid-regional pro-atrial natriuretic peptide (MR-proANP), C-terminal pro-atrial vaso-pressin (CT-proAVP), procalcitonin , C-reactive protein, leucocyte count (WBC) and CRB-65 score were determined on admission. Patients were followed up for 180 days.

Results.—MR-proANP and CT-proAVP levels increased with increasing severity of CAP, classified according to CRB-65 score. In patients who died within 28 and 180 days, median MR-proANP (313.9 vs 80.0 and 277.8 vs 76.0 pmol/l, each p<0.0001) and CT-proAVP (42.6 vs 11.2 and 33.2 vs 10.7 pmol/l, each p<0.0001) levels were significantly higher than the levels in survivors. In receiver operating characteristics analysis for survival at 28 and 180 days, the areas under the curves (AUCs) for CT-proAVP (0.84, 95% CI 0.82 to 0.86 and 0.78, 95% CI 0.76 to 0.80) and MR-proANP (0.81, 95% CI 0.79 to 0.83 and 0.81, 95% CI 0.79 to 0.83) were superior to the AUC of CRB-65 (0.74, 95% CI 0.71 to 0.76 and 0.71, 95% CI 0.69 to 0.74, p<0.05), procalcitonin, C-reactive protein and WBC. In multivari-able Cox proportional hazards regression analyses adjusted for comorbid-ity and pneumonia severity, MR-proANP and CT-proAVP were independent and the strongest predictors of short-term and long-term mortality.

Conclusions.—MR-proANP and CT-proAVP are powerful tools for the prediction of short-term and long-term risk stratification of patients with CAP (Fig 3).

▶ Over the past decade or so, both clinical tools, for example, the pneumonia severity index and confusion, urea nitrogen, respiratory rate, blood pressure, 65 years and older (CURB-65), and its variants and biomarkers, for example, procalcitonin, C-reactive protein, C-terminal proatrial vasopressin (CT-proAVP), and midregional proatrial natriuretic peptide (MR-proANP), have been shown to be helpful in assessing the severity of community-acquired pneumonia on presentation and, in many cases, predicting short-term outcomes. These outcomes that have been looked at are typically 30-day survivals. This study, from a large German network that keeps a database of all patients with standard community-acquired pneumonia criteria from all participating centers and conducts studies using that data, aimed to see if any of the criteria that had been successful in predicting short-term outcomes could also be used to predict further into the future. This is of interest because it has been previously noted that patients who successfully recover from pneu-monia have a higher rate of death than age-matched controls remote from the pneumonia episode. Excessive mortality is highest in the first year but has been reported up to 5 years.[1-3] Identifying predictors of high risk of late death could potentially lead to risk-modification strategies that could improve outcomes. The obvious place to start (the focus of this study) is with the markers that have already been validated for short-term outcomes. Of the markers, CT-proAVP and MR-proANP were most helpful in predicting long-term outcomes. Because this is a database study and followed mortality only to 180 days,

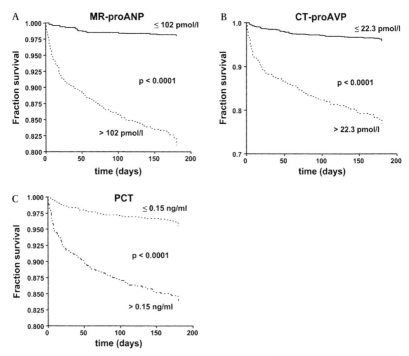

FIGURE 3.—Kaplan–Meier analysis according to (A) mid-regional pro-atrial natriuretic peptide (MR-proANP levels) (groups below (n=998, solid line) and above (n=727, dotted line) a cut-off concentration of 102 pmol/l; p<0.0001, log-rank test); (B) C-terminal pro-atrial vasopressin (CT-proAVP) levels (groups below (n=1270, solid line) and above (n=391, dotted line) a cut-off concentration of 22.3 pmol/l; p<0.0001, log-rank test); (C) procalcitonin (PCT) levels (groups below (n=1037, solid line) and above (n=688, dotted line) a cut-off concentration of 0.15 ng/ml; p<0.0001, log-rank test). (Reprinted from Krüger S, the CAPNETZ Study Group. Pro-atrial natriuretic peptide and pro-vasopressin for predicting short-term and long-term survival in community-acquired pneumonia: results from the German Competence Network CAPNETZ. *Thorax*. 2010;65:208-214, and reproduced/amended with permission from the BMJ Publishing Group.)

clearly prospective studies evaluating these data over a longer time frame are needed.

J. R. Maurer, MD, MBA

References

1. Waterer GW, Kessler LA, Wunderink RG. Medium-term survival after hospitalization with community-acquired pneumonia. *Am J Respir Crit Care Med.* 2004;169: 910-914.
2. Mortensen EM, Coley CM, Singer DE, et al. Causes of death for patients with community-acquired pneumonia: results from the Pneumonia Patient Outcomes Research Team cohort study. *Arch Intern Med.* 2002;162:1059-1064.
3. Brancati FL, Chow JW, Wagener MM, Vacarello SJ, Yu VL. Is pneumonia really the old man's friend? Two-year prognosis after community-acquired pneumonia. *Lancet.* 1993;342:30-33.

Hospital Volume and 30-Day Mortality for Three Common Medical Conditions

Ross JS, Normand S-LT, Wang Y, et al (Mount Sinai School of Medicine, NY; Harvard Med School and Harvard School of Public Health, Boston, MA; Yale-New Haven Hosp, CT; et al)
N Engl J Med 362:1110-1118, 2010

Background.—The association between hospital volume and the death rate for patients who are hospitalized for acute myocardial infarction, heart failure, or pneumonia remains unclear. It is also not known whether a volume threshold for such an association exists.

Methods.—We conducted cross-sectional analyses of data from Medicare administrative claims for all fee-for-service beneficiaries who were hospitalized between 2004 and 2006 in acute care hospitals in the United States for acute myocardial infarction, heart failure, or pneumonia. Using hierarchical logistic-regression models for each condition, we estimated the change in the odds of death within 30 days associated with an increase of 100 patients in the annual hospital volume. Analyses were adjusted for patients' risk factors and hospital characteristics. Bootstrapping procedures were used to estimate 95% confidence intervals to identify the condition-specific volume thresholds above which an increased volume was not associated with reduced mortality.

Results.—There were 734,972 hospitalizations for acute myocardial infarction in 4128 hospitals, 1,324,287 for heart failure in 4679 hospitals, and 1,418,252 for pneumonia in 4673 hospitals. An increased hospital volume was associated with reduced 30-day mortality for all conditions (P<0.001 for all comparisons). For each condition, the association between volume and outcome was attenuated as the hospital's volume increased. For acute myocardial infarction, once the annual volume reached 610 patients (95% confidence interval [CI], 539 to 679), an increase in the hospital volume by 100 patients was no longer significantly associated with reduced odds of death. The volume threshold was 500 patients (95% CI, 433 to 566) for heart failure and 210 patients (95% CI, 142 to 284) for pneumonia.

Conclusions.—Admission to higher-volume hospitals was associated with a reduction in mortality for acute myocardial infarction, heart failure, and pneumonia, although there was a volume threshold above which an increased condition-specific hospital volume was no longer significantly associated with reduced mortality (Fig 1).

▶ Using a 2-year snapshot of the huge Medicare administrative database of fee for service admissions, the authors were able to show that outcomes were significantly better in hospitals that care for higher volumes of patients up to a certain threshold. For community-acquired pneumonia, the threshold was less than half that of either heart failure or myocardial infarction. The authors also found that once the volume of admissions for any of the conditions in a hospital reached 100 patients/year, the morbidity/mortality curves began to

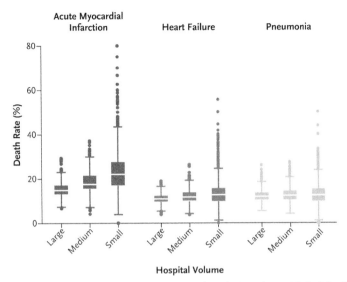

FIGURE 1.—Frequency Distribution of 30-Day Rates of Death, According to Medical Condition and Hospital Volume. The upper boundaries of the boxes represent the 75th percentile, the white horizontal line within each box represents the median or 50th percentile, and the lower boundaries of the boxes represent the 25th percentile. Individual data points represent outliers. The I bars represent the highest and lowest values within 1.5 times the interquartile range. (Reprinted from Ross JS, Normand S-LT, Wang Y, et al. Hospital volume and 30-day mortality for three common medical conditions. *N Engl J Med.* 2010;362:1110-1118, with permission from Massachusetts Medical Society. All rights reserved.)

flatten. Many patients with an acute illness may have access only to a smaller hospital or may prefer to be cared for in a smaller hospital, despite these findings. In fact, the authors of this study found significant heterogeneity among hospitals and noted that a number of small-volume hospitals had excellent outcomes. They further suggest that the study has 2 policy implications. First, those policy makers might wish to regionalize acute care and require that anyone with 1 of the 3 acute illnesses be transferred to hospitals with an appropriate threshold of patients. This does not seem very feasible and will meet with significant patient resistance. The second policy implication suggested is to increase the volumes of some of the smallest hospitals by ensuring that multiple small hospitals do not exist in close proximity to each other, as can be accomplished through state certificate of need regulations, for example. It seems that a simpler and more acceptable approach would be to study the care patterns in the smaller hospitals with excellent outcomes and incentivize the less successful smaller hospitals to implement those approaches.

J. R. Maurer, MD, MBA

A Comparison of Culture-Positive and Culture-Negative Health-Care-Associated Pneumonia

Labelle AJ, Arnold H, Reichley RM, et al (Washington Univ School of Medicine, St Louis, MO; Barnes-Jewish Hosp, St Louis, MO; BJC Healthcare, St Louis, MO)

Chest 137:1130-1137, 2010

Objective.—The aim of this study is to describe the initial antibiotic treatment regimens, severity of illness, and in-hospital mortality among culture-negative (CN) and culture-positive (CP) patients with health-care-associated pneumonia (HCAP).

Methods.—We used a retrospective cohort study, examining adult patients with HCAP from Barnes-Jewish Hospital, a 1,200-bed urban teaching hospital.

Results.—Eight hundred seventy patients with HCAP were identified over a 3-year period (January 2003 through December 2005) of whom 431 (49.5%) were CP. Among the non-CP patients, 290 (66.1%) had no respiratory cultures obtained, and 149 (33.9%) had no growth or nonpathogenic oral flora identified and were classified as CN. CN patients were more likely to have received an initial antibiotic regimen (ceftriaxone ± azithromycin or moxifloxacin) targeting community-acquired pneumonia pathogens compared with CP patients (71.8% vs 25.5%, $P < .001$). Severity of illness as assessed by ICU admission and mechanical ventilation (MV) was statistically lower in CN compared with CP patients (ICU admittance 12.1% vs 48.7%, $P < .001$; MV: 6.7% vs 44.5%, $P < .001$). In-hospital mortality and hospital length of stay were also statistically lower for CN patients (mortality: 7.4% vs 24.6%, $P < .001$; hospital length of stay: 6.7 ± 7.4 days vs 12.1 ± 11.7 days, $P < .001$).

Conclusions.—In this analysis, patients with CN HCAP had lower severity of illness, hospital mortality, and hospital length of stay compared with CP patients. These data suggest that patients with CN HCAP differ substantially from patients with HCAP with positive microbiologic cultures (Fig 2).

▶ Like the study reported in this section by Rello et al,[1] LaBelle and colleagues have tried to better characterize the relatively newly defined entity of health care–associated pneumonia (HCAP).[1] As the authors state, many of the aspects of typical community-acquired pneumonia (CAP) that have been well studied have not yet been addressed in HCAP. They note that most studies of HCAP to date have focused on culture-positive patients; however, HCAP is not defined by culture status or the type of organism cultured but rather by recurrent or extensive association with a health care facility or environment or an immuno-suppressed state, for example, nursing home, hospital, dialysis unit, or under-lying malignancy. The implication is that such patients are likely to have infections by resistant or particularly virulent organisms because of these associations/conditions. But this has not been proven. So in this study, all patients admitted over 3 years to a large hospital who met HCAP criteria

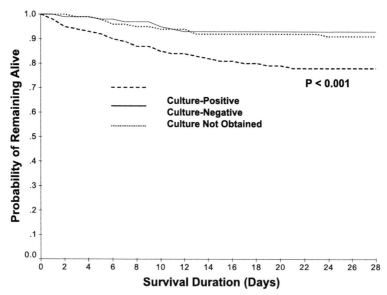

FIGURE 2.—Kaplan-Meier curves depicting the probability of survival in patients with culture-positive (HCAP), patients with culture-negative HCAP, and patients with HCAP and no cultures obtained according to the duration of survival ($P < .001$ by log-rank test comparing culture-positive HCAP to both other groups). (Reprinted from Labelle AJ, Arnold H, Reichley RM, et al. A comparison of culture-positive and culture-negative health-care-associated pneumonia. *Chest*. 2010;137:1130-1137, with permission from American College of Chest Physicians.)

were identified. Slightly more than half the patients were culture negative or had no cultures obtained. Compared with culture-positive patients, the culture-negative patients were less ill, had a shorter length of stay, and had less in-hospital mortality. Culture-negative or no culture patients often were treated as if they had routine CAP rather than organisms associated with HCAP and most did well. This study has many limitations in that it was a retrospective study and subject to all the biases of that methodology. No serologic or molecular studies were done to confirm infecting agents in the culture-negative/no culture patients; if more organisms had been identified, some of these patients might have migrated to the known-organism group and changed the relative mortality rates. Despite the limitations of the study, though, some interesting findings emerge. Certainly this group of patients has a significant risk of routine CAP based on their comorbidities and age, and many, maybe up to half, can probably be successfully treated with the usual approach to CAP. Further, prospective trials are needed to better define this subset of patients with HCAP.

J. R. Maurer, MD, MBA

Reference

1. Rello J, Luján M, Gallego M, et al. Why mortality is increased in health-care-associated pneumonia: lessons from pneumococcal bacteremic pneumonia. *Chest*. 2010;137:1138-1144.

Why Mortality Is Increased in Health-Care-Associated Pneumonia: Lessons From Pneumococcal Bacteremic Pneumonia

Rello J, for the PROCORNEU Study Group (Joan XXIII Univ Hosp, Tarragona, Spain; et al)
Chest 137:1138-1144, 2010

Background.—A cohort of patients with bacteremic *Streptococcus pneumoniae* pneumonia was reviewed to assess why mortality is higher in health-care-associated pneumonia (HCAP) than in community-acquired pneumonia (CAP).

Methods.—A prospective cohort of all adult patients with bacteremic pneumococcal pneumonia attended at the ED was used.

Results.—One hundred eighty-four cases were classified as CAP and 44 (19%) as HCAP. Fifty-two (23%) were admitted to the ICU. Three (1.5%) isolates were resistant to β-lactams, and only two patients received inappropriate therapy. The CAP cohort was significantly younger (median age 68 years, interquartile range [IQR] 42-78 vs 77 years, IQR 67-82, $P < .001$). The HCAP cohort presented a higher Charlson index (2.81 ± 1.9 vs 1.23 ± 1.42, $P < .001$) and had higher severity of illness at admission (altered mental status, respiratory rate > 30/min, Pao_2 /Fio_2 <250, and multi-lobar involvement). HCAP patients had a lower rate of ICU admission (11.3% vs 25.5%, $P < .05$), and a trend toward lower mechanical ventilation (9% vs 19%, $P = .17$) and vasopressor use (9% vs 18.4%, $P = .17$) were documented. More patients in the HCAP cohort presented with a pneumonia severity index score >90 (class IV-V, 95% vs 65%, $P < .001$), and 30-day mortality was significantly higher (29.5% vs 7.6%, $P < .001$). A multivariable regression logistic analysis adjusting for underlying conditions and variables related to severity of illness confirmed that HCAP is an independent variable associated with increased mortality (odds ratio = 5.56; 95% CI, 1.86-16.5).

Conclusions.—Pneumococcal HCAP presents excess mortality, which is independent of bacterial susceptibility. Differences in outcomes were probably due to differences in age, comorbidities, and criteria for ICU admission rather than to therapeutic decisions.

▶ Health care–associated pneumonia (HCAP) has been defined as a subset of pneumonia that occurs in people who have had some ongoing relationship with health care institutions so that they are likely to have had some exposure to resistant or more aggressive organisms than the usual causes of community-acquired pneumonia (CAP). The characteristics of HCAP are still being defined. For instance, as the authors note, it is not yet clear whether the poor outcomes of patients with HCAP are because of comorbidities or a higher rate of antibiotic-resistant bacteria that do not respond to the usual empiric treatment regimens. The point of this study was to try to address some of these issues. To do this the authors decided to concentrate on bacteremic pneumococcal pneumonia in a cohort of all patients presenting to an emergency department with pneumonia over an 8.5-year period. While they were prospectively identified with pneumonia, they were retrospectively assigned a designation of HCAP versus routine CAP. Approximately one-fifth of the patients were classified into this group. Patients with HCAP had higher death rates but lower use of ICUs and more frequently had advance directives around limits on therapy. Only 2 patients, 1 in each group, received inappropriate therapy for their isolate. The patients with HCAP were indeed older, had more comorbidities, and appeared generally sicker. The authors state that the higher mortality in HCAP was possibly because of the decision of the physician and patient to limit the extent of support. Whether the use of ICU care would have affected 30-day mortality is questionable. It certainly would have been much more expensive.

J. R. Maurer, MD, MBA

Determinants of community-acquired pneumonia in children and young adults in primary care

Teepe J, Grigoryan L, Verheij TJM (Univ Med Ctr Utrecht, the Netherlands)
Eur Respir J 35:1113-1117, 2010

Most studies on determinants of community-acquired pneumonia (CAP) in primary care have focused primarily on the elderly. Using a case–control study in four Dutch healthcare centres, determinants of CAP among children and young adults were identified.

Cases included 156 young adults (aged 16–40 yrs) and 107 children (aged 0–15 yrs) diagnosed with CAP during 1999–2008. For each case, three controls were selected from the same age group. Separate logistic regression analyses were used to identify determinants in young adults and children.

Lower age, asthma and previous upper respiratory tract infections (URTIs) were independently associated with CAP in children. Increasing age, asthma, three or more children at home, current smoking and three or more previous URTIs were independent determinants of CAP in young adults.

The present study has three remarkable findings: 1) increasing age was an independent determinant of CAP in young adults; 2) having young children increased the risk of the development of CAP in young adults; and 3) the number of previous URTIs was independently associated with CAP in both children and young adults, possibly due to higher infection susceptibility. Further studies are required in order to better understand the aetiology of CAP and permit better diagnosis and treatment of this serious condition.

▶ So much attention around community-acquired pneumonia is focused on the elderly and very elderly that I think we sometimes forget that it is also a significant cause of morbidity in younger people. The reported incidence of pneumonia in children < 5 years is 36 per 1000 and in young adults, aged 15 to 44 years, the incidence is reported at 1 to 8 per 1000.[1,2] It is also a significant cause of mortality in the very young, accounting for about 20% of deaths in children aged < 5 years.[3] This study is a retrospective case control study in which 3 controls were selected for each case. It is a Dutch study using the Utrecht Health Project database, a database of health information that is gathered from patients visiting 4 health centers near the city of Utrecht. All new patients are asked to register, and currently more than 60% of the area's inhabitants have done so. Because the data used are retrospective and from an administrative database, there are some important limitations. In particular, a set of clinical parameters (signs and symptoms) was used to identify patients with pneumonia along with X-ray findings. However, in an unstated number of cases, radiographs were not done as is the practice of primary care providers in the region. Of the main findings in the study, I think one of the most interesting is the relationship of previous upper respiratory tract infections to episodes of pneumonia. We know that the predisposition to bacterial pneumonia in the wake of influenza may be an untoward effect of resolution of the viral-related inflammation, which leaves an impaired host immune response.[4] Could a similar mechanism be invoked in the wake of multiple upper respiratory tract viral infections? Further prospective studies would be very valuable in providing more perspective on the identified pneumonia risk factors in the younger populations.

J. R. Maurer, MD, MBA

References

1. Jokinen C, Heiskanen L, Juvonen H, et al. Incidence of community-acquired pneumonia in the population of four municipalities in eastern Finland. *Am J Epidemiol.* 1993;137:977-988.
2. Almirall J, Bolíbar I, Vidal J, et al. Epidemiology of community-acquired pneumonia in adults: a population-based study. *Eur Respir J.* 2000;15:757-763.
3. Bryce J, Boschi-Pinto C, Shibuya K, Black RE. WHO estimates of the causes of death in children. *Lancet.* 2005;365:1147-1152.
4. van der Sluijs KF, van der Poll T, Lutter R, Juffermans NP, Schultz MJ. Bench-to-bedside review: bacterial pneumonia with influenza-pathogenesis and clinical implications. *Crit Care.* 2010;14:219.

Association of Community-Acquired Pneumonia With Antipsychotic Drug Use in Elderly patients: A Nested Case–Control Study
Trifirò G, Gambassi G, Sen EF, et al (Erasmus Univ Med Ctr, Rotterdam, the Netherlands; Università Cattolica del Sacro Cuore, Rome, Italy; Universidad de Santiago de Compostela, Spain, et al)
Ann Intern Med 152:418-425, 2010

Background.—According to safety alerts from the U.S. Food and Drug Administration, pneumonia is one of the most frequently reported causes of death in elderly patients with dementia who are treated with antipsychotic drugs. However, epidemiologic evidence of the association between antipsychotic drug use and pneumonia is limited.

Objective.—To evaluate whether typical or atypical antipsychotic use is associated with fatal or nonfatal pneumonia in elderly persons.

Design.—Population-based, nested case–control study.

Setting.—Dutch Integrated Primary Care Information database.

Patients.—Cohort of persons who used an antipsychotic drug, were 65 years or older, and were registered in the IPCI database from 1996 to 2006. Case patients were all persons with incident community-acquired pneumonia. Up to 20 control participants were matched to each case patient on the basis of age, sex, and date of onset.

Measurements.—Risk for fatal or nonfatal community-acquired pneumonia with atypical and typical antipsychotic use. Anti-psychotic exposure was categorized by type, timing, and daily dose, and the association with pneumonia was assessed by using conditional logistic regression.

Results.—258 case patients with incident pneumonia were matched to 1686 control participants. Sixty-five (25%) of the case patients died in 30 days, and their disease was considered fatal. Current use of either atypical (odds ratio [OR], 2.61 [95% CI, 1.48 to 4.61]) or typical (OR, 1.76 [CI, 1.22 to 2.53]) antipsychotic drugs was associated with a dose-dependent increase in the risk for pneumonia compared with past use of antipsychotic drugs. Only atypical antipsychotic drugs were associated with an increase in the risk for fatal pneumonia (OR, 5.97 [CI, 1.49 to 23.98]).

Limitations.—Antipsychotic exposure was based on prescription files. Residual confounding due to unmeasured covariates or severity of disease was possible.

Conclusion.—The use of either atypical or typical antipsychotic drugs in elderly patients is associated in a dose-dependent manner with risk for community-acquired pneumonia.

▶ In 2005, the Food and Drug Administration issued a warning that elderly patients with dementia on atypical antipsychotics were at risk of increased mortality.[1] This warning was extended to include typical antipsychotics in June 2008 after several more observational studies were published.[2] However, still in need of clarification are the actual causes of death that account for the excess mortality in these patients. Because the rate of pneumonia dramatically increases as people age, particularly from age 65 to 90+,[3] as does the rate of dementia. In addition, because patients with dementia are prone to aspiration, it seems intuitive that a significant portion of the excess mortality associated with antipsychotics is related to pneumonia. Certainly this well-designed study supports that theory; however, it does not address potential increased rates of other causes of mortality that require study. Another important finding of this study was that the development of pneumonia was dose dependent. This is an important reminder to health care providers: avoid antipsychotic medication in the elderly population if at all possible, but if that is not possible, use the lowest possible dose of these drugs or adjust to lower doses as soon as possible.

J. R. Maurer, MD, MBA

References

1. US Food and Drug Administration. Public Health Advisory. *Deaths with Antipsychotics In Reply to: Elderly Patients with Behavioral Disturbances.* Available at:. Silver Spring, MD: US Food and Drug Administration; 2005 http://www.fda.gov/Drugs/DrugSafety/PublicHealthAdvisories/ucm053171.htm; 2005.
2. US Food and Drug Administration. *FDA Requests Box Warnings on Older Class of Antipsychotic Drugs.* Available at:. Silver Spring, MD: US Food and Drug Administration; 2008 http://www.fda.gov/NewsEvents/Newsroom/PressAnnouncements/2008/ucm116912.htm; 2008.
3. Kaplan V, Angus DC, Griffin MF, Clermont G, Scott Watson R, Linde-Zwirble WT. Hospitalized community-acquired pneumonia in the elderly: age- and sex-related patterns of care and outcome in the United States. *Am J Respir Crit Care Med.* 2002;165:766-772.

The influence of pre-existing diabetes mellitus on the host immune response and outcome of pneumonia: analysis of two multicentre cohort studies

Yende S, for the GenIMS and Health ABC study (Univ of Pittsburgh, PA; et al)
Thorax 65:870-877, 2010

Background.—Although diabetes mellitus is implicated in susceptibility to infection, the association of diabetes with the subsequent course and outcome is unclear.

Methods.—A retrospective analysis of two multicentre cohorts was carried out. The effect of pre-existing diabetes on the host immune response, acute organ function and mortality in patients hospitalised with community-acquired pneumonia (CAP) in the GenIMS study (n=1895) and on mortality following either CAP or non-infectious hospitalisations in the population-based cohort study, Health ABC (n=1639) was determined. Measurements included the mortality rate within the first year, risk of organ dysfunction, and immune responses, including circulating inflammatory (tumour necrosis factor, interleukin 6, interleukin 10), coagulation (Factor IX, thrombin–antithrombin complexes, antithrombin), fibrinolysis (plasminogen-activator inhibitor-1 and D-dimer) and cell surface markers (CD120a, CD120b, human leucocyte antigen (HLA)-DR, Toll-like receptor-2 and Toll-like receptor-4).

Results.—In GenIMS, diabetes increased the mortality rate within the first year after CAP (unadjusted HR 1.41, 95% CI 1.12 to 1.76, p=0.002), even after adjusting for pre-existing cardiovascular and renal disease (adjusted HR 1.3, 95% CI 1.03 to 1.65, p=0.02). In Health ABC, diabetes increased the mortality rate within the first year following CAP hospitalisation, but not after hospitalisation for non-infectious illnesses (significant interaction for diabetes and reason for hospitalisation (p=0.04); HR for diabetes on mortality over the first year after CAP 1.87, 95% CI 0.76 to 4.6, p=0.16, and after non-infectious hospitalisation 1.16, 95% CI 0.8 to 1.6, p=0.37). In GenIMS, immediate immune response was similar, as evidenced by similar circulating immune marker levels, in the

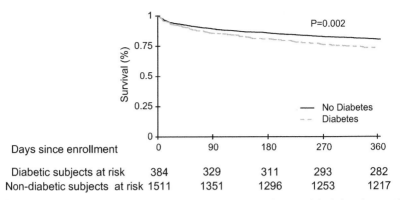

FIGURE 1.—Kaplan–Meier survival curves over 1 year showing higher risk of death for subjects with diabetes compared with those without diabetes following hospitalisation for community-acquired pneumonia in GenIMS. (Reprinted from Yende S, for the GenIMS and Health ABC study. The influence of pre-existing diabetes mellitus on the host immune response and outcome of pneumonia: analysis of two multicentre cohort studies. *Thorax.* 2010;65:870-877, and reproduced/amended with permission from the BMJ Publishing Group.)

emergency department and during the first week. Those with diabetes had a higher risk of acute kidney injury during hospitalisation (39.3% vs 31.7%, p=0.005) and they were more likely to die due to cardiovascular and kidney disease (34.4% vs 26.8% and 10.4% vs 4.5%, p=0.03).

Conclusions.—Pre-existing diabetes was associated with a higher risk of death following CAP. The mechanism is not due to an altered immune response, at least as measured by a broad panel of circulating and cell surface markers, but may be due to worsening of pre-existing cardiovascular and kidney disease (Fig 1).

▶ It is often stated that patients have higher risk of infections, but it is not clear whether infections in patients with diabetes result in higher complication or death rates than in patients without diabetes. This is an increasingly important question because rates of diabetes mellitus are rising dramatically in many countries; if infections such as pneumonia are more common in these patients, more information about the impact of infections is critical to improving management. The authors of this study compared diabetic patients with nondiabetic patients in 2 large observational studies that contained large groups of patients with diabetes. The Genetic and Inflammatory Markers of Sepsis (GenIMS) study included patients presenting to emergency rooms with community-acquired pneumonia from 28 institutions in 4 regions of the United States. In this study, multiple measures of inflammation were measured and that allowed the authors to compare immune responses and mortality in 384 patients with diabetes with those of 1511 nondiabetic patients from the Health, Ageing, and Body Composition (Health ABC) study, a population-based cohort of 70- to 79-year-old well-functioning adults, the authors followed 299 patients with diabetes and 1340 without diabetes who were hospitalized within the first 5 years of follow-up. Several interesting observations came out of this study. First, that immune response as measured by the markers used in GenIMS doesn't seem to be different between patients with diabetes and patients without diabetes, though patients with diabetes clearly have higher mortality rates during the first year after hospitalization for pneumonia, and 20% of all patients with community-acquired pneumonia had diabetes. Interestingly, in the Health ABC study, mortality was higher in the hospitalized diabetes cohort, when the hospitalization was for diabetes and not other causes. Possibly one of the most instructive findings was that the rate of acute kidney injury in patients with diabetes and with pneumonia was 1.3 times that of patients without diabetes. As the authors suggest, the burden of a serious infection could be the tipping point for patients with subclinical microvascular disease. Given the epidemic of diabetes that is occurring in many countries, it is critical to undertake research that will enable us to better understand the impact of diabetes on the pathophysiology and outcome of common acute illnesses such as pneumonia.

J. R. Maurer, MD, MBA

Severity assessment tools for predicting mortality in hospitalised patients with community-acquired pneumonia. Systematic review and meta-analysis
Chalmers JD, Singanayagam A, Akram AR, et al (Univ of Edinburgh, UK; Royal Infirmary of Edinburgh, UK; et al)
Thorax 65:878-883, 2010

Introduction.—International guidelines recommend a severity-based approach to management in community-acquired pneumonia. CURB65, CRB65 and the Pneumonia Severity Index (PSI) are the most widely recommended severity scores. The aim of this study was to compare the performance characteristics of these scores for predicting mortality in community-acquired pneumonia.

Methods.—A systematic review and meta-analysis was conducted according to MOOSE (meta-analysis of observational studies in epidemiology) guidelines. PUBMED and EMBASE were searched (1980–2009). 40 studies reporting prognostic information for the PSI, CURB65 and CRB65 severity scores were identified. Performance characteristics were pooled using a random effects model. Relationships between sensitivity and specificity were plotted using summary receiver operator characteristic (sROC) curves.

Results.—All three scores predicted 30 day mortality. The PSI had the highest area under the sROC curve, 0.81 (SE 0.008), compared with CURB65, 0.80 (SE 0.008), p=0.1, and CRB65, 0.79 (0.01), p=0.09. These differences were not statistically significant. Performance characteristics were similar across comparable cut-offs for low, intermediate and high risk for each score. In identifying low risk patients, PSI (groups I and II) had the best negative likelihood ratio 0.08 (0.06–0.12) compared with CURB65 (score 0–1) 0.21 (0.15–0.30) and CRB65 (score 0), 0.15 (0.10–0.22).

Conclusion.—There were no significant differences in overall test performance between PSI, CURB65 and CRB65 for predicting mortality from community-acquired pneumonia.

▶ Severity indices are frequently used to determine approach to management of patients presenting with community-acquired pneumonia (CAP), both in terms of antibiotic approach and venue of care. The most commonly used indices are the Pneumonia Severity Index (PSI) developed in 1997 following a large number of patients with CAP.[1] It has been widely studied, recommended by several CAP guidelines, and has generally served to steer management of less severe disease to outpatient treatment. Other widely used indices are the CURB index, developed by the British Thoracic Society, and a modification of that index that added age, the CRB65.[2] These indices are also often recommended by CAP management guidelines. This study is a large meta-analysis designed to assess the performance characteristics of the 3 indices, the most commonly used severity scores by treating clinicians. This study provides very useful information because the CURB score is generally easier to use with fewer parameters and a simpler scoring system. It is also easier to use in an outpatient (or emergency room setting). The analysis shows that all 3 predictors were relatively good and not significantly different, though PSI was slightly better at predicting low-risk patients and the CURB/CRB65 slightly better at identifying high-risk patients. The message is that all 3 indices perform well, but because the CURB and CRB65 are easier to use, they may be preferred.

J. R. Maurer, MD, MBA

References

1. Fine MJ, Auble TE, Yealy DM, et al. A prediction rule to identify low-risk patients with community-acquired pneumonia. *N Engl J Med.* 1997;336:243-250.
2. Lim WS, van der Eerden MM, Laing R, et al. Defining community-acquired pneumonia severity on presentation to hospital: an international derivation and validation study. *Thorax.* 2003;58:377-382.

A multicenter analysis of the ED diagnosis of pneumonia

Chandra A, Nicks B, Maniago E, et al (Duke Univ Med Ctr Durham, NC; Wake Forest Univ Baptist Med Ctr, Winston Salem, NC; Staten Island Univ Hosp, NY)
Am J Emerg Med 28:862-865, 2010

Objectives.—The objective of this study was to describe the prevalence of pneumonia-like signs and symptoms in patients admitted from the emergency department (ED) with a diagnosis of community acquired pneumonia (CAP) but subsequently discharged from the hospital with a nonpneumonia diagnosis.

Methods.—A retrospective, structured, chart review of ED patients with CAP at 3 academic hospitals was performed by trained extractors on all adult patients admitted for CAP. Demographic data, Pneumonia Patient Outcomes Research Team scores, and discharge diagnosis data (*International Classification of Diseases, Ninth Revision* [ICD-9] codes) were extracted using a predetermined case report form.

Results.—A total of 800 patients were admitted from the ED with a diagnosis of CAP from the 3 hospitals, and 219 (27.3%; 95% confidence interval [CI], 24-31) ultimately had a nonpneumonia diagnosis upon discharge. Characteristics of this group included a mean age of 62.6 years, 50% female, and a history of congestive heart failure (CHF) (14%) or cancer (12%). After excluding patients with missing data, 123 patients (65%) had an abnormal chest x-ray, and 13% had abnormal oxygen saturation. Cough, sputum production, fever, tachypnea, or leukocytosis were present in 91.5% of this cohort, and 63.8% had at least 2 of these findings. Twenty alternate *ICD-9*s were identified, including non-CAP pulmonary disease (18%; 95% CI, 13-24), renal disease (16%; 95% CI, 13-19), other infections (9%; 95% CI, 7-11), cardiovascular diseases (3%; 95% CI, 2-4), and other miscellaneous diagnosis (28%; 95% CI, 25-31).

Conclusions.—Our data suggest that the ED diagnosis of CAP frequently differs from the discharge diagnosis. This may be due to the fact that a diagnosis of CAP relies on a combination of potentially nonspecific clinical and radiographic features. New diagnostic approaches and tools with better specificity are needed to improve ED diagnosis of CAP.

▶ Data collected from large content management system databases have resulted in the development of quality standards for the acute management of community-acquired pneumonia.[1] One of the most controversial of these standards has been the timing of delivery of the first dose of antibiotic treatment. Because database analysis showed that patients receiving antibiotics early (typically within 4 hours of presentation) had lower mortality rates, antibiotic timing became a critical quality measure. This has led to concerns around several issues. First, clinicians note that patients, especially elderly patients, with congestive heart failure or other conditions may be given unnecessary (and potentially harmful) antibiotics. Second, there is a concern that with the emphasis on early antibiotics, other diagnoses may be overlooked or delayed to the patient's detriment. Third, overuse of antibiotics is both costly and may increase antibiotic resistance. Fourth, there is concern that the use of a retrospective database to inform widespread, prospective, acute care may be treacherous. This study is the latest and a multicenter study that suggests that an emergency room diagnosis of community-acquired pneumonia is wrong at least one-quarter of the time and that currently used signs, symptoms, and tests often do not adequately separate pneumonia from other conditions. I agree with the authors that increased research into more specific means of diagnosis are urgently needed as are studies looking at varied timing of first antibiotic administration.

J. R. Maurer, MD, MBA

Reference

1. Houck PM, Bratzler DW, Nsa W, Ma A, Bartlett JG. Timing of antibiotic administration and outcomes for Medicare patients hospitalized with community-acquired pneumonia. *Arch Intern Med.* 2004;164:637-644.

6 Lung Transplantation

Introduction

In 2010, the Organ Procurement Transplantation Network (OPTN) reported that 1618 lung transplants were performed in the United States.[1] This was slightly fewer than the 1660 performed in 2009, but about 200 more than were performed each year between 2005 and 2008. Another trend worth noting is that there were no living donor transplants reported for 2010. The numbers of this type of transplant peaked in the high 20s per year around 2000, and in the last few years they have fallen to minimal numbers per year.

In 2005, a new algorithm for allocation of donor lungs was put into place. This fundamentally changed the criteria for allocation from one of "longest on the waitlist" to one of "sickest first." An algorithm for criteria of "sickest" (meaning shortest predicted survival) was derived from data of patients who had been known to die on the waitlist and other sources. Formal evaluations of the impact of this change addressing outcomes and costs associated with those outcomes are beginning to appear in the literature. The first 2 papers in this section address the new allocation system.

The next 2 articles in the section address donor quality. Many approaches have been explored over the years to try to increase the number of donors. One of the more recent is using organs from non-heart–beating donors coming from different situations, such as controlled (taken off life support) and noncontrolled (in cardiac arrest on presentation). The article by Erasmus et al reports on use of "controlled" situation donors who appear to be the most viable but also most controversial. A second article suggests that much can be learned about cadaveric donors by analyzing past experience and that there may be significant issues affecting the donor quality that have little to do directly with the lungs.

New information on transplant outcomes is represented in articles by Keating et al and Weiss et al. The Keating study presents outcomes of living lobar donors that were followed up to 3½ years. The Weiss et al study looks at a group of patients surviving 10 years and compares them to patients who survived less than 5 years in terms of causes of death, complications, and other factors.

Bronchiolitis obliterans is always a topic of many studies because it remains the greatest threat to a transplanted lung and is the major underlying factor in deaths. Studies in this edition from 2010 address donor factors associated with the development of bronchiolitis obliterans as well as approaches to treatment that include azithromycin and photophoresis. Progress in addressing underlying factors and in management of this devastating problem remain limited.

The remaining 4 papers in this chapter address 4 different topics: a renewed interest in using silicone stents over metal stents for airway management, the use of invasive biopsies as opposed to transbronchial approaches in assessing certain lung abnormalities post transplant, the potential role of natural killer cells in acute rejection, and a randomized controlled trial using everolimus in patients with developing renal failure.

Janet R. Maurer, MD, MBA

References

1. http://www.unos.org/donation/index.php?topic=data. Accessed February 26, 2011.

The efficacy of photopheresis for bronchiolitis obliterans syndrome after lung transplantation

Morrell MR, Despotis GJ, Lublin DM, et al (Washington Univ School of Medicine/Barnes-Jewish Hosp, St Louis, MO)
J Heart Lung Transplant 29:424-431, 2010

Background.—Extracorporeal photopheresis (ECP) has been used to treat acute and chronic rejection after solid organ transplantation. However, data supporting the use of ECP for bronchiolitis obliterans syndrome (BOS) after lung transplantation are limited.

Methods.—We retrospectively analyzed the efficacy and safety of ECP for progressive BOS at our institution. Between January 1, 2000, and December 31, 2007, 60 lung allograft recipients were treated with ECP for progressive BOS.

Results.—During the 6-month period before the initiation of ECP, the average rate of decline in forced expiratory volume in 1 second (FEV_1) was −116.0 ml/month, but the slope decreased to −28.9 ml/month during the 6-month period after the initiation of ECP, and the mean difference in the rate of decline was 87.1 ml/month (95% confidence interval, 57.3–116.9; $p < 0.0001$). The FEV_1 improved in 25.0% of patients after the initiation of ECP, with a mean increase of 20.1 ml/month.

Conclusions.—ECP is associated with a reduction in the rate of decline in lung function associated with progressive BOS.

▶ Photopheresis is an old treatment for bronchiolitis obliterans (BOS) dating to the mid-1990s.[1] Reports of this treatment in small numbers of patients from poorly designed studies but with encouraging reports (such as this one) keep surfacing every couple of years. So is this a treatment that works, and, if so, why hasn't it caught on? There are several reasons. First, like this article, most studies show in most patients a change in the rate of decline of forced expiratory volume in 1 second but not a change in the rate of death from BOS. Second, this treatment is usually, as in this article, a last approach once BOS is established and other treatments have failed. Thus long-term follow-up is often hard to do because of the high death rate of the patients undergoing the treatments. Third, and possibly an explanation for its late use in BOS, is the cost. At the study institution, the cost of each treatment, which lasts for hours, is $6663, so 24 treatments cost almost $160 000, which is actually greater than the cost of the original transplant in many institutions. Surely this warrants a prospective assessment of photopheresis, compared with other approaches (eg, azithromycin) in early BOS to really establish whether the resource consumption of the approach is warranted.

J. R. Maurer, MD, MBA

Reference

1. Slovis BS, Loyd JE, King LE Jr. Photopheresis for chronic rejection of lung allografts. *N Eng J Med.* 1995;332:962.

Should lung transplantation be performed for patients on mechanical respiratory support? The US experience
Mason DP, Thuita L, Nowicki ER, et al (Cleveland Clinic, OH)
J Thorac Cardiovasc Surg 139:765-773, 2010

Objective.—The study objectives were to (1) compare survival after lung transplantation in patients requiring pretransplant mechanical ventilation or extracorporeal membrane oxygenation with that of patients not requiring mechanical support and (2) identify risk factors for mortality.

Methods.—Data were obtained from the United Network for Organ Sharing for lung transplantation from October 1987 to January 2008. A total of 15,934 primary transplants were performed: 586 in patients on mechanical ventilation and 51 in patients on extracorporeal membrane oxygenation. Differences between nonsupport patients and those on mechanical ventilation or extracorporeal membrane oxygenation support were expressed as 2 propensity scores for use in comparing risk-adjusted survival.

Results.—Unadjusted survival at 1, 6, 12, and 24 months was 83%, 67%, 62%, and 57% for mechanical ventilation, respectively; 72%, 53%, 50%, and 45% for extracorporeal membrane oxygenation, respectively; and 93%, 85%, 79%, and 70% for unsupported patients, respectively ($P < .0001$). Recipients on mechanical ventilation were younger, had lower forced vital capacity, and had diagnoses other than emphysema. Recipients on extracorporeal membrane oxygenation were also younger, had higher body mass index, and had diagnoses other than cystic fibrosis/bronchiectasis. Once these variables, transplant year, and propensity for mechanical support were accounted for, survival remained worse after lung transplantation for patients on mechanical ventilation and extracorporeal membrane oxygenation.

Conclusion.—Although survival after lung transplantation is markedly worse when preoperative mechanical support is necessary, it is not dismal. Thus, additional risk factors for mortality should be considered when selecting patients for lung transplantation to maximize survival. Reduced survival for this high-risk population raises the important issue of balancing maximal individual patient survival against benefit to the maximum number of patients.

▶ At its most extreme in terms of prioritizing the sickest patients for lung transplant, the Lung Allocation Score model introduced in 2005 as the means of allocation of donor lungs to waiting recipients identifies those patients on mechanical ventilation or extracorporeal membrane oxygenation (ECMO) at the top of the waitlist (receive the highest scores). But what are the outcomes of these patients? Like the more generic article by Russo et al (included in this section), clearly the sickest patients have the worst outcomes. This particular study, using the same United Network for Organ Sharing database as the Russo et al study, broke down the sickest patients into those on mechanical ventilation and those on ECMO. Overall, these were younger patients than the overall transplant population (mean age 38-39 years) and most had diagnoses of either pulmonary fibrosis or cystic fibrosis. Nevertheless, the survivals, especially in the early posttransplant period and especially on patients supported by ECMO, were significantly worse than unsupported patients. In addition, the medical resources consumed are highest in the ECMO group, which had the lowest survivals. This again highlights the ethical issue, as the authors note, of "balancing maximal individual patient survival against benefit to the maximum number of patients," an issue that requires careful thought and fairness and will not be easy to resolve.

J. R. Maurer, MD, MBA

Factors indicative of long-term survival after lung transplantation: A review of 836 10-year survivors
Weiss ES, Allen JG, Merlo CA, et al (The Johns Hopkins Med Insts, Baltimore, MD)
J Heart Lung Transplant 29:240-246, 2010

Introduction.—Despite 20 years of lung transplantation (LTx), factors influencing long-term survival remain largely unknown. The United Network for Organ Sharing (UNOS) data set provides an opportunity to examine long-term LTx survivors.

Methods.—We conducted a case-control study embedded within the prospectively collected UNOS LTx cohort to identify 836 adults from 1987 to 1997 who survived ≥10 years after first LTx. LTx patients within the same era and surviving 1 to 5 years served as controls. Multivariable logistic regression with incorporation of spline terms evaluated the odds of being a 10-year survivor. Two separate models were constructed. Model A incorporated pre-operative, operative, and donor-specific factors. Model B incorporated the factors used in Model A with post-operative covariates. Additional outcomes evaluated included hospitalizations for infection, rejection, and bronchiolitis obliterans.

Results.—Of 4,818 LTx patients from 1987 to 1997, 836 (17.3%) survived ≥10 years with a mean follow-up of 148.8 ± 21.6 months. Mean follow-up for 1,657 controls was 34.0 ± 13.9 months. The distribution of 10-year survivors by disease was cystic fibrosis, 170 (20%); chronic obstructive pulmonary disease, 254 (30%); and idiopathic pulmonary fibrosis, 92 (11%). On multivariable logistic regression, significant factors influencing 10-year survival included age ≤35 years (odds ratio [OR] 1.07, 95% confidence interval [CI], 1.03–1.11; $p = 0.01$), bilateral LTx (OR. 1.71; 95% CI, 1.25–2.34; $p = 0.001$), and hospitalizations for infections (OR, 1.40; 95% CI, 1.27–1.54; $p < 0.001$) and for rejection (OR, 0.55; 95% CI, 0.48–0.65; $p < 0.001$).

Conclusions.—Examination of a cohort of long-term LTx survivors in the UNOS data set indicates that bilateral LTx and fewer hospitalizations for rejection may portend improved long-term survival after LTx.

▶ Are there specific characteristics or events around or after transplant that impact long-term survival? Or is it mostly luck? We have not previously had enough patients in the 10-year survival group to learn about this. For this study 10-year survivors (transplanted between 1987 and 1997) were compared with a control group of patients who were transplanted during the same 10-year period but survived only 1 to 5 years. Interestingly, the number of 10-year survivors increased dramatically between 1987 and 1990 but remained constant for the next 7 years. More than 60% of 10-year survivors had bronchiolitis obliterans syndrome (BOS) compared with about 45% of the controls; however, the controls died more often of BOS. Ten-year survivors were more likely to die of nonspecific respiratory failure or malignancy. Possibly, the most important finding in this analysis was the significant impact of bilateral transplant. In patients surviving at least a year, the impact of receiving a bilateral transplant instead of a unilateral transplant was to double the odds of surviving for 10 years. While many centers have routinely adopted bilateral transplant for most candidates for a variety of reasons, this objective finding suggests substantial utility to this approach and may have implications for overall lung transplant policy decisions.

J. R. Maurer, MD, MBA

Long-term outcomes of cadaveric lobar lung transplantation: Helping to maximize resources

Keating DT, Marasco SF, Negri J, et al (Alfred Hosp, Prahran, Victoria, Australia)
J Heart Lung Transplant 29:439-444, 2010

Background.—Cadaveric lobar lung transplantation (CLLTx) represents a potential opportunity to address the bias against smaller recipients, especially children, on transplant waiting lists. The widespread use of CLLTx is hindered by the paucity of outcome data with respect to early complications and long-term lung function and survival.

Methods.—We looked at the long-term outcomes in 9 patients undergoing CLLTx since May 2003, including early surgical complications, pulmonary function tests, and survival. Patients were analyzed by whether the decision to perform CLLTx was elective (made at the time of listing) or emergent (surgical decision).

Results.—The incidence of early complications in the entire group was low, with the most common being atrial arrhythmias and prolonged thoracostomy tube. Lung function at 1 and 2 years (mean forced expiratory volume in 1 second % predicted ± standard deviation of 73 ± 18 and 60.5 ± 27, respectively) was equivalent to living lobar transplant results. Overall survival was similar to 199 patients who received conventional cadaveric LTx during the same period.

Conclusion.—This study suggests that CLLTx has a low complication rate with acceptable lung function and long-term survival, especially in cases where consideration has been given to CLLTx at the time of listing. CLLTx warrants consideration more often for patients of smaller physique to improve their chance of receiving LTx.

► The option of lung transplantation for end-stage disease remains limited by donor scarcity despite relaxed standards for acceptance of donor organs and occasional use of living lobar donors. This article describes reasonable survival rates in patients followed up to 3.5 years who received cadaveric lobar transplants. Living lobar transplantation has been quite limited because it usually is performed using 2 donors who each donate a lobe. Cadaveric lobar transplantation has not become more widespread either probably because of the lack of long-term outcomes reported and because this is typically performed using only one lobe and therefore is an option only for smaller adult patients and pediatric patients. Nevertheless, the survivals reported here suggest a role for this approach. Increased use of cadaveric lobar transplant could increase the donor pool in that lobes could be recovered from cadaveric lungs that otherwise are not useable because of localized lesions.

J. R. Maurer, MD, MBA

Azithromycin is associated with increased survival in lung transplant recipients with bronchiolitis obliterans syndrome

Jain R, Hachem RR, Morrell MR, et al (Washington Univ School of Medicine, St Louis, MO)

J Heart Lung Transplant 29:531-537, 2010

Background.—Previous studies have suggested that azithromycin improves lung function in lung transplant recipients with bronchiolitis obliterans syndrome (BOS). However, these studies did not include a non-treated BOS control cohort or perform survival analysis. This study was undertaken to estimate the effect of azithromycin treatment on survival in lung transplant recipients with BOS.

Methods.—We conducted a retrospective cohort study of consecutive lung transplant recipients who developed BOS between 1999 and 2007. An association between azithromycin treatment and death was assessed using univariate and multivariate time-dependent Cox regression analysis.

Results.—Of the 178 recipients who developed BOS in our study, 78 did so after 2003 and were treated with azithromycin. The azithromycin-treated and untreated cohorts had similar baseline characteristics. Univariate analysis demonstrated that azithromycin treatment was associated with a survival advantage and this beneficial treatment effect was more pronounced when treatment was initiated during BOS Stage 1. Multivariate analysis demonstrated azithromycin treatment during BOS Stage 1 (adjusted hazard ratio $= 0.23$, $p = 0.01$) and absolute forced expiratory volume in 1 second (FEV_1) at the time of BOS Stage 1 (adjusted hazard ratio $= 0.52$, $p = 0.003$) were both associated with a decreased risk of death.

Conclusions.—In lung transplant recipients with BOS Stage 1, azithromycin treatment initiated before BOS Stage 2 was independently associated with a significant reduction in the risk of death. This finding supports the need for a randomized, controlled trial to confirm the impact of azithromycin on survival in lung transplant recipients.

▶ Azithromycin is a hot drug in the prevention and management of bronchiolitis obliterans syndrome (BOS). Theoretically, there are very good reasons for thinking it might be useful. As the authors note, it is a macrolide antibiotic that not only inhibits interleukin-8–mediated inflammation and is antimicrobial but is also prokinetic in the gastrointestinal tract. Thus, it potentially helps combat lymphocytic bronchiolitis as well as aspiration, both of which appear to be risk factors for BOS. Unfortunately, the quality of studies published to date are not generally of high quality in that they have small numbers, do not have control groups, and have short follow-up periods. The gold standard would be a prospective, randomized double-blinded trial in which azithromycin would be compared with placebo. Because many of the studies published so far, though poor in quality, tend to show increases or maintenance of lung function, it may be difficult to convince centers to do a true randomized controlled trial. This study is not a prospective trial; it is a retrospective cohort study designed in this way. Almost 300 consecutive lung transplants performed at a single center over a 6-year period were entered into the study. Then 78 patients who had or developed BOS in 2003 when azithromycin use was initiated for BOS in this population were divided into 2 cohorts: those with BOS stage 2 or greater and those with BOS stage 1 or less. The control comparator was a group of patients who developed BOS before 2003 when azithromycin was not being used for treatment. Data are presented only in terms of risk of death in the different groups, not in any parameter relative to movement from one stage of BOS to another or other interim changes; so we lack detail of the impact of azithromycin, particularly in terms of differences within the population. While this is a valiant attempt to improve the study methodology, in the end, the groups remain small and all the inherent biases of retrospective studies remain. Because of the widespread use of azithromycin now, even as a preventive drug, it is likely that the most useful data about its impact on BOS will come from historical trends in large databases of transplant recipients.

J. R. Maurer, MD, MBA

A retrospective study of silicone stent placement for management of anastomotic airway complications in lung transplant recipients: Short- and long-term outcomes

Dutau H, Cavailles A, Sakr L, et al (Université de la Méditerrannée, Marseille, France)

J Heart Lung Transplant 29:658-664, 2010

Background.—Airway anastomotic complications remain a major cause of morbidity and mortality after lung transplantation (LT). Few data are available with regard to the use of silicone stents for these airway disorders. The aim of this retrospective study was to evaluate the clinical efficacy and safety of silicone stents for such an indication.

Methods.—Data of adult lung transplant recipients who had procedures performed between January 1997 and December 2007 at our institution were reviewed retrospectively. We included patients with post-transplant airway complications who required bronchoscopic intervention with a silicone stent.

Results.—In 17 of 117 (14.5%) LT recipients, silicone stents were inserted at a mean time of 165 (range 5 to 360) days after surgery in order to palliate 23 anastomotic airway stenoses. Symptomatic improvement was noted in all patients, and mean forced expiratory volume in 1 second (FEV1) increased by 672 ± 496 ml ($p < 0.001$) after stent insertion. The stent-related complication rate was 0.13/patient per month. The latter consisted of obstructive granulomas ($n = 10$), mucus plugging ($n = 7$) and migration ($n = 7$), which were of mild to moderate severity and were successfully managed endoscopically. Mean stent duration was 266 days (range 24 to 1,407 days). Successful stent removal was achieved in 16 of 23 cases (69.5%) without recurrence of stenosis. Overall survival was similar in patients with and without airway complications ($p = 0.36$).

Conclusions.—Silicone stents allow clinical and lung function improvement in patients with LT-related airway complications. Stent-related complications were of mild to moderate severity, and were appropriately managed endoscopically. Permanent resolution of airway stenosis was obtained in most patients, allowing definitive stent removal without recurrence.

▶ Airway complications have always plagued lung transplantation. The complications, which are usually attributed to relative ischemia of the bronchus, range from dehiscence to stenosis to malacia. They occur to a degree requiring intervention, in most series, in 15% to 20% of patients. Dilatation or other measures are often temporary successes unfortunately, and many patients will go on to require stents. In the 1980s silicone stents were often used but had problems with migration, infection, and granuloma formation. With the advent of metal mesh stents, these became almost universally used. Metal stents rarely migrated but had some drawbacks, including significant granuloma formation, infection, and rare migration. The biggest drawback, however, was that once a metal stent is placed, it is very hard to remove, especially after a few weeks. And complications typically have to be managed with the stent in place. Thus, for most patients, once a metal stent is in place, it is there for life. In 2005, the Food and Drug Administration issued a public health advisory about the complications of metal stents used to treat benign airway problems.[1] This has made the use of metal stents less popular and some lung transplant programs have reverted to using silicone stents. This article suggests that the complications related to silicone stents are no greater than those associated with metal stents and most can be permanently removed after varying periods.

J. R. Maurer, MD, MBA

Reference

1. FDA Public Health Notification: Complications from Metallic Tracheal Stents in Patients with Benign Airway Disorders. http://www.fda.gov/MedicalDevices/Safety/AlertsandNotices/PublicHealthNotifications/ucm062115.htm. Accessed April 5, 2011.

Invasive biopsy is effective and useful after lung transplant
Burdett CL, Critchley RJ, Black F, et al (Newcastle Univ, UK; The Freeman Hosp, High Heaton, Newcastle upon Tyne, UK)
J Heart Lung Transplant 29:759-763, 2010

Background.—Transbronchial biopsy (TBB) is widely used after lung transplant but may not be diagnostic. Our group has used invasive approaches, open lung biopsy (OLB) or video-assisted thoracoscopy (VAT), to establish a definitive diagnosis in unexplained clinical deterioration. We sought to demonstrate the risks and benefits of this approach.

Methods.—A retrospective review was made of the case notes of the patients undergoing OLB or VAT during a 12-year period from August 1996.

Results.—During a 12-year period in 442 recipients, there were 51 invasive biopsies in 45 patients (6 had 2 procedures), of which 41 (80%) were OLB and 10 (20%) were VAT. Time of biopsy ranged from 7 days to 11 years after transplant. Thirty-seven (73%) took place in the first year, including 12 (24%) within the first 30 days. Nine patients died within 30 days of biopsy; 7 of them were already ventilated. Overall, biopsy provided a new unsuspected diagnosis in 37% of patients and confirmed the diagnostic suspicion in 47%. In only 16% of patients did it fail to provide a result that was clinically useful. The results of 29 (57%) biopsies led to a change in treatment. Sixty-three percent of new diagnoses and 71% where clinical suspicion was confirmed resulted in a treatment change. In all but 2 cases, a change was made to medication.

Conclusions.—In this large series of invasive biopsies, there was a high rate of useful results, with a frequent change in treatment. Invasive biopsies are a safe intervention in ambulatory patients.

▶ Transplant physicians are often reluctant to resort to open procedures on lung transplant recipients to get a diagnosis. There are concerns (not well documented) about bleeding or prolonged air leaks due to complicated pleural spaces resulting from the original transplant surgery and possibly a fear of worsening of the clinical picture because of the invasive procedure. Thus, transbronchial biopsy or even repeated transbronchial biopsy have been the only paths pursued for diagnosis with the result often of an uncertain diagnosis and a shotgun approach to therapy. In this instructive report of more than 50 open procedures, both video-assisted thoracoscopy and open-lung biopsies, there were 19 cases in which a previously unknown diagnosis was established. Most of the biopsies that were clinically helpful were done within 1 month of transplant; however, 3 biopsies taken greater than 5 years from transplant also yielded useful clinical information. Complications primarily were prolonged ventilation and prolonged air leak. Though 9 patients died within 30 days of the procedure, none of the deaths were thought related to the procedure. This experience suggests an early role for open biopsy in lieu of shotgun therapy, particularly if initial transbronchial biopsy is equivocal or nondiagnostic.

J. R. Maurer, MD, MBA

Lung Transplantation from Nonheparinized Category III Non-Heart-Beating Donors. A Single-Centre Report
Erasmus ME, Verschuuren EAM, Nijkamp DM, et al (Univ of Groningen, The Netherlands; et al)
Transplantation 89:452-457, 2010

Background.—Despite the increasing use of extended lung donors, the shortage of lung donors remains. Usage of non-heart-beating (NHB) lung donors contributes to fight this shortage. We describe our experience in 21 consecutive adult lung transplantations using nonheparinized category III NHB donors and standard flush preservation.

Methods.—From January 2005 to December 2008, we collected donor and recipient data of all NHB category III lung transplantations performed in our center. For comparison, we also collected the data of all heart-beating (HB) lung transplantations in the same period. We focused on data describing the donor, the donor procedure, the recipient's primary graft dysfunction, survival, rejection episodes, and the lung graft function.

Results.—Twenty-one NHB and 77 HB lung transplantations were performed. Circulation arrest occurred after 14 (4–62) min and warm ischemia time was 30 (19–44) min. Occurrence of primary graft dysfunction, acute rejection episodes, development of bronchiolitis obliterans syndrome was equal to the HB cohort as was the 2 years survival of 95% in the NHB group compared with 86% in the HB group. Lung graft function during the first 2 years tended to be better preserved in the NHB group.

Conclusion.—Category III NHB lung donation is a good alternative in addition to HB lung donation. Using nonheparinized category III NHB donors and standard ante- and retrograde, flush perfusion resulted in good lung graft function and survival. NHB donation offers a great opportunity to reduce the burden of donor lung shortage.

▶ This is one in an increasing number of reports on the use of lungs from nonheart beating donors, a rapidly growing approach to enlarging the donor pool. The use of nonheart beating donors became a research focus in the late 1990s but really gained momentum in the last decade when preliminary success in clinical transplant began to be reported.[1,2] Five different types of nonheart beating donors are recognized (modified Maastricht classification): category 1 are dead on arrival donors; category 2 are those who have failed resuscitation; category 3 are donors who are removed from life support, and organs are retrieved some period after vital signs cease; category 4 are brainstem dead donors who experience cardiac arrest; and category 5 are critically ill donors who experience unexpected cardiac arrest.[3] Most series, including this study, report on the use of category 3 donors as retrieving these donors can be done in much more controlled situations. The outcomes of recipients receiving organs from category 3 donors have been very similar to those of the standard heart-beating donors. Ongoing discussion focuses on ethical issues surrounding this type of donor. Clearly, the transplant team can have no involvement in the decision to actually remove life support. Other questions. such as whether medication to improve organ quality can be given before removal of life support or how long retrieval teams must wait after vital signs cease. are the topics of ongoing discussions and refinement.

J. R. Maurer, MD, MBA

References

1. Steen S, Sjöberg T, Pierre L, Liao Q, Eriksson L, Algotsson L. Transplantation of lungs from a non-heart beating donor. *Lancet.* 2001;357:825-829.

2. Butt TA, Aitchison JD, Corris PA, et al. Lung transplantation from deceased donors without pretreatment. *J Heart Lung Transplant.* 2007;26:s110.
3. Ridley S, Bonner S, Bray K, Falvey S, Mackay J, Manara A, Intensive Care Society's Working Group on Organ and Tissue Donation. UK guidance for non-heart-beating donation. *Br J Anaesth.* 2005;95:592-595.

High Lung Allocation Score Is Associated With Increased Morbidity and Mortality Following Transplantation

Russo MJ, Iribarne A, Hong KN, et al (Columbia Univ, NY; et al)
Chest 137:651-657, 2010

Background.—The lung allocation score (LAS) was initiated in May 2005 to allocate lungs based on medical urgency and posttransplant survival. The purpose of this study was to determine if there is an association between an elevated LAS at the time of transplantation and increased postoperative morbidity and mortality.

Methods.—The United Network for Organ Sharing provided de-identified patient-level data. Analysis included lung transplant recipients aged ≥ 12 years who received transplants between April 5, 2006, and December 31, 2007 (n = 3,836). Recipients were stratified into three groups: LAS < 50 (n = 3,161, 83.87%), LAS 50 to 75 (n = 411, 10.9%), and LAS ≥ 75 (n = 197, 5.23%), referred to as low LAS (LLAS), intermediate LAS (ILAS), and high LAS (HLAS), respectively. The primary outcome was posttransplant graft survival at 1 year. Secondary outcomes included length of stay and in-hospital complications.

Results.—HLAS recipients had significantly worse actuarial survival at 90 days and 1 year compared with LLAS recipients. When transplant recipients were stratified by disease etiology, a trend of decreased survival with elevated LAS was observed across all major causes of lung transplant. HLAS recipients were more likely to require dialysis or to have infections compared with LLAS recipients ($P < .001$). In addition, length of stay was higher in the HLAS group when compared with the LLAS group ($P < .001$).

Conclusions.—HLAS is associated with decreased survival and increased complications during the transplant hospitalization. Whereas the LAS has improved organ allocation through decreased waiting list deaths and waiting list times, lower survival and higher morbidity among HLAS recipients suggests that continued review of LAS scoring is needed to ensure optimal long-term transplant survival (Fig 2).

▶ In May 2005, the United Network for Organ Sharing adopted a new system for allocation of donor lungs to waiting recipients. This new system was based on a model designed to prioritize waiting recipients such that those likely to receive the most benefit rose to the top of the waiting list.[1] The measure used to determine "most benefit" is likelihood of survival to 1 year posttransplant. This was quite different from the traditional model that prioritized potential

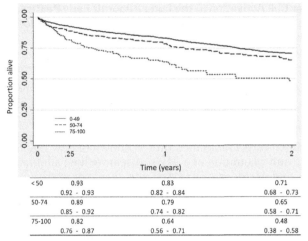

< 50	0.93	0.83	0.71
	0.92 - 0.93	0.82 - 0.84	0.68 - 0.73
50-74	0.89	0.79	0.65
	0.85 - 0.92	0.74 - 0.82	0.58 - 0.71
75-100	0.82	0.64	0.48
	0.76 - 0.87	0.56 - 0.71	0.38 - 0.58

FIGURE 2.—Kaplan-Meier survival curve of patients transplanted by LAS. (Reprinted from Russo MJ, Iribarne A, Hong KN, et al. High lung allocation score is associated with increased morbidity and mortality following transplantation. *Chest.* 2010;137:651-657, with permission from American College of Chest Physicians.)

recipients according to time on the waiting list. As predicted, the initial impact of the new model was to create a shift in the numbers of different diagnoses receiving transplants; ie, those with more rapidly progressive disease, such as idiopathic pulmonary fibrosis, were more often prioritized for transplant. Now, several years after the implementation of the new model, data on survival are being analyzed with interesting results. This article and 2 others document that patients with high to very high scores in the new allocation system have poorer survivals than patients with lower scores, and they consume higher levels of medical resources in the peritransplant period.[2,3] Very scarce resources, such as donor organs, should be allocated in a way that aims to achieve a societal goal of optimal cost-effective benefit. It could be argued that the current allocation system is not achieving that goal and that some revision of the model that better achieves "most benefit" should be undertaken as argued in the article by Gries et al.

J. R. Maurer, MD, MBA

References

1. Egan TM, Murray S, Bustami RT, et al. Development of the new lung allocation system in the United States. *Am J Transplant.* 2006;6:1212-1227.
2. Gries CJ, Rue TC, Heagerty PJ, Edelman JD, Mulligan MS, Goss CH. Development of a model for long-term survival after lung transplantation and implications for the lung allocation score. *J Heart Lung Transplant.* 2010;29:731-738.
3. Liu V, Zamora MR, Dhillon GS, Weill D. Increasing lung allocation scores predict worsened survival among lung transplant recipients. *Am J Transplant.* 2010;10: 915-920.

Natural Killer Cell Activation in the Lung Allograft Early Posttransplantation

Meehan AC, Sullivan LC, Mifsud NA, et al (Monash Univ, Melbourne, Victoria, Australia; Univ of Melbourne, Victoria, Australia)
Transplantation 89:756-763, 2010

Background.—In addition to their known antiviral and host defense functions, emerging evidence suggests that natural killer (NK) cells may influence allograft outcomes after solid organ transplantation. Although it is accepted that NK cells are activated in the absence of self-major histocompatibility complex (MHC) class I molecules, little is known of how NK cell dynamics change after transplantation of a MHC disparate lung allograft.

Materials and Methods.—To assess this, we characterized longitudinal changes in NK cell frequency and phenotype, using flow cytometry, both in the peripheral blood and lung allograft in 34 patients undergoing lung transplantation.

Results.—NK cell frequency decreased with time from transplant with mature NK cells being replaced by a population of less differentiated NK cells expressing lower levels of killer cell immunoglobulin-like receptors. In contrast to peripheral blood, NK cells within the allograft consisted of a greater proportion of CD56^{bright} cells, expressed less killer cell immunoglobulin-like receptors, and demonstrated an activated phenotype. In clinically stable recipients, peripheral blood NK cells were not activated, however, this contrasted markedly with a small subset of patients experiencing acute allograft rejection or cytomegalovirus reactivation, whose NK cells demonstrated a more activated profile.

Conclusions.—Our studies suggest that NK cells become activated after MHC-mismatched lung transplantation.

▶ Natural killer (NK) cells are part of the innate immunity and do not require previous antigen exposure for an effector response. They provide a first-line defense against pathogens and can directly secrete chemokines, cytokines, or be cytoxic. Their role in lung transplant immunology is beginning to be explored, but little data is currently available. Studies in other solid organ transplant have shown varying results, including influence both on graft survival and graft dysfunction depending on the complex immune influence of NK cells on tolerance or rejection pathways. On one hand, NK cells could interact with donor-derived antigen presenting cells to inhibit allopresentation and participate in tolerance induction. But on the other hand, NK cells in the graft can potentially become activated when there are no self-major histocompatibility complex (MHC) molecules present. In this study, activated NK cells were found in patients receiving MHC-mismatched grafts and were more activated in patients experiencing acute rejection or viral infection. However, role of an NK cell in these episodes is not clear. In other recent studies, NK cells were also associated with chronic rejection, likely a very different process from acute rejection.[1] The role of an NK cell in lung transplant outcomes is likely very complex and will require much more study to be fully understood.

J. R. Maurer, MD, MBA

Reference

1. Fildes JE, Yonan N, Tunstall K, et al. Natural killer cells in peripheral blood and lung tissue are associated with chronic rejection after lung transplantation. *J Heart Lung Transplant.* 2008;27:203-207.

Everolimus With Reduced Calcineurin Inhibitor in Thoracic Transplant Recipients With Renal Dysfunction: A Multicenter, Randomized Trial

Gullestad L, Iversen M, Mortensen S-A, et al (Univ of Oslo, Norway; Rigshospitalet, Copenhagen, Denmark; et al)

Transplantation 89:864-872, 2010

Background.—The proliferation signal inhibitor everolimus offers the potential to reduce calcineurin inhibitor (CNI) exposure and alleviate CNI-related nephrotoxicity. Randomized trials in maintenance thoracic transplant patients are lacking.

Methods.—In a 12-month, open-labeled, multicenter study, maintenance thoracic transplant patients (glomerular filtration rate ≥ 20 mL/min/1.73 m^2 and <90 mL/min/1.73 m^2) >1 year posttransplant were randomized to continue their current CNI-based immunosuppression or start everolimus with predefined CNI exposure reduction.

Results.—Two hundred eighty-two patients were randomized (140 everolimus, 142 controls; 190 heart, 92 lung transplants). From baseline to month 12, mean cyclosporine and tacrolimus trough levels in the everolimus cohort decreased by 57% and 56%, respectively. The primary endpoint, mean change in measured glomerular filtration rate from baseline to month 12, was 4.6 mL/min with everolimus and −0.5 mL/min in controls (P<0.0001). Everolimus-treated heart and lung transplant patients in the lowest tertile for time posttransplant exhibited mean increases of 7.8 mL/min and 4.9 mL/min, respectively. Biopsy-proven treated acute rejection occurred in six everolimus and four control heart transplant patients (P=0.54). In total, 138 everolimus patients (98.6%) and 127 control patients (89.4%) experienced one or more adverse event (P=0.002). Serious adverse events occurred in 66 everolimus patients (46.8%) and 44 controls (31.0%) (P=0.02).

Conclusion.—Introduction of everolimus with CNI reduction offers a significant improvement in renal function in maintenance heart and lung transplant recipients. The greatest benefit is observed in patients with a shorter time since transplantation (Fig 4).

▶ This study is important for a couple of reasons. First, prospective, randomized controlled clinical trials are difficult to do in thoracic transplant (especially lung transplant) because they require close cooperation between multiple centers with multiple researchers and are time consuming. Second, it has a different result than a previous study of lung transplants in which everolimus was compared with azathioprine with respect to whether or not it could delay

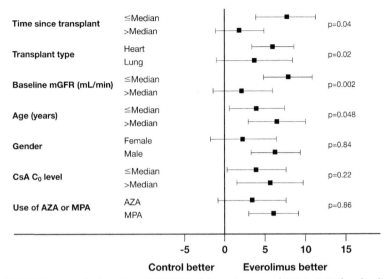

FIGURE 4.—Analysis of covariance(ANCOVA) of change in measured GFR (mGFR) from baseline to month 12 in different patient subpopulations. Values shown represent the mean between-group difference (everolimus–controls) with 95% confidence interval (CI), of change in mGFR from baseline to month 12, i.e., a positive value shows a benefit in the everolimus cohort vs. controls. Median time posttransplant, 51 months; median baseline mGFR, 48.5 mL/min; median age 60.6 years. (Reprinted from Gullestad L, Iversen M, Mortensen S-A, et al. Everolimus with reduced calcineurin inhibitor in thoracic transplant recipients with renal dysfunction: a multicenter, randomized trial. *Transplantation*. 2010;89:864-872, with permission from Lippincott Williams & Wilkins.)

progression of bronchiolitis obliterans.[1] Unfortunately in that study, worsening renal function was such a problem that many of the patients dropped from the everolimus arm.

In this study, everolimus seems to have at least reduced the rate of progression of renal failure. Theoretically, this makes sense because the mechanism of action of everolimus is similar to sirolimus (inhibitors of the kinase mammalian target of rapamycin [mTOR]) and is significantly less nephrotoxic than calcineurin inhibitors. It is known, though, that when used together, calcineurin inhibitors and mTOR inhibitors can act synergistically to worsen renal function. In the trial by Snell et al, the amounts of calcineurin inhibitor used with everolimus were apparently high enough that many patients in fact left the trial because of worsening renal function. The other important finding was that institution of the renal-saving approach earlier in the patient's course appeared to have more impact. With respect to the issue of bronchiolitis obliterans, the authors found no difference between the 2 groups but that may be because the follow-up period was too short. Hopefully, the investigators will continue to report on the pulmonary function of the control and everolimus groups so that we can learn more about the impact on bronchiolitis obliterans.

J. R. Maurer, MD, MBA

Reference

1. Snell GI, Valentine VG, Vitulo P, et al. Everolimus versus azathioprine in maintenance lung transplant recipients: an international randomized, double-blind clinical trial. *Am J Transplant*. 2006;6:169-177.

Guidelines for Donor Lung Selection: Time for Revision?
Reyes KG, Mason DP, Thuita L, et al (Cleveland Clinic, OH)
Ann Thorac Surg 89:1756-1765, 2010

Background.—Few data support current guidelines for donor selection in lung transplantation. We determined degree of compliance with current donor guidelines, effect of these and variances on survival, and other donor factors predicting survival.

Methods.—From July 1999 to June 2008, 10,333 primary transplants were performed in the US, with United Network for Organ Sharing data available for age, ABO type, chest radiograph, arterial difference in partial pressure of oxygen (Pao$_2$) greater than 300 on 100% fraction of inspired oxygen, smoking, absence of aspiration/sepsis, and purulent secretions. Multivariable survival methods were used to determine relevance of these and new variables, adjusted for recipient risk factors.

Results.—In 56% of transplants, variance from at least one guideline was observed: chest radiograph, 41%; smoking, 21%; and Pao$_2$, 18%; but rarely ABO compatibility (0.06%). Practice within guidelines was not associated with increased mortality. Common variances from guidelines; eg, Pao$_2$/fraction of inspired oxygen down to 230, were not associated with increased mortality, but smoking ($p = 0.02$) was. New donor variables associated with increased mortality were diabetes ($p = 0.001$), presence of cytomegalovirus antibodies ($p < 0.0001$), recent smoking history ($p = 0.02$), African-American ($p = 0.005$), blood type A ($p = 0.02$), death other than from head trauma ($p = 0.02$), and gender ($p = 0.02$), race ($p = 0.03$), and size ($p = 0.002$) discordances.

Conclusions.—Variance from current donor guidelines for lung transplantation is frequent; analysis suggests that donor Pao$_2$ ranges can be widened and a suspicious chest radiograph, evidence of sepsis, and purulent bronchial secretions ignored. Older age and smoking history appear to have a minor impact. New and possibly important factors identified suggest the need to better understand the impact of a wider range of donor variables on recipient outcomes.

▶ Since the 1980s when lung transplant became successful, a set of criteria has been used to assess the quality of donor lungs. These criteria—lack of infiltrates, high PaO$_2$ on oxygen challenge, lack of airway purulence, little or no smoking history, and absence of aspiration/sepsis—have been used to accept or reject organs. Strict adherence to the criteria results in rejection of most potential donor organs. Thus, in the late 1990s, transplant teams began to relax these criteria to reduce the number of lungs rejected for transplant, generally with acceptable survival results in recipients.[1,2] This article takes a different approach; the authors were able to get United Network for Organ Sharing data on donor characteristics and the traditional donor lung criteria from more than 10 000 lung donors. Not only did they find that in practice, at least one of the traditional donor graft quality criteria was broached, without an impact on mortality except when current smoking was noted, but more importantly, that other nongraft donor information may be very important. Possibly the most interesting of these was the significant reduction in survival of recipients who received grafts from donors with diabetes. The message of this study seems to be that a more comprehensive approach to donor assessment/ acceptance may be an important factor in the overall survival of transplant recipients. Further prospective studies of more general patient characteristics may be difficult to perform but could provide very valuable information.

J. R. Maurer, MD, MBA

References

1. Sundaresan S, Semenkovich J, Ochoa L, et al. Successful outcome of lung transplantation is not compromised by the use of marginal donor lungs. *J Thorac Cardiovasc Surg.* 1995;109:1075-1080.
2. Aigner C, Winkler G, Jaksch P, et al. Extended donor criteria for lung transplantation—a clinical reality. *Eur J Cardiothorac Surg.* 2005;27:757-761.

Donor Factors Are Associated With Bronchiolitis Obliterans Syndrome After Lung Transplantation

Hennessy SA, Hranjec T, Swenson BR, et al (Univ of Virginia, Charlottesville)
Ann Thorac Surg 89:1555-1562, 2010

Background.—Bronchiolitis obliterans syndrome (BOS) is the major hurdle preventing long-term success in lung transplantation, and is the primary reason for the 50% 5-year survival. Recipient and perioperative risk factors have been investigated in BOS, but less is known about donor factors. Therefore, we investigated what donor factors are important in the development of BOS.

Methods.—We performed a retrospective review of the United Network for Organ Sharing lung transplant database from 1987 to 2008. Lung transplant recipients had yearly follow-up. Donor factors were evaluated for their influence on BOS development. Kaplan-Meier plots of BOS-free survival were compared for each donor factor and a multivariate Cox proportional hazard model for BOS was created with donor factors.

Results.—A total of 17,222 lung transplant recipients were identified; 6,991 recipients had sufficient follow-up BOS data. Of these recipients 57% (n = 3,984) developed BOS within 5 years. Recipients who received lungs from donors who were younger, without an active pulmonary infection, or those without current tobacco use had longer BOS-free survival. Recipients who received lungs with higher partial pressures of oxygen in arterial blood (Pao$_2$) developed more BOS ($p < 0.0001$). Donor high Pao$_2$, older age, and current tobacco use were independent predictors of BOS in lung transplant recipients.

Conclusions.—Donor factors and donor management strategies are important contributors to development of recipient BOS. Identification of these factors may help limit BOS and may identify recipients at high risk. Surprisingly, high Pao$_2$ in the donor is an independent predictor of BOS development.

▶ Bronchiolitis obliterans syndrome (BOS) remains the principal cause of morbidity and mortality in lung transplant recipients in the intermediate and long term. A number of risk factors and potential risk factors have been identified in recipients, for example, numbers and severity of acute rejection episodes, lymphocytic bronchial infiltrates, and viral respiratory infections, that predict onset of BO. Less investigation has centered on donor and donor organ characteristics that may factor into the development of this dreaded complication.[1] This study used the extensive United Network for Organ Sharing database of organ donor and donor organ characteristics to try to identify any donor factor that might correlate with BO. Though more than 17 000 transplant recipients were included in the database, only about 7000 had sufficient follow-up data to use. Of those, however, 57% had developed BOS within 5 years, which is consistent with most reports of lung transplant survivals. Some of the donor factors associated with BOS development are not surprising, for example, older donor age and current tobacco use; however, the finding of high PaO$_2$ is surprising. In fact, high PaO$_2$ only became a factor in predicting BOS at hyperoxic ranges. High fraction of inspired oxygen (FiO$_2$) has been associated with the development of oxygen radicals and acute lung injury, but this has not previously been recognized as an issue in potential donors. The findings of this study suggest that those managing potential donors should avoid using high FiO$_2$ when possible, as this may have significant impact on the long-term outcome of the recipient.

J. R. Maurer, MD, MBA

Reference

1. Sharples LD, McNeil K, Stewart S, Wallwork J. Risk factors for bronchiolitis obliterans: a systematic review of recent publications. *J Heart Lung Transplant.* 2002; 21:271-281.

7 Sleep Disorders

Introduction

This year's Sleep Disorders articles are great! In this chapter, you will find a variety of articles on obstructive sleep apnea. We continue to learn about the consequences of sleep apnea and diabetes, including the impact of untreated sleep apnea in type 2 diabetes and the effect of continuous positive airway pressure (CPAP) on insulin sensitivity. Studies on obstructive sleep apnea and hypertension examine the effect of CPAP on blood pressure in patients with resistant hypertension and another of this year's selections examines the reduction of blood pressure versus valsartan.

I have included sleep articles on a variety of other sleep-related problems. Be sure to read the article on the association of obstructive sleep apnea with asthma control. I believe this topic is an area of much-needed research. The article on maternal and neonatal morbidities associated with obstructive sleep apnea is the largest to date in this population, to my knowledge. I particularly like the article that examines outcomes in patients with both obstructive sleep apnea and chronic obstructive pulmonary disease. This article provides useful information that clinicians can use when discussing the importance of CPAP use in these patients. I have also included an article examining outcomes of adenotonsillectomy for treatment of obstructive sleep apnea in children, and this will make you reexamine this practice.

The selected articles on insomnia and sleep in the psychiatric patient are very interesting. The longitudinal study on insomnia and outcomes on mortality deserves a read. Sleep physicians who are not in the field of psychiatry will enjoy a review of the spectrum of sleep abnormalities in schizophrenia, anxiety, cognitive disorders, and substance abuse.

I hope you enjoy these selections.

Shirley F. Jones, MD, FCCP

Consequences of Sleep-Disordered Breathing

Maternal and neonatal morbidities associated with obstructive sleep apnea complicating pregnancy

Louis JM, Auckley D, Sokol RJ, et al (Case Western Reserve Univ School of Medicine, Cleveland, OH; Wayne State Univ School of Medicine, Detroit, MI)
Am J Obstet Gynecol 202:261.e1-261.e5, 2010

Objective.—The objective of the study was to estimate the maternal and neonatal morbidities associated with obstructive sleep apnea (OSA) in pregnancy.

Study Design.—Women delivering between 2000–2008 with confirmed OSA in an academic center were included. Normal-weight and obese controls were randomly selected at a 2:1 ratio. Maternal and neonatal morbidities were compared between the groups. Multivariate analyses were performed to evaluate maternal morbidity and preterm birth (PTB).

Results.—The analysis included 57 pregnancies complicated by OSA. Compared with normal-weight (n = 114) controls, OSA patients had more preeclampsia (PET) (19.3% vs 7.0%; $P = .02$) and PTB (29.8% vs 12.3%; $P = .007$). Controlling for comorbid conditions, OSA was associated with an increased risk of PTB (odds ratio [OR], 2.6; 95% confidence interval [CI], 1.02–6.6), mostly secondary to PET (63%). Cesarean delivery (OR, 8.1; 95% CI, 2.9–22.1) and OSA were associated with maternal morbidity (OR, 4.6; 95% CI, 1.5–13.7).

Conclusion.—Pregnancies complicated by OSA are at increased risk for preeclampsia, medical complications, and indicated PTB.

▶ Limited data exist examining perinatal complications of obstructive sleep apnea (OSA) to mother and baby. Theoretically, the periods of oxygen desaturation experienced during apneic and hypopneic events may lead to complications, including preeclampsia, growth restriction, and stillbirth. The lack of an accurate diagnosis (via polysomnography) in previous studies contributes to the lack of evidence in this field. The authors performed a retrospective study of 57 pregnant women with known OSA (diagnosis made through polysomnography) and compared outcomes in these patients with pregnant obese women without known OSA and pregnant women of normal weight. The mean body mass index in the OSA group was 46. This group also had more cases of hypertension, diabetes, asthma, depression, and history of preterm delivery compared with the obese and normal weight groups. Patients with OSA had more preeclampsia and preterm birth compared with normal patients, but this was not significantly higher than the obese group. In addition, cesarean delivery was more common in the OSA group. Cesarean delivery and OSA were both associated with composite maternal morbidity (odds ratio [OR] 4.6 and 8.1, respectively). Furthermore, the OR of preterm birth was 2.6 with OSA, second only to diabetes (OR 4.3). Though there are a number of limitations with this study that the authors point out, to my knowledge this retrospective study of pregnant patients with OSA is the largest. Hopefully, this study will lead to further investigation of OSA, pregnancy, and morbidity. Additional studies examining effect of continuous positive airway pressure on morbidity are needed.

S. F. Jones, MD

Outcomes in Patients with Chronic Obstructive Pulmonary Disease and Obstructive Sleep Apnea: The Overlap Syndrome

Marin JM, Soriano JB, Carrizo SJ, et al (Hospital Universitario Miguel Servet and Instituto Aragones de Ciencias de la Salud, Zaragoza, Spain; CIBER in Respiratory Diseases (CIBERES), Madrid, Spain; et al)

Am J Respir Crit Care Med 182:325-331, 2010

Rationale.—Patients with chronic obstructive pulmonary disease (COPD) and obstructive sleep apnea (OSA) (overlap syndrome) are more likely to develop pulmonary hypertension than patients with either condition alone.

Objectives.—To assess the relation of overlap syndrome to mortality and first-time hospitalization because of COPD exacerbation and the effect of continuous positive airway pressure (CPAP) on these major outcomes.

Methods.—We included 228 patients with overlap syndrome treated with CPAP, 213 patients with overlap syndrome not treated with CPAP, and 210 patients with COPD without OSA. All were free of heart failure, myocardial infarction, or stroke. Median follow-up was 9.4 years (range, 3.3–12.7). End points were all-cause mortality and first-time COPD exacerbation leading to hospitalization.

Measurements and Main Results.—After adjustment for age, sex, body mass index, smoking status, alcohol consumption, comorbidities, severity of COPD, apnea-hypopnea index, and daytime sleepiness, patients with overlap syndrome not treated with CPAP had a higher mortality (relative risk, 1.79; 95% confidence interval, 1.16–2.77) and were more likely to suffer a severe COPD exacerbation leading to hospitalization (relative risk, 1.70; 95% confidence interval, 1.21–2.38) versus the COPD-only group. Patients with overlap syndrome treated with CPAP had no increased risk for either outcome compared with patients with COPD-only.

Conclusions.—The overlap syndrome is associated with an increased risk of death and hospitalization because of COPD exacerbation. CPAP treatment was associated with improved survival and decreased hospitalizations in patients with overlap syndrome.

▶ This is a great study. Investigators longitudinally followed 3 groups of patients: (1) chronic obstructive pulmonary disease (COPD) without obstructive sleep apnea (OSA), (2) COPD with untreated OSA, and (3) COPD with treated OSA. Follow-up occurred for 9 years, and primary outcome was time to death from any cause. Secondary outcome was time to a first severe

COPD exacerbation. There are 3 important findings in this study. First, the overlap syndrome is associated with higher mortality compared with COPD alone. Second, treatment of OSA in the overlap syndrome mitigates the increase in mortality. Third, use of continuous positive airway pressure (CPAP) in patients with overlap syndrome reduces COPD exacerbations. Although the exact mechanism is unknown, the authors do suggest some possibilities.

I think that this study has sound implications. We need to evaluate for concomitant OSA in patients with COPD. These patients are more likely to have daytime hypoxemia and higher pulmonary pressures. Furthermore, promotion of use and adherence to CPAP should be emphasized in those patients with the overlap syndrome. The findings in this article can be used to strengthen the support and education of CPAP use in these patients.

S. F. Jones, MD

Impact of Untreated Obstructive Sleep Apnea on Glucose Control in Type 2 Diabetes

Aronsohn RS, Whitmore H, Van Cauter E, et al (Univ of Chicago, IL)
Am J Respir Crit Care Med 181:507-513, 2010

Rationale.—Obstructive sleep apnea (OSA), a treatable sleep disorder that is associated with alterations in glucose metabolism in individuals without diabetes, is a highly prevalent comorbidity of type 2 diabetes. However, it is not known whether the severity of OSA is a predictor of glycemic control in patients with diabetes.

Objectives.—To determine the impact of OSA on hemoglobin A1c (HbA1c), the major clinical indicator of glycemic control, in patients with type 2 diabetes.

Methods.—We performed polysomnography studies and measured HbA1c in 60 consecutive patients with diabetes recruited from outpatient clinics between February 2007 and August 2009.

Measurements and Main Results.—A total of 77% of patients with diabetes had OSA (apnea–hypopnea index [AHI] $\geq$5). Increasing OSA severity was associated with poorer glucose control, after controlling for age, sex, race, body mass index, number of diabetes medications, level of exercise, years of diabetes and total sleep time. Compared with patients without OSA, the adjusted mean HbA1c was increased by 1.49% ($P = 0.0028$) in patients with mild OSA, 1.93% ($P = 0.0033$) in patients with moderate OSA, and 3.69% ($P < 0.0001$) in patients with severe OSA ($P < 0.0001$ for linear trend). Measures of OSA severity, including total AHI ($P = 0.004$), rapid eye movement AHI ($P = 0.005$), and the oxygen desaturation index during total and rapid eye movement sleep ($P = 0.005$ and $P = 0.008$, respectively) were positively correlated with increasing HbA1c levels.

Conclusions.—In patients with type 2 diabetes, increasing severity of OSA is associated with poorer glucose control, independent of adiposity and other confounders, with effect sizes comparable to those of widely used hypoglycemic drugs.

▶ The authors set out to examine the association between obstructive sleep apnea (OSA) and hemoglobin A1c (a marker of glycemic control). In a sample of 60 patients with a known diagnosis of diabetes, polysomnography was performed. The findings are interesting in a number of ways. First, 77% of subjects had polysomnography-proven OSA (apnea-hypopnea index [AHI] ≥5). The mean AHI in patients with OSA was 19.2 ± 14.8 versus 2.0 ± 1.2 in subjects who did not have OSA. The high prevalence of OSA in the diabetic population is in stark contrast to the general population, which is reported to be 2% to 4%. Of course, the body mass index of subjects in this study is increased. Second, nearly 90% of patients in this study had *not* been previously evaluated for OSA. Only one-third of the subjects reported snoring; I am unsurprised, since this symptom often elicits further suspicion of OSA on the doctor's part. Nevertheless, I think it is important that we recognize the amount of undiagnosed OSA in this at-risk population. Third—and the biggest finding—is that increasing severity of OSA was associated with poorer glucose control after adjusting for covariates. The difference between adjusted mean hemoglobin A1c in mild, moderate, and severe OSA when compared with those without OSA was 1.49%, 1.93%, and 3.69%, respectively. The authors introduce an interesting idea in the discussion. Because many diabetic medications are associated with side effects of weight gain, this may impact the severity of OSA or promote its development. The authors' work supports the hypothesis that improving OSA would improve glycemic control. One step further... nonpharmacologic treatment of OSA may improve glycemic control. At the present time, a diagnosis of diabetes is not factored into the decision to treat OSA, which is in contrast to hypertension, coronary artery disease, and stroke in which the threshold to treat OSA is lower (AHI ≥ 5 events per hour). With the significance of this work, maybe it should be factored.

S. F. Jones, MD

Consequences of Comorbid Sleep Apnea in the Metabolic Syndrome—Implications for Cardiovascular Risk
Trombetta IC, Somers VK, Maki-Nunes C, et al (Univ of São Paulo Med School, Brazil; Mayo Clinic and Foundation, Rochester, MN)
Sleep 33:1193-1199, 2010

Study Objectives.—Metabolic syndrome (MetSyn) increases overall cardiovascular risk. MetSyn is also strongly associated with obstructive sleep apnea (OSA), and these 2 conditions share similar comorbidities. Whether OSA increases cardiovascular risk in patients with the MetSyn has not been investigated. We examined how the presence of OSA in patients with MetSyn affected hemodynamic and autonomic variables associated with poor cardiovascular outcome.

Design.—Prospective clinical study.

Participants.—We studied 36 patients with MetSyn (ATP-III) divided into 2 groups matched for age and sex: (1) MetSyn+OSA (n = 18) and (2) MetSyn-OSA (n = 18).

Measurements.—OSA was defined by an apnea-hypopnea index (AHI) > 15 events/hour by polysomnography. We recorded muscle sympathetic nerve activity (MSNA - microneurography), heart rate (HR), and blood pressure (BP - Finapres). Baroreflex sensitivity (BRS) was analyzed by spontaneous BP and HR fluctuations.

Results.—MSNA (34 ± 2 vs 28 ± 1 bursts/min, P = 0.02) and mean BP (111 ± 3 vs. 99 ± 2 mm Hg, P = 0.003) were higher in patients with MetSyn+OSA versus patients with MetSyn-OSA. Patients with MetSyn+ OSA had lower spontaneous BRS for increases (7.6 ± 0.6 vs 12.2 ± 1.2 msec/mm Hg, P = 0.003) and decreases (7.2 ± 0.6 vs 11.9 ± 1.6 msec/mm Hg, P = 0.01) in BP. MSNA was correlated with AHI (r = 0.48; P = 0.009) and minimum nocturnal oxygen saturation (r = −0.38, P = 0.04).

Conclusion.—Patients with MetSyn and comorbid OSA have higher BP, higher sympathetic drive, and diminished BRS, compared with patients with MetSyn without OSA. These adverse cardiovascular and autonomic consequences of OSA may be associated with poorer outcomes in these patients. Moreover, increased BP and sympathetic drive in patients with MetSyn+OSA may be linked, in part, to impairment of baroreflex gain.

▶ In this prospective case-control study, the authors set out to examine differences in the hemodynamic and autonomic variables in patients with metabolic syndrome and obstructive sleep apnea and compare them with metabolic syndrome patients without obstructive sleep apnea. The authors report that baroreflex sensitivity (spontaneous heart rate and blood pressure fluctuation) was significantly lower in subjects with metabolic syndrome and obstructive sleep apnea. In addition, muscle sympathetic nerve activity and mean blood pressure were higher. Increased sympathetic activity correlated with the severity of the obstructive sleep apnea and the nadir of the oxygen saturation. The authors suggest 2 possible mechanisms for the enhanced sympathetic activation: sleep-related hypoxia or an impaired baroreflex sensitivity. Both plausible mechanisms support the available evidence of increased cardiovascular risk in those with obstructive sleep apnea. It is already known that metabolic syndrome alone is associated with increased cardiovascular risk. This study suggests that those with both conditions may be at an even higher risk. Additional important and much needed areas of research should focus on whether treatment of obstructive sleep apnea reduces the risk in this group and whether increased risk is still seen in those subjects being treated for metabolic syndrome.

S. F. Jones, MD

Association of Obstructive Sleep Apnea Risk With Asthma Control in Adults

Teodorescu M, Polomis DA, Hall SV, et al (William S. Middleton Memorial Veterans Hosp, Madison, WI; Pulmonary and Critical Care Medicine, Madison, WI; et al)
Chest 138:543-550, 2010

Background.—Unrecognized obstructive sleep apnea (OSA) may lead to poor asthma control despite optimal therapy. Our objective was to evaluate the relationship between OSA risk and asthma control in adults.

Methods.—Patients with asthma seen routinely at tertiary-care clinic visits completed the validated Sleep Apnea Scale of the Sleep Disorders Questionnaire (SA-SDQ) and Asthma Control Questionnaire (ACQ). An ACQ score of ≥ 1.5 defined not-well-controlled asthma, and an SA-SDQ score of ≥ 36 for men and ≥ 32 for women defined high OSA risk. Logistic regression was used to model associations of high OSA risk with not-well-controlled asthma (ACQ full version and short versions).

Results.—Among 472 subjects with asthma, the mean $\pm$ SD ACQ (full version) score was 0.87 ± 0.90, and 80 (17%) subjects were not well controlled. Mean SA-SDQ score was 27 ± 7, and 109 (23%) subjects met the definition of high OSA risk. High OSA risk was associated, on average, with 2.87-times higher odds for not-well-controlled asthma (ACQ full version) (95% CI, 1.54-5.32; $P < .0009$) after adjusting for obesity and other factors known to worsen asthma control. Similar independent associations were seen when using the short ACQ versions.

Conclusions.—High OSA risk is significantly associated with not-well-controlled asthma independent of known asthma aggravators and regardless of the ACQ version used. Patients who have difficulty achieving adequate asthma control should be screened for OSA.

▶ Very little literature is available on the link between obstructive sleep apnea (OSA) and asthma. This is reflective of the grade level of recommendation (expert panel) for the evaluation of OSA in patients with inadequately controlled asthma[1] and highlights the need for further research in this area.

The authors hypothesized that high OSA risk will independently predict a higher likelihood for not-well-controlled asthma. They performed a cross-sectional observational study in an allergy clinic in a tertiary health care system. Most of subjects (95%) had rhinitis, 17% had asthma that was not well controlled, and 23% had high risk for OSA. The results of the study indicate that high risk for OSA was associated with a 2.87 higher odds of not-well-controlled asthma. This was after adjustment for factors that are well known to worsen asthma control. While the cross-sectional design of the study does not allow for cause and effect analysis, this study contributes to the much-needed area between asthma and OSA. What I find particularly interesting in this article is the inverse relationship between rhinitis and not-well-controlled asthma, probably reflective that most patients were on treatment and followed up in the allergy clinic. There is another article that suggests that patients with nonallergic rhinitis are more likely to have greater disease impact with more severe apnea, despite having only mild and intermittent symptoms.[2] I wonder if those patients in this study with high risk for OSA had nonallergic rhinitis. I encourage you to read that article as well.

S. F. Jones, MD

References

1. Kalpaklioğlu AF, Kavut AB, Ekici M. Allergic and nonallergic rhinitis: the threat for obstructive sleep apnea. *Ann Allergy Asthma Immunol.* 2009;103:20-25.
2. US Department of Health and Human Services: National Institutes of Health; National Heart, Lung and Blood Institute; National Asthma Education and Prevention Program. Expert panel report 3 (EPR-3): Guideline for the diagnosis and management of asthma. Full report 2007. http://www.nhlbi.nih.gov/guidelines/asthma/asthgdln.pdf. Accessed November 30, 2010.

Sleepiness, Quality of Life, and Sleep Maintenance in REM versus non-REM Sleep-disordered Breathing

Chami HA, Baldwin CM, Silverman A, et al (Boston Univ School of Medicine, MA; Arizona State Univ College of Nursing and Health Innovation, Phoenix; MedStar Res Inst, Hyattsville, MD; et al)

Am J Respir Crit Care Med 181:997-1002, 2010

Rationale.—The impact of REM-predominant sleep-disordered breathing (SDB) on sleepiness, quality of life (QOL), and sleep maintenance is uncertain.

Objective.—To evaluate the association of SDB during REM sleep with daytime sleepiness, health-related QOL, and difficulty maintaining sleep, in comparison to their association with SDB during non-REM sleep in a community-based cohort.

Methods.—Cross-sectional analysis of 5,649 Sleep Heart Health Study participants (mean age 62.5 [SD = 10.9], 52.6% women, 22.6% ethnic minorities). SDB during REM and non-REM sleep was quantified using polysomnographically derived apnea-hypopnea index in REM (AHI_{REM}) and non-REM ($AHIN_{REM}$) sleep. Sleepiness, sleep maintenance, and QOL were respectively quantified using the Epworth Sleepiness Scale (ESS), the Sleep Heart Health Study Sleep Habit Questionnaire, and the physical and mental composites scales of the Medical Outcomes Study Short Form (SF)-36.

Measurements and Main Results.—AHI_{REM} was not associated with the ESS scores or the physical and mental components scales scores of the SF-36 after adjusting for demographics, body mass index, and $AHIN_{REM}$. AHI_{REM} was not associated with frequent difficulty maintaining sleep or early awakening from sleep. $AHIN_{REM}$ was associated with the ESS score ($\beta = 0.25$; 95% confidence interval [CI], 0.16 to 0.34) and the physical ($\beta = -0.12$; 95% CI, -0.42 to -0.01) and mental ($\beta = -0.20$; 95% CI, -0.20 to -0.01) components scores of the SF-36 adjusting for demographics, body mass index, and AHI_{REM}.

Conclusions.—In a community-based sample of middle-aged and older adults, REM-predominant SDB is not independently associated with daytime sleepiness, impaired health-related QOL, or self-reported sleep disruption.

▶ Many of us have seen rapid eye movement (REM)-predominant sleep-disordered breathing in our practice. We have probably also pondered its significance. The authors bring us closer in our understanding of the relationship between REM-predominant sleep-disordered breathing, sleepiness, quality of life, and sleep maintenance. Previous studies have shown mixed results and examined clinic populations, a source of referral bias. The authors performed a cross-sectional analysis of the Sleep Heart Health Study, a large community-based study whose primary objective is to examine the cardiovascular effects of sleep-disordered breathing. The authors did not find a significant association between REM-predominant sleep-disordered breathing and the dependent measures of Epworth sleepiness score, health-related quality of life as assessed by the Short Form 36, and subjective measures of sleep disruption. This makes sense. REM is approximately 25% to 30% of total sleep time in normal individuals, while non-REM (NREM) sleep is 70% to 75%, so fewer disruptions in the total sleep time would be generated in individuals with REM-predominant sleep-disordered breathing compared with sleep-disordered breathing that involved NREM sleep. There are some limitations, which the authors addressed nicely. Other questions that arise out of this study (and need to be addressed in future research) are the association of REM-predominant sleep-disordered breathing in other outcomes, such as cardiovascular disease, mortality, etc, and whether its treatment with continuous positive airway pressure alters these outcomes.

S. F. Jones, MD

CPAP Treatment and Benefits

Continuous positive airway pressure treatment in sleep apnea patients with resistant hypertension: a randomized, controlled trial
Lozano L, Tovar JL, Sampol G, et al (Hosp Mútua de Terrassa, Spain; Universitat Autònoma de Barcelona (UAB), Spain)
J Hypertens 28:2161-2168, 2010

Objectives.—This controlled trial assessed the effect of continuous positive airway pressure (CPAP) on blood pressure (BP) in patients with obstructive sleep apnea (OSA) and resistant hypertension (RH).

Methods.—We evaluated 96 patients with resistant hypertension, defined as clinic BP at least 140/90 mmHg despite treatment with at least three drugs at adequate doses, including a diuretic. Patients underwent a polysomnography and a 24-h ambulatory BP monitoring (ABPM). They were classified as consulting room or ABPM-confirmed resistant hypertension, according to 24-h BP lower or higher than 125/80 mmHg. Patients with an apnea-hypopnea index at least 15 events/h ($n = 75$) were randomized to receive either CPAP added to conventional treatment

($n = 38$) or conventional medical treatment alone ($n = 37$). ABPM was repeated at 3 months. The main outcome was the change in systolic and diastolic BP.

Results.—Sixty-four patients completed the follow-up. Patients with ABPM-confirmed resistant hypertension treated with CPAP ($n = 20$), unlike those treated with conventional treatment ($n = 21$), showed a decrease in 24-h diastolic BP (-4.9 ± 6.4 vs. 0.1 ± 7.3 mmHg, $P = 0.027$). Patients who used CPAP > 5.8 h showed a greater reduction in daytime diastolic BP $\{-6.12$ mmHg [confidence interval (CI) $-1.45; -10.82$], $P = 0.004\}$, 24-h diastolic BP (-6.98 mmHg [CI $-1.86; -12.1$], $P = 0.009$) and 24-h systolic BP (-9.71 mmHg [CI $-0.20; -19.22$], $P = 0.046$). The number of patients with a dipping pattern significantly increased in the CPAP group (51.7% vs. 24.1%, $P = 0.008$).

Conclusion.—In patients with resistant hypertension and OSA, CPAP treatment for 3 months achieves reductions in 24-h BP. This effect is seen in patients with ABPM-confirmed resistant hypertension who use CPAP more than 5.8 h.

▶ Available literature supports that blood pressure reductions can be seen in patients with resistant hypertension who are on multiple medications with use of continuous positive airway pressure (CPAP). The authors of this article performed a randomized controlled trial to evaluate this. Improvements were seen only in patients who had defined resistant hypertension based on 24-hour ambulatory blood pressure monitoring. CPAP generated significant reductions in 24-hour diastolic blood pressure. Additional significant reductions in blood pressure were associated with longer durations of CPAP usage.

The population studied primarily included patients with severe obstructive sleep apnea (mean apnea-hypopnea index 52.67 events per hour). While the degree of blood pressure improvement in patients with resistant hypertension has been questioned (please refer to the article by Pépin et al, which I have also commented on), I believe that this article lends profound strength to the theory that there is an additive role of CPAP to conventional therapy, especially in patients with severe obstructive sleep apnea and resistant hypertension, despite multiple antihypertensive medications.

S. F. Jones, MD

A telemedicine intervention to improve adherence to continuous positive airway pressure: a randomised controlled trial
Sparrow D, Aloia M, DeMolles DA, et al (VA Boston Healthcare System, MA; Natl Jewish Health, Denver, CO)
Thorax 65:1061-1066, 2010

Background.—Continuous positive airway pressure (CPAP) is the most widely prescribed treatment for obstructive sleep apnoea syndrome (OSAS). Although it has been shown to improve the symptoms of

OSAS, many patients have difficulty adhering to this treatment. The purpose of this study was to investigate the effectiveness of an automated telemedicine intervention to improve adherence to CPAP.

Methods.—A randomised clinical trial was undertaken in 250 patients being started on CPAP therapy for OSAS. Patients were randomly assigned to use a theory-driven interactive voice response system designed to improve CPAP adherence (telephone-linked communications for CPAP (TLC-CPAP), n = 124) or to an attention placebo control (n = 126) for 12 months. TLC-CPAP monitors patients' self-reported behaviour and CPAP-related symptoms and provides feedback and counselling through a structured dialogue to enhance motivation to use CPAP. A Sleep Symptoms Checklist, the Functional Outcomes of Sleep Questionnaire, the Center for Epidemiological Studies Depression Scale and the Psychomotor Vigilance Task were administered at study entry and at 6-month and 12-month follow-up. Hours of CPAP usage at effective mask pressure were measured by the CPAP device stored in its memory and retrieved at each visit.

Results.—Median observed CPAP use in patients randomised to TLC-CPAP was approximately 1 h/night higher than in the control subjects at 6 months and 2 h/night higher at 12 months. Using generalised estimating equation modelling, the intervention had a significant effect on CPAP adherence. For secondary analysis, the effect of CPAP adherence on the secondary outcomes was analysed. CPAP adherence was significantly associated with a greater reduction in sleep apnoea symptoms and depressive symptoms and a greater improvement in functional status. No significant association was observed between CPAP adherence and reaction time.

Conclusions.—The TLC-CPAP intervention resulted in improved CPAP adherence, which was associated with improved functional status and fewer depressive symptoms.

Clinical trial.gov: NCT00232544.

▶ We (both patients and health care providers) are all still trying to deal with the issues surrounding continuous positive airway pressure (CPAP) adherence. Intensive CPAP support, which includes at-home education, extra nights in the laboratory to address problems with CPAP, and follow-up home visits, is effective in increasing CPAP adherence, but shortages of medical personnel to deliver this type of intervention may be lacking, and its cost-effectiveness is unclear. These authors examined the effectiveness of an automated telemedicine intervention versus placebo to improve CPAP adherence in a randomized controlled trial. The intervention group received telephone calls using digitalized human speech to inquire about the patients' perceptions and experiences with obstructive sleep apnea and CPAP and self-reported CPAP use. Patients could respond to questions using the telephone keypad. Automated feedback was given to the patients depending on their responses. Patients called weekly for the first month and then on a monthly basis. The authors examined a number of outcome variables, including sleep symptoms, depression, functional outcomes, psychomotor vigilance, self-efficacy, and decisional balance (the latter 2 measure motivations).

I admit that the idea of using an automated telephone-delivered intervention is a novel idea and would likely be of low cost and low maintenance. While the authors were able to demonstrate a significant degree of improvement in functional outcomes, symptoms, and depression in the intervention group, unfortunately, most of the patients did not meet the definition of CPAP adherence (median use in intervention group of 2.4 hours/night at 6 months and 2.98 hours/night at 12 months, both well below the Medicare definition of 4 hours of use per night). The authors addressed the possibilities for this finding.

At my institution, we use an automated telephone system to remind patients of their scheduled appointments. Patients are more likely to attend appointments when a person calls to remind them. However, the number of patients reached with an automated system is much higher. So there are obviously pros and cons to both. I believe an automated telephone delivery system to improve CPAP adherence may be helpful, and perhaps a different approach to its use may prove this.

S. F. Jones, MD

A randomised controlled trial of nasal continuous positive airway pressure on insulin sensitivity in obstructive sleep apnoea
Lam JCM, Lam B, Yao TJ, et al (The Univ of Hong Kong, SAR, China; et al)
Eur Respir J 35:138-145, 2010

The effects of treatment of obstructive sleep apnoea (OSA) on glucose metabolism have been investigated previously with conflicting results. This study evaluated the impact of nasal continuous positive airway pressure (nCPAP) treatment of OSA on insulin sensitivity.

Males with moderate/severe OSA and no significant comorbidity were randomised to a therapeutic or sham nCPAP treatment group for 1 week and then reassessed. Those who received therapeutic nCPAP were further evaluated at 12 weeks. Insulin sensitivity (Kitt) was estimated by the short insulin tolerance test. Other evaluations included blood pressure, metabolic profile, urinary catecholamines and intra-abdominal fat.

In total, 61 Chinese subjects were randomised. 31 subjects receiving therapeutic nCPAP showed an increase in Kitt (6.6 ± 2.9 to 7.6 ± 3.2 %· min^{-1}; p = 0.017), while the 30 patients on sham CPAP had no significant change, and the changes in Kitt were different between the two groups (p = 0.022). At 12 weeks, improvement in Kitt was seen in 20 subjects with BMI ≥ 25 kg·m^{-2} (median (interquartile range) 28.3 (26.6–31.5); p = 0.044), but not in the nine subjects with BMI<25 kg·m^{-2}, or the entire group.

The findings indicate that therapeutic nCPAP treatment of OSA for 1 week improved insulin sensitivity in nondiabetic males, and the improvement appeared to be maintained after 12 weeks of treatment in those with moderate obesity.

▶ Previous studies have implicated that obstructive sleep apnea is associated with insulin resistance. As many patients with obstructive sleep apnea are obese, its confounding effect is difficult to control. Furthermore, studies examining the effects of continuous positive airway pressure (CPAP) on insulin resistance have been mixed.

The authors performed a randomized, double-blinded, controlled trial of therapeutic nasal or sham CPAP in males with moderate to severe obstructive sleep apnea (OSA) (apnea/hypopnea index > 15). After 1 week, insulin sensitivity using the short insulin tolerance test was performed. Those randomized to therapeutic CPAP were reassessed at 12 weeks for insulin sensitivity. The authors controlled for confounding variables by targeting a population without significant medical history, who were not on medication, and who were not obese. There were no significant changes to abdominal obesity or body mass index (BMI) during the 12 weeks. A significant improvement in insulin sensitivity was seen in subjects receiving therapeutic CPAP at 1 week, and who this effect was maintained at 12 weeks in subjects with BMI > 25. This study suggests a causal link between OSA and insulin resistance, and that treatment with CPAP may alter this dysfunction.

Further investigations should include a more general population, but if the findings are reproducible, may enhance the clinical relevance of CPAP use in diabetics, a population at high risk for atherosclerotic disease and its complications.

S. F. Jones, MD

Comparison of Continuous Positive Airway Pressure and Valsartan in Hypertensive Patients with Sleep Apnea

Pépin J-L, Tamisier R, Barone-Rochette G, et al (Grenoble Univ Hosp, France)
Am J Respir Crit Care Med 182:954-960, 2010

Rationale.—Randomized controlled trials (RCTs) have shown that continuous positive airway pressure (CPAP) treatment of obstructive sleep apnea (OSA) reduces blood pressure (BP). CPAP treatment has never been compared with antihypertensive medications in an RCT.

Objectives.—To assess the respective efficacy of CPAP and valsartan in reducing BP in hypertensive patients with OSA never treated for either condition.

Methods.—In this 8-week randomized controlled crossover trial, 23 hypertensive patients (office systolic BP/diastolic BP: 155 ± 14/102 ± 11 mm Hg) with OSA (age, 57 ± 8 yr; body mass index, 28 ± 5 kg/m^2; apnea–hypopnea index, 29 ± 18/h) were randomized first to either CPAP or valsartan (160 mg). The second 8-week period consisted of the alternative treatment (crossover) after a 4-week washout period.

Measurements and Main Results.—Office BP and 24-hour BP were measured before and at the end of the two active treatment periods. Twenty-four-hour mean BP was the primary outcome variable. There was an overall significant difference in 24-hour mean BP between treatments: the change in 24-hour mean BP was -2.1 ± 4.9 mm Hg ($P < 0.01$) with CPAP, and -9.1 ± 7.2 mm Hg with valsartan ($P < 0.001$), with a difference of -7.0 mm Hg (95% confidence interval, -10.9 to -3.1 mm Hg; $P < 0.001$). The difference was significant not only during daytime but also during night-time: the change in nighttime mean BP with CPAP was -1.3 ± 4.6 mm Hg (not significant), and -7.4 ± 8.4 mm Hg with valsartan ($P < 0.001$), with a difference of -6.1 mm Hg ($P < 0.05$) (95% confidence interval, -10.8 to -1.4 mm Hg).

Conclusions.—In an RCT, although the BP decrease was significant with CPAP treatment, valsartan induced a fourfold higher decrease in mean 24-hour BP than CPAP in untreated hypertensive patients with OSA.

Clinical trial registered with www.clinicaltrials.gov (NCT00409487).

▶ We already know that the literature supports significant blood pressure reduction with use of continuous positive airway pressure (CPAP), but this is the first study to compare efficacy of CPAP versus valsartan on blood pressure. Again, findings show that blood pressure reduction with CPAP alone is significant but not to the degree of reduction as seen with the use of valsartan. Furthermore, the authors found additive reductions in blood pressure with a combination of both CPAP and valsartan in a subset of patients in whom blood pressure was still uncontrolled with either CPAP or valsartan alone.

We should take caution before we extrapolate the evidence provided by this article. The numbers were small in this study. The intention-to-treat analysis included 23 patients in the comparison between CPAP and valsartan. Furthermore, the comparisons made between combination and single agent alone were only made based on 11 patients. Measures of effects on blood pressure in the CPAP group were made at 8 weeks. This short duration of CPAP therapy may have underestimated CPAP's effect on blood pressure.

The authors suggest use of valsartan for blood pressure control in patients who do not adhere to CPAP therapy. While the reductions in blood pressure with valsartan are significant, a randomized controlled trial comparing other agents, including β-blockers, diuretics, angiotensin-converting enzyme inhibitors, and angiotensin receptor blockers should be performed. I have seen patients who have had reductions in blood pressure with use of CPAP alone or with CPAP in addition to antihypertensive medication. I also have patients who are averse to the idea of taking medication and would prefer to use CPAP if it allows optimal blood pressure control.

S. F. Jones, MD

Non-CPAP Treatment of Sleep-Disordered Breathing

Predictors for Treating Obstructive Sleep Apnea With an Open Nasal Cannula System (Transnasal Insufflation)

Nilius G, Wessendorf T, Maurer J, et al (Univ Witten-Herdecke, Germany; Ruhrlandklinik, Essen, Germany; HNO-Klinik der Universität, Mannheim, Germany; et al)
Chest 137:521-528, 2010

Background.—Obstructive sleep apnea (OSA) is a disorder that is associated with increased morbidity and mortality. Although continuous positive airway pressure effectively treats OSA, compliance is variable because of the encumbrance of wearing a sealed nasal mask throughout sleep. In a small group of patients, it was recently shown that an open nasal cannula (transnasal insufflation [TNI]) can treat OSA. The aim of this larger study was to find predictors for treatment responses with TNI.

Methods.—Standard sleep studies with and without TNI were performed in 56 patients with a wide spectrum of disease severity. A therapeutic response was defined as a reduction of the respiratory disturbance index (RDI) below 10 events/h associated with a 50% reduction of the event rate from baseline and was used to identify subgroups of patients particularly responsive or resistant to TNI treatment.

Results.—For the entire group (N = 56), TNI decreased the RDI from 22.6 ± 15.6 to 17.2 ± 13.2 events/h ($P < .01$). A therapeutic reduction in the RDI was observed in 27% of patients. Treatment responses were similar in patients with a low and a high RDI, but were greater in patients who predominantly had obstructive hypopneas or respiratory effort-related arousals and in patients who predominantly had rapid eye movement (REM) events. The presence of a high percentage of obstructive and central apneas appears to preclude efficacious treatment responses.

Conclusion.—TNI can be used to treat a subgroup of patients across a spectrum from mild-to-severe sleep apnea, particularly if their sleep-disordered breathing events predominantly consist of obstructive hypopneas or REM-related events but not obstructive and central apneas.

▶ We all know that continuous positive airway pressure (CPAP) is not acceptable for some patients and that adherence can be problematic for others. In a small study performed by McGinley et al,[1] an open nasal cannula system with nasal insufflations delivering humidified and warmed air at 20 L/min was able to reduce sleep-disordered breathing. In this study, the authors examined predictors of sleep that were associated with an improved treatment response. Approximately one-fourth of the subjects had an adequate treatment response with the nasal insufflation. Review of the polysomnographic data at baseline showed that there was a heterogenous response to the nasal insufflations across all subjects, but those with predominant hypopneas and respiratory effort–related arousals and those with predominant rapid eye movement–related disease had the best treatment response. The severity of the obstructive sleep apnea was moderate on average in those studied. A study examining efficacy and treatment adherence of nasal insufflation versus CPAP is still needed. Studies including a more general population (women, children, obese) are needed before recommending use of this therapy at current time. I expect more studies in the future.

S. F. Jones, MD

Reference

1. McGinley BM, Patil SP, Kirkness JP, Smith PL, Schwartz AR, Schneider H. A nasal cannula can be used to treat obstructive sleep apnea. *Am J Respir Crit Care Med.* 2007;176:194-200.

Adenotonsillectomy Outcomes in Treatment of Obstructive Sleep Apnea in Children: A Multicenter Retrospective Study

Bhattacharjee R, Kheirandish-Gozal L, Spruyt K, et al (Univ of Louisville, KY; et al)
Am J Respir Crit Care Med 182:676-683, 2010

Rationale.—The overall efficacy of adenotonsillectomy (AT) in treatment of obstructive sleep apnea syndrome (OSAS) in children is unknown. Although success rates are likely lower than previously estimated, factors that promote incomplete resolution of OSAS after AT remain undefined.

Objectives.—To quantify the effect of demographic and clinical confounders known to impact the success of AT in treating OSAS.

Methods.—A multicenter collaborative retrospective review of all nocturnal polysomnograms performed both preoperatively and postoperatively on otherwise healthy children undergoing AT for the diagnosis of OSAS was conducted at six pediatric sleep centers in the United States and two in Europe. Multivariate generalized linear modeling was used to assess contributions of specific demographic factors on the post-AT obstructive apnea-hypopnea index (AHI).

Measurements and Main Results.—Data from 578 children (mean age, 6.9 ± 3.8 yr) were analyzed, of which approximately 50% of included children were obese. AT resulted in a significant AHI reduction from 18.2 ± 21.4 to 4.1 ± 6.4/hour total sleep time ($P < 0.001$). Of the 578 children, only 157 (27.2%) had complete resolution of OSAS (i.e., post-AT AHI <1/h total sleep time). Age and body mass index z-score emerged as the two principal factors contributing to post-AT AHI ($P < 0.001$), with modest contributions by the presence of asthma and magnitude of pre-AT AHI ($P < 0.05$) among nonobese children.

Conclusions.—AT leads to significant improvements in indices of sleep-disordered breathing in children. However, residual disease is present in a large proportion of children after AT, particularly among older (>7 yr) or obese children. In addition, the presence of severe OSAS in nonobese children or of chronic asthma warrants post-AT nocturnal polysomnography, in view of the higher risk for residual OSAS.

▶ Obstructive sleep apnea (OSA) syndrome affects 2% to 3% of children.[1] While most clinicians, in keeping with the American Academy of Pediatrics, recommend adenotonsillectomy as the first line of treatment, we really do not know its efficacy. Traditionally, very high cure rates of 90% or more are cited. These particular authors challenge that exact notion. Many of us have seen children with residual OSA after adenotonsillectomy and have been curious about its risk factors (age, body mass index [BMI], and severity of presurgical OSA). This article examines the success of adenotonsillectomy in children and aims to delineate the factors that may contribute to residual OSA post surgery. The investigators performed a multicenter retrospective review of all nocturnal polysomnograms (preadenotonsillectomy and postadenotonsillectomy) performed in healthy children for OSA. This study included 578 children from 8 centers in the United States and Europe. The authors found that curative rates of adenotonsillectomy are not as good as expected. Though most children had a significant reduction in the severity of OSA with adenotonsillectomy, only 27.2% of children has postoperative apnea-hypopnea index (AHI) < 1 per hour, and 21.6% had postoperative AHI > 5 per hour. Examination of risk factors indicates that age > 7 years and increasing BMI were the most predictive of residual OSA. Over half of the children studied meet the criteria for obesity. Presence of asthma and severity of preoperative OSA were also predictive, though to a lesser degree, particularly in nonobese children.

There is a significant degree of criticism surrounding the methods of this study (retrospective, most patients from 2 of the 8 sites, possible selection bias, and lack of standardization of polysomnographic practices between sites). All of these are addressed by the authors. This article certainly generates thought and suggests which patients may need postoperative polysomnography (age > 7 years, obese, and severity of preoperative AHI or presence of asthma in nonobese children). Until a prospective study is performed, the efficacy of adenotonsillectomy should be refuted.

S. F. Jones, MD

Reference

1. Mitki T, Pillar G. Absence of positional effect in children with moderate-severe obstructive sleep apnea syndrome. *Harefuah*. 2009;148:300-303.

Non-Pulmonary Sleep

Attention, Learning, and Arousal of Experimentally Sleep-restricted Adolescents in a Simulated Classroom

Beebe DW, Rose D, Amin R (Univ of Cincinnati College of Medicine, OH)
J Adolesc Health 47:523-525, 2010

Purpose.—To experimentally test whether chronic sleep restriction, which is common among adolescents, is causally related to poor learning, inattentive behaviors, and diminished arousal in a classroom-like situation.

Methods.—Sixteen healthy adolescents underwent a sleep manipulation that included, in counterbalanced order, five consecutive nights of sleep deprivation ($6\frac{1}{2}$ hours in bed) versus five nights of healthy sleep duration (10 hours in bed). At the end of each condition, participants viewed educational films and took related quizzes in a simulated classroom. Eight participants also underwent video and electroencephalography monitoring to assess levels of inattentive behaviors and arousal, respectively.

Results.—As compared with the healthy sleep condition, sleep-deprived participants had lower quiz scores ($p = .05$), more inattentive behaviors ($p < .05$), and lower arousal ($p = .08$).

Conclusions.—These pilot data complement previous correlational reports by showing that chronic sleep restriction during adolescence can cause inattention, diminished learning, and lowered arousal in a simulated classroom.

▶ Sleep deprivation is very common in adolescents, with many sleeping less than 7 hours per night. This is an accepted practice for a number of reasons (part-time jobs to make extra money, late-night studying, etc) or even less accepted practices (staying up late texting friends, use of computer to socialize, etc); whatever the reason, this is generating a society full of sleep-deprived adolescents. These practices are likely to be carried over to young adulthood. Clinicians see this all the time in our practices. Encouraging adolescents to get enough sleep (nearly 10 hours of time in bed) is often met with rebuttals.

I like this article because of its relative simplicity of study design. The authors examined quiz and inattention behaviors in 20 adolescents who all underwent sleep-deprived and healthy duration sleep periods. Detailed electroencephalograms were obtained on a subset. Getting approximately 6 hours of sleep per night was associated with more inattention and worse quiz scores compared with those who got a little more than 9 hours of sleep.

While there are some problems with the validity measuring inattention (observer reporting) and the small sample size that affects the generalizabilty of this study, it is intriguing and should be reproduced. Changes in school start times and an increased public awareness of sleep deprivation in adolescents can be easily argued if additional studies support these findings.

S. F. Jones, MD

Acute Care Surgery Performed by Sleep Deprived Residents: Are Outcomes Affected?
Yaghoubian A, Kaji AH, Ishaque B, et al (Harbor-UCLA Med Ctr, Torrance)
J Surg Res 163:192-196, 2010

Background.—The Institute of Medicine recently recommended further reductions in resident duty hours, including a 5-h rest time for on-call residents after 16 h of work. This recommendation was purportedly intended to better protect patients against fatigue-related errors made by physician trainees. Yet no data are available regarding outcomes of operations performed by surgical trainees working without rest beyond 16 h in the current 80-h workweek era.

Methods.—A retrospective review of all laparoscopic cholecystectomies (LC) and appendectomies performed by surgery residents at a public teaching hospital from July 2003 through March 2009. Operations after 10 PM were performed by residents who began their shift at 6 AM and had thus been working 16 or more hours. An outcomes comparison between time periods was conducted for operations performed between 6 AM and 10 PM (daytime) and 10 PM and 6 AM (nighttime). Outcome measures were rates of total complications, bile duct injury, conversion to open operation, length of surgery, and mortality.

Results.—Over the 7-y study period, 2908 LC and 1726 appendectomies were performed. Appendectomies were performed laparoscopically in 73% of cases in patients for both time periods. There were no differences in rates of overall morbidity and mortality for operations when performed in nighttime compared with daytime. On multivariable analysis, there were no differences in outcomes between the two groups.

Conclusion.—The two most commonly performed general surgical operations performed at night by unrested residents have favorable outcomes similar to those performed during the day. Instituting a 5-h rest period at night is unlikely to improve the outcomes for these commonly performed operations.

▶ Changes to the resident duty hours continue to evolve. It is hard to believe that 7 years ago the 80-hour workweek was adopted. Recently, the Institute of Medicine has recommended additional refinement to the resident duty hours with the aim of reducing errors in care because of fatigue. The current recommendation is to allow for a 5-hour rest time for on-call residents after 16 hours of duty. If you serve on resident education and advisory committees, these recommendations have set forth construction of task forces designed to strategize the implementation of these forthcoming changes.

Fatigue-related errors are real. Need we be reminded about national and international catastrophies (Challenger, Valdez, etc) traced back to fatigue? Despite this, there is little available evidence examining outcomes in patient care because of sleep deprivation. The authors performed a retrospective study examining outcomes in patients who underwent cholecystectomy and appendectomy during daytime versus nighttime hours. The authors state that the nighttime surgeries were performed by residents who had started call by 6 AM that morning (16 hours of duty). They report that the predictor of complications was not the time of day in which the surgery was performed but rather patient-related factors (presence of perforation, gender, and age) and length of duration of surgery. The authors make arguments for how the new changes will affect resident education negatively.

Will patient-centered outcomes be improved with reduction in resident duty hours as suggested by the Institute of Medicine? This is not something where we can perform a randomized controlled trial because 1 negative outcome is too many. As the authors discuss, I believe that there may be some downsides but also some positives. I included this article just for some thought provocation.

S. F. Jones, MD

Insomnia with Short Sleep Duration and Mortality: The Penn State Cohort
Vgontzas AN, Liao D, Pejovic S, et al (Pennsylvania State Univ College of Medicine, Hershey)
Sleep 33:1159-1164, 2010

Study Objectives.—Because insomnia with objective short sleep duration is associated with increased morbidity, we examined the effects of this insomnia subtype on all-cause mortality.

Design.—Longitudinal.

Setting.—Sleep laboratory.

Participants.—1,741 men and women randomly selected from Central Pennsylvania.

Measurements.—Participants were studied in the sleep laboratory and were followed-up for 14 years (men) and 10 years (women). "Insomnia" was defined by a complaint of insomnia with duration $\geq$ 1 year. "Normal sleeping" was defined as absence of insomnia. Polysomnographic sleep duration was classified into two categories: the "normal sleep duration group" subjects who slept $\geq$ 6 h and the "short sleep duration group" subjects who slept < 6 h. We adjusted for age, race, education, body mass index, smoking, alcohol, depression, sleep disordered breathing, and sampling weight.

Results.—The mortality rate was 21% for men and 5% for women. In men, mortality risk was significantly increased in insomniacs who slept less than 6 hours compared to the "normal sleep duration, no insomnia" group, (OR = 4.00, CI 1.14-13.99) after adjusting for diabetes, hypertension, and other confounders. Furthermore, there was a marginally significant trend (P = 0.15) towards higher mortality risk from insomnia and short sleep in patients with diabetes or hypertension (OR = 7.17, 95% CI 1.41-36.62) than in those without these comorbid conditions (OR = 1.45, 95% CI 0.13-16.14). In women, mortality was not associated with insomnia and short sleep duration.

Conclusions.—Insomnia with objective short sleep duration in men is associated with increased mortality, a risk that has been underestimated.

▶ We have known for a while that obstructive sleep apnea increases morbidity of hypertension and cardiovascular disease. On the contrary, our knowledge of insomnia has been its association with comorbid psychiatric disease but lack of association with the same morbidities is seen with obstructive sleep apnea. The authors of this study used objective criteria of sleep duration and long duration of follow-up (up to 14 years), both of this study's strong points. After adjustment for a number of conditions, which included depression and sleep disordered breathing, the results indicate that insomnia was associated with a higher risk of mortality, particularly in men who slept less than 6 hours. Particular attention should be focused on patients with chronic insomnia and comorbid diabetes or hypertension in which an odds ratio for mortality of 7.17 is reported. More studies should be done to confirm these findings in particular.

Overall, this study sheds light on the poor outcomes associated with insomnia and challenges the current knowledge of this common sleep disorder. Future studies corroborating these findings are likely to make a tremendous impact on the management of insomnia.

S. F. Jones, MD

Sleep in Psychiatric Disorders: Where Are We Now?
Lee EK, Douglass AB (Univ of Ottawa, Ontario, Canada)
Can J Psychiatry 55:403-412, 2010

Although the precise function of sleep is unknown, decades of research strongly implicate that sleep has a vital role in central nervous system (CNS) restoration, memory consolidation, and affect regulation. Slow-wave sleep (SWS) and rapid eye movement (REM) sleep have been of significant interest to psychiatrists; SWS because of its putative role in CNS energy recuperation and cognitive function, and REM sleep because of its suggested involvement in memory, mood regulation, and possible emotional adaptation. With the advent of the polysomnogram, researchers are now beginning to understand some of the consequences of disrupted sleep and sleep deprivation in psychiatric disorders. The same neurochemistry that controls the sleep–wake cycle has also been implicated in the pathophysiology of numerous psychiatric disorders. Thus it is no surprise that several psychiatric disorders have prominent sleep symptoms. This review will summarize normal sleep architecture, and then examine sleep abnormalities and comorbid sleep disorders seen in schizophrenia, as well as anxiety, cognitive, and substance abuse disorders.

▶ This article provides a great review of the sleep abnormalities associated with schizophrenia, anxiety, cognitive, and substance abuse disorders. There is a nice review and table of drugs used in schizophrenia and the polysomnographic effects of their use. Prevalence data for sleep disorders is included in this review. There is a nice discussion of posttraumatic stress disorders and nightmares. A review of aging and sleep is included along with discussions of movement disorders and parasomnias in the elderly. The authors nicely describe the effects of substance abuse (acute, chronic, and withdrawal) on sleep. Overall, this is a very nice review of comorbid sleep disorders in a psychiatric population. There is a lot of high-yield information in this article and is useful for both the practicing psychiatrist who may have limited involvement in sleep medicine and the sleep medicine specialist who does not practice psychiatry.

S. F. Jones, MD

Pediatric Sleep-Disordered Breathing

B-Type Natriuretic Peptide and Cardiovascular Function in Young Children With Obstructive Sleep Apnea

Goldbart AD, Levitas A, Greenberg-Dotan S, et al (Soroka Univ Med Ctr, Beer-Sheva, Israel)
Chest 138:528-535, 2010

Objective.—N-terminal pro-B-type natriuretic peptide (NT-proBNP), a marker of ventricular strain, and C-reactive protein (CRP), a marker of inflammation, are reportedly elevated in school-aged children with obstructive sleep apnea (OSA). We hypothesized that cardiovascular morbidity affects circulating markers and their echocardiographic and polysomnographic (PSG) correlates in young children with OSA.

Methods.—We assessed young children undergoing adenotonsillectomy (TA) for OSA by polysomnography, echocardiography, and serum CRP and NT-proBNP levels.

Results.—A total of 90 children with OSA (mean age 19 ± 7 months; 71.2% male; BMI, $z \pm 0.62 \pm 1.04$) and 45 age- and sex-matched controls were included. Three months following TA, 72 children were reassessed for NT-proBNP and CRP. NT-proBNP level (pg/mL) was higher in subjects with OSA (189.1 ± 112.7) vs control subjects (104.8 ± 49.5; $P = .006$). Both NT-proBNP (187.8 ± 114 vs 86 ± 32.6; $P = .002$) and CRP levels (mg %) (0.49 ± 0.41 vs 0.1 ± 0.17; $P < .05$) decreased following TA. Doppler pulse wave measuring tricuspid regurgitation (TR), a reflection of pulmonary hypertension, correlated with CRP ($r = 0.61$, $P < .01$) but not NT-proBNP ($r = -0.14$, $P = .53$) levels. Left ventricle end-diastolic diameter (LVEDD) was at the maximal normal range (0.91 ± 0.11), but did not correlate with CRP or NT-proBNP levels. Both CRP level and TR correlated with PSG variables reflecting nocturnal hypoxemia, whereas NT-proBNP level and LVEDD did not. Echocardiography in 40 children (out of 90) showed a decline in TR that was abnormal before TA and correlated with the decrease in CRP following TA.

Conclusions.—NT-proBNP levels are increased in children with OSA and decrease following TA. Echocardiographic parameters suggesting increased pulmonary pressure in young children with OSA are related to nocturnal hypoxemia and systemic inflammation, which also decrease following therapy.

▶ The authors examined markers of inflammation (C-reactive protein [CRP]) and cardiac strain (N-terminal pro-B-type natriuretic peptide [NT-proBNP]) before and after tonsillectomy in young children with obstructive sleep apnea. Echocardiography was also performed pre- and postsurgery. The gold standard of polysomnography was used to identify obstructive sleep apnea and all cases had apnea-hypopnea index > 5. Their finding that inflammation correlates with hypoxia and echocardiographic findings of tricuspid regurgitation is unique. The surprising part is that the mean age of cases was 19 months ± 7. Why the other marker of inflammation, NT-proBNP, did not correlate is unknown to me. Perhaps not enough cardiac strain was generated? There are some limitations to this study that are significant, the small sample size is probably the biggest limitation.

If markers of inflammation and hemodynamic cardiac changes can be seen in such a young age with obstructive sleep apnea, the consequences of untreated disease are something we must reckon with. Longitudinal studies may be helpful to determine if these findings reduce the occurrence of disease entities associated with pediatric obstructive sleep apnea—cognitive changes, growth problems, etc.

S. F. Jones, MD

Risk Factors and Pathophysiology of Sleep-Disordered Breathing

Allergic and nonallergic rhinitis: the threat for obstructive sleep apnea
Kalpaklıoğlu AF, Kavut AB, Ekici M (Kirikkale Univ Faculty of Medicine, Turkey)
Ann Allergy Asthma Immunol 103:20-25, 2009

Background.—Although allergic rhinitis (AR) is accepted as a risk factor for obstructive sleep apnea syndrome (OSAS), the role of nonallergic rhinitis (NAR) is unknown.

Objective.—To compare OSAS in patients with AR vs NAR.

Methods.—We performed an observational study in 48 adults with AR and NAR that included a review of rhinitis and sleep symptoms, skin prick test results, self-administered questionnaire (Epworth Sleepiness Scale and 36-Item Short Form Health Survey) findings, and all-night polysomnography records.

Results.—The most frequent sleep symptom was snoring. Patients with AR had a significantly longer sleep duration and better sleep efficiency than did those with NAR. Both groups had frequent arousals. OSAS was diagnosed in 36% of patients with AR and in 83% of those with NAR ($P = .001$). Severe OSAS existed only in the NAR group. NAR showed a high correlation with OSAS (odds ratio, 6.4) and with apneas (odds ratio, 0.2). Body mass index, sex, and coexisting asthma did not have any predictable effect on OSAS, but age was correlated with OSAS. The impairment in quality of life was similar in both groups.

Conclusions.—Both AR and NAR are risk factors for a high apnea-hypopnea index, and both can predispose to sleep apnea. However, NAR seems to have a greater risk according to impaired polysomnography results and higher Epworth Sleepiness Scale scores. Therefore, patients with rhinitis should be treated not only for nasal symptoms but also for a better quality of sleep.

▶ In practice, patients frequently ask if rhinitis causes obstructive sleep apnea. This article is something to share with your patients and is straightforward. The authors investigated the impact of allergic versus nonallergic rhinitis on health-related quality of life and sleep disturbances using the 36-Item Short Form Health Survey and polysomnography, respectively. Subjects with allergic rhinitis (AR) were classified as moderate to severe seasonal and persistent symptoms, whereas those with nonallergic rhinitis (NAR) had mild perennial and intermittent symptoms. I find it interesting that this classification of symptom severity did not have any bearing on objective measures of sleep. The NAR group had a higher apnea-hypopnea index (12.2 vs 6.5 events/h), sleep duration, and poorer sleep efficiency than those subjects with AR. The Epworth sleepiness score was much higher in the NAR group, indicating greater daytime sleepiness. The mean body mass index in this study was 26—nonobese. This study shows that both AR and NAR are risk factors for obstructive sleep apnea, but those with the NAR are more likely to have greater disease impact and more severe apnea despite having only mild and intermittent symptoms.

S. F. Jones, MD

Miscellaneous

A Compromise Circadian Phase Position for Permanent Night Work Improves Mood, Fatigue, and Performance
Smith MR, Fogg LF, Eastman CI (Rush Univ Med Ctr, Chicago, IL)
Sleep 32:1481-1489, 2009

Study Objective.—To assess night shift improvements in mood, fatigue, and performance when the misalignment between circadian rhythms and a night shift, day sleep schedule is reduced.

Design.—Blocks of simulated night shifts alternated with days off. Experimental subjects had interventions to delay their circadian clocks to partially align with a night shift schedule. Control subjects had no interventions. Subjects were categorized according to the degree of circadian realignment independent of whether they were in the experimental or control groups. Twelve subjects were categorized as not re-entrained, 21 as partially re-entrained, and 6 as completely re-entrained.

Setting.—Home sleep and laboratory night shifts.

Participants.—Young healthy adults.

Interventions.—Experimental subjects had intermittent bright light pulses during night shifts, wore dark sunglasses outside, and had scheduled sleep episodes in darkness.

Measurements and Results.—A computerized test battery was administered every 2 hours during day and night shifts. After about one week on the night shift schedule, which included a weekend off, the partially and completely re-entrained groups had markedly improved mood, fatigue, and performance compared to the group that was not re-entrained. The completely and partially re-entrained groups were similar to each other and had levels of mood, fatigue, and performance that were close to daytime levels.

Conclusions.—Partial re-entrainment to a permanent night shift schedule, which can be produced by feasible, inexpensive interventions, is associated with greatly reduced impairments during night shifts.

▶ Shift work describes work schedules that are outside the day work hours and includes permanent night work. These individuals are at risk for shift work disorder and impairments in performance and alertness. These impairments can result in faulty errors in judgment and reaction time and be detrimental to safety. Methods to improve performance and alertness include timed light therapy, napping, caffeine, and modafinil. Re-entrainment of the circadian rhythm to night work and daytime sleep using bright light therapy is a slow process. Despite its usefulness, night shift workers may not be likely to adapt to this new schedule because of social limitations and may revert back to nighttime sleep on their days off work. These investigators examined a sleep schedule compromise or partial re-entrainment. The propensity to sleep is delayed until daytime on workdays and maintained near the end of nighttime sleep on days off. Mood, fatigue, and performance levels were improved in the partially re-entrained group and similar to those completely re-entrained. Circadian rhythm re-entrainment occurred with use of 4 to 5 timed pulses of bright light therapy, scheduled sleep-wake periods, and dark sunglasses worn outside. While this study was performed in healthy individuals under simulation in the laboratory and needs to be repeated in field studies and in those with shift work disorder, its application could spell numerous benefits: inexpensive, improved performance and alertness (which could translate into improved safety for both the work and public), and yet be more socially acceptable.

S. F. Jones, MD

Assessing the Prioritization of Primary Care Referrals for Polysomnograms
Thornton JD, Chandriani K, Thornton JG, et al (Case Western Reserve Univ, Cleveland, OH; et al)
Sleep 33:1255-1260, 2010

Study Objective.—The mortality attributed to obstructive sleep apnea (OSA) is comparable to that of breast cancer and colon cancer. We sought to determine if patients at high risk for OSA were less likely to be referred by their primary care physician for polysomnograms (PSG) than mammograms or endoscopies.

Design.—Prospective cohort study; patients were recruited between January 2007 and April 2007.

Setting.—Academic public hospital system.

Patients.—395 patients waiting for family or internal medicine primary care appointments were administered the Berlin questionnaire. Chart abstraction or interview determined demographics; insurance and employment status; body mass index (BMI); comorbidities; and prior PSG, mammography, or endoscopy referrals.

Results.—Mean BMI was $30 \pm 7.4 \, kg/m^2$; 187 (47%) patients had high-risk Berlin scores. Overall, 19% of patients with high-risk Berlin scores were referred for PSG, compared to 63% of those eligible for mammograms and 80% of those eligible for endoscopies. Women (OR = 2.9, P = 0.02), COPD (OR = 4.6, P = 0.03), high-risk Berlin scores (OR = 3.4, P = 0.009), and higher BMI (OR = 1.1, P < 0.001) were positively associated with PSG referrals. Privately insured patients were less likely to be referred than uninsured patients (OR = 0.3, P = 0.04). There was no significant difference in referrals among those with other forms of insurance. Race was not associated with PSG referrals.

Conclusion.—In a public hospital, primary care patients were less likely to be referred for PSG compared to mammogram and endoscopy. Uninsured patients were more likely to be referred for PSG than those with private insurance. Further studies are needed to address the low PSG referral rates in high-risk populations.

▶ There is still underrecognition of the importance of identifying obstructive sleep apnea (OSA) in the primary care setting, despite increasing available evidence that severe OSA is associated with higher risk of all-cause mortality. In a recent article by Punjabi et al,[1] mortality from OSA is as high as 20 deaths per 1000 person-years. The investigators sought to determine if patients at high risk for OSA were less likely to be referred by their primary care physician for polysomnograms than mammographies or endoscopies. Breast cancer and colon cancer were selected because of similar mortality rates compared with OSA. Nearly 400 patients were screened for OSA using the Berlin questionnaire, and notice of high-risk status was made to the patient's respective primary care physician. Within 2 years of notification, only 19% of patients with high-risk Berlin scores had been referred for polysomnograms. Rates of referrals for mammography and endoscopy were much higher (63% and 80%, respectively). The insurance status of the patient had no bearing on referrals for polysomnography.

While this study does not examine causes of low referral rates, the authors do suggest possibilities, which deserve consideration. How frequently do primary care physicians discuss sleep with their patients? Are public awareness campaigns for breast cancer and OSA more effective than sleep awareness campaigns? Are there too many time constraints placed on our primary care physicians so it is not possible to discuss OSA? In my opinion, the rising numbers of obese patients will in turn force primary care physicians to increase awareness and recognition. Perhaps even quality initiative will be put into place in the future. Quality measures are already underway with chronic obstructive pulmonary disease. OSA may see similar efforts.

S. F. Jones, MD

Reference

1. Punjabi NM, Caffo BS, Goodwin JL, et al. Sleep-disordered breathing and mortality: a prospective cohort study. *PLoS Med.* 2009;6:e1000132.

Changes in brain morphology in patients with obstructive sleep apnoea
Morrell MJ, Jackson ML, Twigg GL, et al (Imperial College, London, UK; Washington State Univ, Spokane; et al)
Thorax 65:908-914, 2010

Background.—Obstructive sleep apnoea (OSA) is a common disease that leads to daytime sleepiness and cognitive impairment. Attempts to investigate changes in brain morphology that may underlie these impairments have led to conflicting conclusions. This study was undertaken to aim to resolve this confusion, and determine whether OSA is associated with changes in brain morphology in a large group of patients with OSA, using improved voxel-based morphometry analysis, an automated unbiased method of detecting local changes in brain structure.

Methods.—60 patients with OSA (mean apnoea hypopnoea index 55 (95% CI 48 to 62) events/h, 3 women) and 60 non-apnoeic controls (mean apnoea hypopnoea index 4 (95% CI 3 to 5) events/h, 5 women) were studied. Subjects were imaged using T1-weighted 3-D structural MRI (69 subjects at 1.5 T, 51 subjects at 3 T). Differences in grey matter were investigated in the two groups, controlling for age, sex, site and intracranial volume. Dedicated cerebellar analysis was performed on a subset of 108 scans using a spatially unbiased infratentorial template.

Results.—Patients with OSA had a reduction in grey matter volume in the right middle temporal gyrus compared with non-apnoeic controls ($p<0.05$, corrected for topological false discovery rate across the entire brain). A reduction in grey matter was also seen within the cerebellum, maximal in the left lobe VIIIb close to XI, extending across the midline into the right lobe.

Conclusion.—These data show that OSA is associated with focal loss of grey matter that could contribute to cognitive decline. Specifically, lesions in the cerebellum may result in both motor dysfunction and working memory deficits, with downstream negative consequences on tasks such as driving.

▶ This is a cross-sectional study comparing structural brain changes in patients with obstructive sleep apnea and controls. The authors report loss of gray matter in 2 areas of the brain. The left cerebellum functions in attention-related tasks and working memory, both needed in performance of driving. Though functional aspects of these morphological changes were not addressed in this particular study, inclusion of these measurements will be important in further studies.

S. F. Jones, MD

A Candidate Gene Study of Obstructive Sleep Apnea in European Americans and African Americans
Larkin EK, Patel SR, Goodloe RJ, et al (Vanderbilt Univ Med Ctr, Nashville, TN; Case Western Reserve Univ, Cleveland, OH; et al)
Am J Respir Crit Care Med 182:947-953, 2010

Rationale.—Obstructive sleep apnea (OSA) is hypothesized to be influenced by genes within pathways involved with obesity, craniofacial development, inflammation, and ventilatory control.

Objectives.—We conducted the first candidate gene study of OSA using family data from European Americans and African Americans, selecting biologically plausible genes from within these pathways.

Methods.—A total of 1,080 single nucleotide polymorphisms (SNPs) were genotyped in 729 African Americans and 505 SNPs were genotyped in 694 European Americans. Coding for SNPs additively, association testing on the apnea-hypopnea index (AHI) as a continuous trait, and OSA as a dichotomous trait (AHI $\geq$ 15) was conducted using methods that account for familial correlations in models adjusted for age, age-squared, and sex, with and without body mass index.

Measurements and Main Results.—In European Americans, variants within C-reactive protein (CRP) and glial cell line–derived neurotrophic factor (GDNF) were associated with AHI (CRP: $\beta = 4.6$; SE $= 1.1$; $P = 0.0000402$) (GDNF: $\beta = 4.3$; SE $= 1$; $P = 0.0000201$) and with the dichotomous OSA trait (CRP: odds ratio $= 2.4$; 95% confidence interval, 1.5–3.9; $P = 0.000170$) (GDNF: odds ratio $= 2$; 95% confidence interval, 1.4–2.89; $P = 0.0000433$). In African Americans, rs9526240 within serotonin receptor 2a (HTR2A: odds ratio $= 2.1$; 95% confidence interval, 1.5–2.9; $P = 0.00005233$) was associated with OSA.

Conclusions.—This candidate gene analysis identified the potential role of genes operating through intermediate disease pathways to influence sleep apnea phenotypes, providing a framework for focusing future replication studies.

▶ There is a strong genetic component in obstructive sleep apnea (OSA). Having a first-degree relative with sleep-disordered breathing increases the risk > 1.5-fold.[1] This is the largest candidate gene study to date. A strong aspect of this study is that it includes African Americans, a group with high risk for OSA. All subjects had polysomnography-confirmed OSA, either portable or in laboratory. The authors examined genetic variants associated with the obesity, ventilatory control, inflammation, and craniofacial morphology. Significant associations between severity of OSA and its presence were identified in cell lines responsible for inflammation and neural control of breathing in European Americans. In African Americans, polymorphisms with the serotonin receptor were associated with OSA. The results from this study will lead to further investigation with emphasis on polymorphisms in these focused areas.

S. F. Jones, MD

Reference

1. Redline S, Tishler PV, Tosteson TD, et al. The familial aggregation of obstructive sleep apnea. *Am J Respir Crit Care Med.* 1995;151:682-687.

8 Critical Care Medicine

Introduction

Critical Care literature continues to be more refined and to ever increase in knowledge base. Gaps in knowledge base and care continue to fill in. Airway pressure release ventilation (APRV) is a commonly used mode of ventilation that appears to be efficacious. However, randomized controlled trials (RCTs) and scientific proof have been sparse to date. Maxwell and colleagues report the results of a well-done RCT on APRV versus acute respiratory distress syndrome (ARDS) net protocol in trauma patients. Results appear equivalent and thus those of us who use this modality frequently now have some science to match our practice.

Two articles on important topics in pregnant women with respiratory failure are included. These high-risk ARDS patients are very complex. One summarizes nicely the severity of H1N1 influenza in this subgroup of patients. The other discusses the rare but potentially fatal presentation of metastatic choriocarcinoma (molar pregnancy). We just had one of these tragic cases at our institution, and this discussion was certainly prescient.

Obstructive sleep apnea is of course quite common both here and abroad. Hang et al have a nice description of results and outcomes of these patients (in Taiwan) when admitted to critical care. In addition, I found the article by Serrano and Rabinstein regarding acute neuromuscular respiratory failure to be both fascinating and practically useful. Their results seem in line with my own experience. Please read on!

Heliox remains a treatment looking for a disease. Its use in COPD is discussed herein. This is an important article since many practioners widely use it, and there is expected to be an international shortage soon.

Some excellent airway and technique articles are discussed in this chapter. This area of our practice continues to be refined and made safer.

Two neat articles for neurocritical care are included. One, by Ward et al, further expands our knowledge base in the critically ill stroke patient. These patients are known to have high rates of pneumonia and insufficient cough. The physiology and reflexes are discussed very nicely by the authors of this study. A giant in the field of neurocritical care, Eelco

Wijdicks, makes a very cogent argument AGAINST doing tests other than physical examination and apnea studies for the diagnosis of brain death.

Every article included in this chapter has practical value for intensivists. Be sure to read the article by Sareyyupoglu et al on surgical approach to acute pulmonary embolism. This likely heralds an important paradigm shift for us in this too-often fatal disease.

Happy Reading!

James A. Barker, MD

Acute Respiratory Disorder Syndrome

A Randomized Prospective Trial of Airway Pressure Release Ventilation and Low Tidal Volume Ventilation in Adult Trauma Patients With Acute Respiratory Failure
Maxwell RA, Green JM, Waldrop J, et al (Univ of Tennessee College of Medicine, Chattanooga; Carolinas Med Ctr, Charlotte, NC; et al)
J Trauma 69:501-511, 2010

Background.—Airway pressure release ventilation (APRV) is a mode of mechanical ventilation, which has demonstrated potential benefits in trauma patients. We therefore sought to compare relevant pulmonary data and safety outcomes of this modality to the recommendations of the Adult Respiratory Distress Syndrome Network.

Methods.—Patients admitted after traumatic injury requiring mechanical ventilation were randomized under a 72-hour waiver of consent to a respiratory protocol for APRV or low tidal volume ventilation (LOVT). Data were collected regarding demographics, Injury Severity Score, oxygenation, ventilation, airway pressure, failure of modality, tracheostomy, ventilator-associated pneumonia, ventilator days, length of stay (LOS), pneumothorax, and mortality.

Results.—Sixty-three patients were enrolled during a 21-month period ending in February 2006. Thirty-one patients were assigned to APRV and 32 to LOVT. Patients were well matched for demographic variables with no differences between groups. Mean Acute Physiology and Chronic Health Evaluation II score was higher for APRV than LOVT (20.5 ± 5.35 vs. 16.9 ± 7.17) with a p value $= 0.027$. Outcome variables showed no differences between APRV and LOVT for ventilator days (10.49 days ± 7.23 days vs. 8.00 days ± 4.01 days), ICU LOS (16.47 days ± 12.83 days vs. 14.18 days ± 13.26 days), pneumothorax (0% vs. 3.1%), ventilator-associated pneumonia per patient (1.00 ± 0.86 vs. 0.56 ± 0.67), percent receiving tracheostomy (61.3% vs. 65.6%), percent failure of modality (12.9% vs. 15.6%), or percent mortality (6.45% vs. 6.25%).

Conclusions.—For patients sustaining significant trauma requiring mechanical ventilation for greater than 72 hours, APRV seems to have a similar safety profile as the LOVT. Trends for APRV patients to have increased ventilator days, ICU LOS, and ventilator-associated pneumonia may be explained by initial worse physiologic derangement demonstrated by higher Acute Physiology and Chronic Health Evaluation II scores.

▶ I applaud these authors for this very nice study. Airway pressure release ventilation (APRV) is commonly used in adult respiratory distress syndrome (ARDS) and patients with acute lung injury (ALI). Likewise, it is commonly used in patients with trauma. However, there are little data available as to proof of efficacy. The goals of ventilation are clearly different for this mode (pressure targeted, focused on oxygenation, perhaps at the expense of ventilation, and not focused on tidal volume size) as compared with the ARDS Network protocol with which we are all familiar. (Recall that ARDS Network protocol is volume limited with tidal volume 5-6 cc/kg ideal body weight of the patient along with moderate positive and expiratory pressure and high ventilator rate.)

The results of this study are important: there was no difference in any significant parameters such as survival or ventilator days amongst the 2 groups. So at least for patients with trauma with ALI/ARDS, APRV can be considered equally safe and efficacious as to the ARDS Network protocol. Our armamentarium of ventilator strategies can thus be expanded!

The authors noted that CO_2 clearance was better with APRV despite a lower minute ventilation rate. This is a surprise finding and one that I believe should be further investigated. Is it better clearance through the long breath hold? Or is it the dump cycle? Or perhaps is it because the patients can freely breathe throughout any APRV cycle? The physiology questions are intriguing.

J. A. Barker, MD

A 29-Year-Old Female at 33 Weeks' Gestation With Respiratory Failure
Gayle RB, Dorsey DA, Cole MA, et al (William Beaumont Army Med Ctr, El Paso, TX)
Chest 137:1474-1478, 2010

Background.—The influenza A (H1N1) pandemic occurring in the United States between August and November 2009 included 26,315 laboratory-confirmed influenza-associated hospitalizations and 1049 influenza-associated deaths, according to the Centers for Disease Control and Prevention (CDC). Younger patients, age 27 to 44 years, were particularly susceptible, along with pregnant women, who are at a fourfold to fivefold increased risk of severe illness or hospitalization when infected with influenza. A young pregnant patient came for treatment after a syncopal episode associated with rhinorrhea and cough, myalgia, lethargy, fever, and progressive dyspnea.

Case Report.—Woman, 29, at 33 weeks' gestation complained of rhinorrhea, cough, myalgias, lethargy, fever, and progressive dyspnea, for which she was given albuterol, azithromycin, and

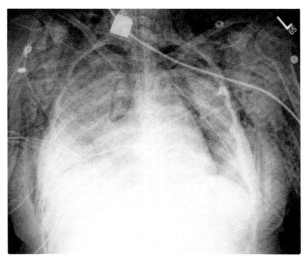

FIGURE 2.—Chest radiograph from hospital day 6 showing dense bilateral alveolar infiltrates with air bronchograms, subcutaneous emphysema, and left thoracostomy tube. (Reprinted from Gayle RB, Dorsey DA, Cole MA, et al. A 29-year-old female at 33 weeks' gestation with respiratory failure. *Chest.* 2010;137:1474-1478.)

acetaminophen. With progressive dyspnea and a syncopal episode 2 days later, she was admitted to the hospital. Her coughing produced nonbloody yellowish sputum and her fever was as high as 39.4°C. Her history showed no ill contacts and no chronic medical problems, but she had had breast augmentation and previous dilatation and curettage for a spontaneous abortion with retained products of conception. She did not smoke or use illicit drugs and rarely consumed alcohol.

Physical examination revealed mild tachycardia, heart rate of 114 beats/min, normotension, fever of 38.4°C, tachypnea, and oxygen saturation of 89% while breathing 5 L via nasal cannula. She appeared ill but alert and oriented and had rhonchi and wheezing bilaterally. Her white blood cell count was 4.1×10^3 cells/μL with 89% neutrophils and 9% lymphocytes. Platelet count was 91×10^3 cells/μL. Sodium was 133 mEq/L and potassium 2.8 mEq/L; other blood chemistry values were normal. Mild elevations of aspartate aminotransferase and myoglobin levels were noted. The chest radiograph showed bilateral alveolar infiltrates and a dense region of consolidation in the left hilar area.

The patient's respiratory status grew worse, leading to admission to the intensive care unit (ICU). She was intubated after an arterial blood gas test revealed a pH of 7.44, partial pressure of carbon dioxide (Pco_2) of 25 mm Hg, and partial pressure of oxygen

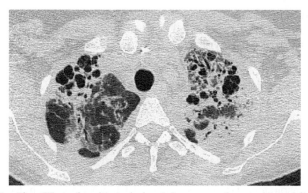

FIGURE 3.—Chest CT scan from late in the hospital course reveals severe bilateral fibrotic changes with traction bronchiectasis and airspace disease. (Reprinted from Gayle RB, Dorsey DA, Cole MA, et al. A 29-year-old female at 33 weeks' gestation with respiratory failure. *Chest.* 2010;137:1474-1478.)

(Po_2) of 61 mm Hg while receiving 100% inspired oxygen fraction (FIO_2) delivered through a non-rebreather mask. Her rapid influenza antigen test was negative, but a real-time reverse transcriptase-polymerase chain reaction (rFT-PCR) test was positive for influenza A (H1N1).

Management included oseltamivar and broad-spectrum antibiotics to guard against possible secondary infection, corticosteroids for fetal lung maturity, and an emergency cesarean section. Airway pressure release ventilation stabilized her hypoxemia for about a week, then refractory hypoxemia developed. High-frequency oscillatory ventilation was begun, along with inhaled nitric oxide, which eventually stabilized her hypoxemic respiratory failure. The patient then developed severe fibrotic acute respiratory distress syndrome (ARDS). Her oxygenation index (OI) was monitored throughout her hospitalization. The prolonged ICU stay was complicated by bilateral pneumothoraces and a methicillin-resistant *Staphylococcus aureus* ventilator-associated pneumonia, but the patient finally recovered and was transferred to a rehabilitation facility. Both patient and baby are now doing well.

Conclusions.—It is important to have a high index of suspicion for influenza A (H1N1) in patients who complain of fever and respiratory distress. The diagnosis of influenza cannot be made on the basis of a rapid influenza diagnostic test, which is unable to distinguish between virus subtypes and has a low sensitivity. rRT-PCR tests are the most sensitive and specific tests currently available but require 48 to 96 hours for processing. Patients who are hospitalized with suspected, probable, or confirmed influenza can be managed effectively with oxeltamivir or zanamivir. ARDS secondary to influenza A (H1N1) often produces severe hypoxemia that requires lung rescue therapies. Pregnant patients with ARDS must be managed with consideration of both the patient and the fetus. A multidisciplinary team, including an intensivist, maternal fetal medicine specialist, anesthesiologist, and neonatologist, will provide optimal care in these cases (Figs 2 and 3).

▶ This case report nicely outlines the severe illness that we just endured in epidemic form, namely H1N1 influenza. As outlined here, there was a predilection for pregnant and otherwise healthy patients. This influenza strain seemed to be particularly pulmonary virulent in some patients leading, to a hemorrhagic process similar to that previously described with *Hantavirus*.

The progression of ventilation that occurred here is identical to what ours would be and, I suspect, to that of most centers. The patient was first treated with acute respiratory distress syndrome NET low VT approach. Next she was changed to airway pressure release ventilation (APRV) when oxygenation worsened and then moved over to high frequency oscillation ventilation when oxygenation did not hold with APRV. She did not progress to the need for extracorporeal membrane oxygenation, but in many centers that was required for survival of these patients.

Likewise, it is illustrated that she developed methicillin-resistant *Staphylococcus aureus* pneumonia as a complication. *S aureus* pneumonia is unfortunately a common sequelae of severe influenzae.

Fortunately for our patient here, survival occurred!

Unfortunately, it requires an epidemic such as H1N1 to push us to learn how to improve our armamentarium of preparedness for epidemics as well as to stretch out and improve our acute respiratory distress syndrome care.

J. A. Barker, MD

Acute Respiratory Failure

Clinical characteristics and outcomes of patients with obstructive sleep apnoea requiring intensive care

Hang LW, Chen W, Liang SJ, et al (China Med Univ Hosp, Taichung, Taiwan)
Anaesth Intensive Care 38:506-512, 2010

We reviewed the clinical characteristics, required intervention and short- and long-term outcomes in obstructive sleep apnoea (OSA) patients requiring intensive care. A retrospective, single-centre, observational cohort study was undertaken in a multidisciplinary teaching medical and surgical intensive care unit. Adult patients with OSA (apnoea-hypopnoea index of 5 or higher) requiring intensive care from January 2000 to January 2005 were included. Thirty-seven OSA patients (age: 58 ± 14 years, male:female 27:10) were admitted due to respiratory (n=12, 32%), cerebrovascular (n=8, 22%), cardiovascular (n=16, 43%) and infectious events (n=1, 2.7%). Comparing the clinical features, polysomnographic data and outcome among these groups, we found that OSA patients admitted due to respiratory events had significantly higher Acute Physiology and Chronic Health Evaluation II scores, lower arterial blood gas pH, higher $PaCO_2$, a higher incidence of respiratory failure (92%) and required non-invasive ventilation after extubation (73%), and higher intensive care unit readmission rates than patients admitted due to cerebrovascular events and cardiovascular events (P <0.05). No difference was found in the in-hospital and long-term mortality rate.

The most common reason for intensive care unit admission in critically ill OSA patients was a cardiovascular event, followed by respiratory and cerebrovascular events. The baseline polysomnographic data of the OSA patients were not correlated with their clinical features and outcomes in the intensive care unit. A more complicated clinical course and higher intensive care unit readmission rate were encountered in OSA patients admitted due to respiratory events. Further studies would be required to evaluate the efficacy of non-invasive ventilation for facilitation of extubation in OSA patients presenting with hypercapnic respiratory failure.

▶ As the population ages and the obesity epidemic widens, it will behoove us to understand this growing (pun intended!) subgroup of patients in the ICU. Obstructive sleep apnea really does appear to predispose people to cardiovascular and cerebrovascular events. Patients with sleep apnea who are admitted to ICU are more ill in general than other patients. Consequently, their respiratory health is more complex. Over 70% require noninvasive ventilation after extubation. This study collates some very useful information.

J. A. Barker, MD

Causes and Outcomes of Acute Neuromuscular Respiratory Failure
Serrano MC, Rabinstein AA (Mayo Clinic, Rochester, MN)
Arch Neurol 67:1089-1094, 2010

Objective.—To identify the spectrum of causes, analyze the usefulness of diagnostic tests, and recognize prognostic factors in patients with acute neuromuscular respiratory failure.

Methods.—We evaluated 85 patients admitted to the intensive care unit (ICU) at Mayo Clinic, Rochester, between 2003 and 2009 with acute neuromuscular respiratory failure, defined as a need for mechanical ventilation owing to primary impairment of the peripheral nervous system. Outcome was assessed at hospital discharge and at last follow-up. Poor outcome was defined as a modified Rankin score greater than 3.

Results.—The median age was 66 years; median follow-up, 5 months. The most frequent diagnoses were myasthenia gravis, Guillain-Barré syndrome, myopathies, and amyotrophic lateral sclerosis (27, 12, 12, and 12 patients, respectively). Forty-seven patients (55%) had no known neuromuscular diagnosis before admission, and 36 of them (77%) had poor short-term outcomes. In 10 patients (12%), the diagnosis remained unknown on discharge; only 1 (10%) had regained independent function. Older age was associated with increased mortality during hospitalization.

TABLE 1.—Final Diagnoses of Patients Admitted to the ICU With Acute Neuromuscular Respiratory Failure

Final Diagnosis	Patients, No. (%)
Myasthenia	27 (32)
GBS	12 (14)
Myopathies	12 (14)
Dermatomyositis	2
α-sarcoglycanopathy	1
Toxic necrotizing myopathy	1
Hypernatremic myopathy	1
Myotonic dystrophy	1
Myopathy with anti-SRP antibodies	1
Undetermined	5
ALS	12 (14)
Postpolio syndrome	3 (4)
CIDP	2 (2)
West Nile infection polyradiculoneuropathy	2 (2)
Amyloid polyradiculoneuropathy	1 (1)
Kennedy syndrome	1 (1)
Congenital myasthenic syndrome	1 (1)
Pseudocholinesterase deficiency	1 (1)
Myelopathy	1 (1)
Unknown	10 (12)

Abbreviations: ALS, amyotrophic lateral sclerosis; CIDP, chronic inflammatory demyelinating polyradiculoneuropathy; GBS, Guillain-Barré syndrome; ICU, intensive care unit; SRP, signal recognition particle.

Longer mechanical ventilation times and ICU stays were associated with poor outcome at discharge but not at the last follow-up. Patients without a known neuromuscular diagnosis before admission had longer duration of mechanical ventilation, longer ICU stays, and worse outcomes at discharge. Electromyography was the most useful diagnostic test in patients without previously known neuromuscular diagnoses. The presence of spontaneous activity on needle insertion predicted poor short-term outcome regardless of final diagnosis. Coexistent cardiopulmonary diseases also predicted poor long-term outcome.

Conclusions.—Among patients with neuromuscular respiratory failure, those without known diagnosis before admission have poorer outcomes. Patients whose diagnoses remain unclear at discharge have the highest rates of disability (Tables 1 and 2).

▶ I definitely recommend this article to intensivists who practice in general medical-surgical ICUs. Respiratory failure can occur for myriad reasons. Primary lung disease is not a sine qua non. I have found a number of new cases of amyotrophic lateral sclerosis (ALS) and myasthenia gravis in investigating patients who appear with respiratory failure of apparent neuromuscular cause.

The authors characterize their experience here in Table 1. Of interest, ALS was the second most common diagnosis in those admitted without a known neurologic diagnosis (Table 2).

The authors herein found electromyography (EMG) as the most useful tool in differentiating these patients and disorders. This is an important pearl.

TABLE 2.—Final Diagnoses in Patients Without Known Neuromuscular Disease at Admission

Final Diagnosis	Patients, No.
GBS	12
ALS	8
Myasthenia	4
Myopathies	4
Hypernatremic myopathy	1
Toxic necrotizing myopathy	1
Myopathy with anti-SRP antibodies	1
Undetermined	1
CIDP	2
West Nile polyradiculoneuropathy	2
Postpolio syndrome	1
Kennedy disease	1
Pseudocholinesterase deficiency	1
Probable botulism	1
Amyloidosis	1
Unknown	10

Abbreviations: ALS, amyotrophic lateral sclerosis; CIDP, chronic inflammatory demyelinating polyradiculoneuropathy; GBS, Guillain-Barré syndrome; SRP, signal recognition particle.

Neurologic colleagues have usually declined to do EMGs in ICUs where I have worked, citing concerns about portable machines and high degrees of electrical interference.

Clearly the experiences at Mayo Clinic will not necessarily mirror other practices. However, I believe this article offers important epidemiologic and prognostic information for all of us who practice in adult medical critical care.

J. A. Barker, MD

A multicenter, randomized trial of noninvasive ventilation with helium-oxygen mixture in exacerbations of chronic obstructive lung disease
Maggiore SM, Richard J-CM, Abroug F, et al (Università Cattolica del Sacro Cuore, Rome, Italy; Charles Nicolle Univ Hosp, Rouen, France; F Bourguiba Univ Hosp, Monastir, Tunisia; et al)
Crit Care Med 38:145-151, 2010

Objective.—To assess the effect of a helium-oxygen mixture on intubation rate and clinical outcomes during noninvasive ventilation in acute exacerbation of chronic obstructive pulmonary disease.

Design.—Multicenter, prospective, randomized, controlled trial.

Setting.—Seven intensive care units.

Patients.—A total of 204 patients with known or suspected chronic obstructive pulmonary disease and acute dyspnea, $Paco_2 > 45$ mm Hg and two among the following factors: pH <7.35, $Paco_2 < 50$ mm Hg, respiratory rate >25/min.

Interventions.—Noninvasive ventilation randomly applied with or without helium (inspired oxygen fraction 0.35) via a face mask.

Measurements and Main Results.—Duration and complications of NIV and mechanical ventilation, endotracheal intubation, discharge from intensive care unit and hospital, mortality at day 28, adverse and serious adverse events were recorded. Follow-up lasted until 28 days since enrollment. Intubation rate did not significantly differ between groups (24.5% vs. 30.4% with or without helium, $p = .35$). No difference was observed in terms of improvement of arterial blood gases, dyspnea, and respiratory rate between groups. Duration of noninvasive ventilation, length of stay, 28-day mortality, complications and adverse events were similar, although serious adverse events tended to be lower with helium (10.8% vs. 19.6%, $p = .08$).

Conclusions.—Despite small trends favoring helium, this study did not show a statistical superiority of using helium during NIV to decrease the intubation rate in acute exacerbation of chronic obstructive pulmonary disease.

▶ Heliox is like religion for some. It just makes sense that it would work in acute respiratory failure, right? It makes respirable gas lighter. Work of breathing is less.

Yet there was no benefit in this study. This is important information. Heliox is cumbersome, expensive, and has risk (can't control FiO_2 as easily as with regular blended oxygen). There is therefore no role for combined noninvasive ventilation and heliox. Perhaps any benefit to the lighter gas has already occurred because of the muscle rest from noninvasive ventilation.

J. A. Barker, MD

A 24-Year-Old Pregnant Patient With Diffuse Alveolar Hemorrhage

Venkatram S, Muppuri S, Niazi M, et al (Bronx Lebanon Hosp Ctr, NY)
Chest 138:220-223, 2010

Background.—Choriocarcinoma is a highly aggressive germ cell tumor identifiable by the secretion of Human Chorionic Gonadotropin (HCG) and hematogenous metastasis. It may be seen after a hydatiform mole, spontaneous abortion, or ectopic pregnancy, but also occurs at a rate of 1 in 40,000 term pregnancies. A young pregnant woman was diagnosed with diffuse alveolar hemorrhage (DAH) that was eventually attributed to choriocarcinoma.

> *Case Report.*—Woman, 24, at 33 weeks' gestation was admitted to the hospital complaining of dyspnea of 2 weeks' duration and a mild dry cough. She had experienced multiple spontaneous abortions caused by cervical incompetence, so prophylactic cerclage had been performed during this pregnancy. She reported no chest pain, fever, hemoptysis, night sweats, arthralgias, rash, anorexia,

abdominal pain, nausea, vomiting, toxic habits, or travel history. Her tuberculin test 6 months previously was negative. Physical examination showed her heart rate at 125 beats/min, blood pressure 110/65 mm Hg, temperature 36.6°C, and respiratory rate 28 breaths/min. No cardiac abnormalities were noted, nor was there jugular venous distention. Rales were noted bilaterally over the lung bases. Her white blood cell count was 8400 cells/mm^3, hematocrit 24%, and platelet count 219 cells/mm^3. Bilateral diffuse nodular infiltrates were seen on the chest radiograph, but her electrolytes, creatinine, liver function tests, and coagulation profile were normal.

The acute hypoxic respiratory failure was managed in the intensive care unit (ICU) with antibiotics given for suspected community-acquired pneumonia and infective endocarditis. The second day her respiratory status deteriorated, requiring a higher inspired oxygen fraction (FIO$_2$). Worsening pulmonary infiltrates were found on the third day, leading to intubation, after which she developed moderate hemoptysis, requiring emergency fiberoptic bronchoscopy. Blood was oozing diffusely from all lung segments. An elective cesarean section produced a viable fetus. Lavage cleared the fluid, which yielded a negative result on Gram staining and culturing. No malignant cells were found. The patient developed acute respiratory distress syndrome (ARDS), septic shock, and multiple organ failure. β-HCG levels fell from 71,139 to 40,331 IU/L after the infant's delivery. Hemosiderin-laden macrophages were found on a second fiberoptic bronchoscopy for hemoptysis, but cytologic and microbiologic analyses remained negative for pathogens. The patient maintained normal heart function, but remained in critical condition with refractory ARDS, managed with high oxygen concentrations and positive end-expiratory pressure. Doctors were unable to perform a surgical lung biopsy because of her critical state. After 13 days the patient died. Autopsy findings indicated choriocarcinoma.

Conclusions.—Rarely does choriocarcinoma cause DAH in pregnancy, so clinicians must have a high index of suspicion to detect it. The diagnosis should be considered in pregnant patients with nodular pulmonary lesions. β-HCG levels should be followed closely after delivery to ensure they decline as expected. Early diagnosis of choriocarcinoma is possible by inspecting the placenta of postpartum patients with lung nodules, especially when lung biopsy is not possible. High cure rates, even in advanced metastatic disease, are achievable with chemotherapy. Early diagnosis is essential.

▶ I wish I had seen this case report a few months ago! We had an identical case here in Texas. I learned about molar pregnancy during MS3 clerkship many years ago. All I knew was that it was pregnancy dedifferentiated into cancer but one that was curable. Of course, much has changed in 30 years since then. β-human chorionic gonadotropin (β-HCG) is now routinely used as is ultrasound imaging in pregnancy. Likewise, diffuse pulmonary hemorrhage is now much more treatable. However, as is illustrated in this nicely done case report, even being young and vigorously healthy may not prevent mortality in the face of diffuse metastatic malignancy.

Major take-home points I would emphasize from this case:

(1) Think of this possibility in those young women who are fertile.

(2) Consider β-HCG plus ultrasound to confirm pregnancy versus molar pregnancy/cancer. Realize that in both pregnancy and this malignancy that β-HCG may be quite high.

(3) Include metastatic malignancy in the differential diagnosis of patients with diffuse alveolar hemorrhage.

(4) When in doubt, a biopsy is in order.

(5) Diffuse metastatic disease with respiratory failure portends a poor prognosis even in previously healthy patients.

J. A. Barker, MD

Airway Management

3,423 Emergency Tracheal Intubations at a University Hospital: Airway Outcomes and Complications
Martin LD, Mhyre JM, Shanks AM, et al (Univ of Michigan Med School, Ann Arbor)
Anesthesiology 114:42-48, 2011

Background.—There are limited outcome data regarding emergent nonoperative intubation. The current study was undertaken with a large observational dataset to evaluate the incidence of difficult intubation and complication rates and to determine predictors of complications in this setting.

Methods.—Adult nonoperating room emergent intubations at our tertiary care institution from December 5, 2001 to July 6, 2009 were reviewed. Prospectively defined data points included time of day, location, attending physician presence, number of attempts, direct laryngoscopy view, adjuvant use, medications, and complications. At our institution, a senior resident with at least 24 months of anesthesia training is the first responder for all emergent airway requests. The primary outcome was a composite airway complication variable that included aspiration, esophageal intubation, dental injury, or pneumothorax.

Results.—A total of 3,423 emergent nonoperating room airway management cases were identified. The incidence of difficult intubation was 10.3%. Complications occurred in 4.2%: aspiration, 2.8%; esophageal intubation, 1.3%; dental injury, 0.2%; and pneumothorax, 0.1%.

TABLE 2.—Complications Overall Compared with Complications for Resident-Only
Intubations

Complication	All Intubations (n = 3,423)	Senior Residents Only (n = 2,284)	P Value*
Aspiration	95 (2.8)	69 (3.0)	0.57
Esophageal intubation	46 (1.3)	26 (1.1)	0.50
Dental injury	6 (0.2)	4 (0.2)	1.00
Pneumothorax	4 (0.1)	1 (0.04)	0.65
Composite complication†	144 (4.2)	96 (4.2)	1.00

Data are given as number (percentage) of each group.
Some patients experienced more than one complication.
*Calculated using the Pearson chi-square or Fisher exact test.
†Denotes the total number of patients experiencing a complication.

A bougie introducer was used in 12.4% of cases. Among 2,284 intubations performed by residents, independent predictors of the composite complication outcome were as follows: three or more intubation attempts (odds ratio, 6.7; 95% CI, 3.2–14.2), grade III or IV view (odds ratio, 1.9; 95% CI, 1.1–3.5), general care floor location (odds ratio, 1.9; 95% CI, 1.2–3.0), and emergency department location (odds ratio, 4.7; 95% CI, 1.1–20.4).

Conclusions.—During emergent nonoperative intubation, specific clinical situations are associated with an increased risk of airway complication and may provide a starting point for allocation of experienced first responders (Table 2).

▶ This is a very useful article. The authors analyzed a very large number of emergent hospital intubations. The conditions were realistic compared with my own experience in teaching hospitals: two-thirds of the intubations were done by upper-level anesthesia residents and one-third had a staff anesthesiologist present. The incidence of complications is higher than I was aware of and should change my practice. In other words, I think I probably should pay much more attention to these high-risk people now after intubations.

The widespread use of many adjunctive techniques is fascinating and demonstrates that the field continues to evolve. Difficult airway techniques are very much in use. (See Fig 1 in the original article for the breakdown.)

Table 2 has probably the most important data outlined. Namely, there is no statistical difference in results or complications when attendings join the upper-level residents in the procedures. Difficult airways are apparently difficult for everyone!

J. A. Barker, MD

Acute ischaemic hemispheric stroke is associated with impairment of reflex in addition to voluntary cough

Ward K, Seymour J, Steier J, et al (King's College London School of Medicine, UK; et al)
Eur Respir J 36:1383-1390, 2010

Cough function is impaired after stroke; this may be important for protection against chest infection. Reflex cough (RC) intensity indices have not been described after stroke. RC, voluntary cough (VC) and respiratory muscle strength were studied in patients within 2 weeks of hemispheric infarct. The null hypotheses were that patients with cortical hemisphere stroke would show the same results as healthy controls on: 1) objective indices of RC and VC intensity; and 2) respiratory muscle strength tests.

Peak cough flow rate (PCFR) and gastric pressure (P_{ga}) were measured during maximum VC and RC. Participants also underwent volitional and nonvolitional respiratory muscle testing. Nonvolitional expiratory muscle strength was assessed by measuring P_{ga} increase after magnetic stimulation over the T_{10} nerve roots (twitch T_{10} P_{ga}). Stroke severity was scored using the National Institutes of Health Stroke Scale (NIHSS; maximum = 31).

18 patients (mean ± SD age 62 ± 15 yrs and NIHSS score 14 ± 8) and 20 controls (56 ± 16 yrs) participated. VC intensity was impaired in patients (PCFR 287 ± 171 *versus* 497 ± 122 L·min^{-1}) as was VC P_{ga} (98.5 ± 61.6 *versus* 208.5 ± 61.3 cmH$_2$O; p<0.001 for both). RC PCFR was reduced in patients (204 ± 111 *versus* 379 ± 110 L·min^{-1}; p<0.001), but RC P_{ga} was not significantly different from that of controls (179.0 ± 78.0 *versus* 208.0 ± 77.4 cmH$_2$O; p=0.266). Patients exhibited impaired volitional respiratory muscle tests, but twitch T_{10} P_{ga} was normal.

VC and RC are both impaired in hemispheric stroke patients, despite preserved expiratory muscle strength. Cough coordination is probably cortically modulated and affected by hemispheric stroke.

▶ We all know how important this topic is. Stroke is a major debility that occurs at increasing frequency with aging. Many patients in fact will state that they would rather die than have a major stroke. In addition, as pulmonologists and intensivists, we are well acquainted with the high rate of pneumonia (quoted here as 30% of patients) that occurs in new stroke patients.

Clearly, cough is impaired. I completely agree with these investigators that to study the mechanism is an important clue to as to how to change pneumonia rates and improve morbidity and mortality.

The results found are of interest. Namely, the expiratory muscle strength is normal. However, the reflexes for both voluntary and involuntary cough are diminished. The authors admit that functional residual capacity is not known. Indeed, I wonder if much of the problem isn't in breath volume up to total lung capacity leading to inadequate volume and, therefore, inadequate flow against the closed glottis that is so very important in generating a powerful and effective cough. See Fig 1 in the original article for the sequence that occurs in cough.

Note that some of the patients (two or more) had essentially no cough and were thus excluded from analysis. This is a small but important study that is a good start on this important problem.

J. A. Barker, MD

A new maneuver for endotracheal tube insertion during difficult glidescope intubation

Walls RM, Samuels-Kalow M, Perkins A (Brigham and Women's Hosp, Boston, MA; Brigham and Women's Hosp/Massachusetts General Hosp, Boston)
J Emerg Med 39:86-88, 2010

Background.—The GlideScope® Video Laryngoscope (Verathon, Bothell, WA) is a video laryngoscopy system that can be used for routine intubation, but is also commonly used as an alternative for difficult or failed airways. Previous reports have identified a very high incidence of grade 1 and grade 2 Cormack-Lehane glottic views, but despite these high-grade views, intubation is sometimes difficult due to the angle of insertion and shape of the endotracheal tube. Several maneuvers have been reported to increase the likelihood of successful endotracheal tube placement in these uncommon cases of failure.

Case Report.—We report the case of a patient who could not be intubated with the GlideScope® despite an easily obtained grade 1 laryngoscopic view. The impediment to intubation was identified as a sharp angulation of the trachea with respect to the larynx, such that the trachea formed a steep posterior angle with the laryngeal/glottic axis. Intubation was achieved using a previously unreported maneuver, in which the endotracheal tube with a sharply curved malleable stylet was inserted through the glottis, and then rotated 180° to permit passage down the trachea.

Discussion and Conclusion.—We believe that this maneuver may be useful in other cases of failed GlideScope® intubation, when a high-grade laryngeal view is obtained but tube passage is not possible due to a sharp posterior angulation of the trachea.

▶ The GlideScope has made intubation in an academic setting wonderful. We can now observe the trainee's technique and positioning as well as giving useful advice. The wide blade has features of both Miller (straight blade usually placed on the tongue and epiglottis) and the McIntosh blade (curved blade placed into the vallecula and thus may have a less obvious view of the larynx). But like any other new technology, there will be human moments when it still isn't possible for the round tube to go into the round hole. The technique described here appears to work and has an excellent rationale. A diving trachea is likely more common than we realize.

J. A. Barker, MD

Advanced Airway Management Does Not Improve Outcome of Out-of-hospital Cardiac Arrest

Arslan Hanif M, Kaji AH, Niemann JT (Harbor-UCLA Med Ctr, Torrance; the Los Angeles Biomedical Res Inst at Harbor-UCLA Med Ctr, Torrance; the David Geffen School of Medicine at UCLA)
Acad Emerg Med 17:926-931, 2010

Background.—The goal of out-of-hospital endotracheal intubation (ETI) is to reduce mortality and morbidity for patients with airway and ventilatory compromise. Yet several studies, mostly involving trauma patients, have demonstrated similar or worse neurologic outcomes and survival-to-hospital discharge rates after out-of-hospital ETI. To date, there is no study comparing out-of-hospital ETI to bag-valve-mask (BVM) ventilation for the outcome of survival to hospital discharge among nontraumatic adult out-of-hospital cardiac arrest (OOHCA) patients.

Objectives.—The objective was to compare survival to hospital discharge among adult OOHCA patients receiving ETI to those managed with BVM.

Methods.—In this retrospective cohort study, the records of all OOHCA patients presenting to a municipal teaching hospital from November 1, 1994, through June 30, 2008, were reviewed. The type of field airway provided, age, sex, race, rhythm on paramedic arrival, presence of bystander cardiopulmonary resuscitation (CPR), whether the arrest was witnessed, site of arrest, return of spontaneous circulation (ROSC), survival to hospital admission, comorbid illnesses, and survival to hospital discharge were noted. A univariate odds ratio (OR) was first computed to describe the association between the type of airway and survival to hospital discharge. A multivariable logistic regression analysis was performed, adjusting for rhythm, bystander CPR, and whether the arrest was witnessed.

Results.—A cohort of 1,294 arrests was evaluated. A total of 1,027 (79.4%) received ETI, while 131 (10.1%) had BVM, 131 (10.1%) had either a Combitube or an esophageal obturator airway, and five (0.4%) had incomplete prehospital records. Fifty-five of 1,294 (4.3%) survived to hospital discharge; there were no survivors in the Combitube/esophageal obturator airway cohort. Even after multivariable adjustment for age, sex, site of arrest, bystander CPR, witnessed arrest, and rhythm on paramedic arrival, the OR for survival to hospital discharge for BVM versus ETI was 4.5 (95% confidence interval [CI] = 2.3–8.9; p<0.0001).

Conclusions.—In this cohort, when compared to BVM ventilation, advanced airway methods were associated with decreased survival to hospital discharge among adult nontraumatic OOHCA patients.

▶ This is another surprising article. Apparently, the new advanced cardiac life support (ACLS) guidelines really are on to something. What do I mean by that? ACLS no longer recommends early intubation but instead there is an emphasis on high quality and early cardiopulmonary resuscitation (CPR). Early defibrillation remains paramount as well. The reasoning is that chest compressions deliver the most blood flow to the brain in early cardiac arrest and that CPR should never or rarely be interrupted. This very large retrospective study shows worse outcomes for those patients intubated in the field. Apparently, a bag valve mask delivers just as much oxygen in these patients with minimal circulation, and of course, CPR is never delayed for endotracheal intubation placement.

An important caveat to notice, however, is the very poor overall survival to discharge: 4%. This is dismal survival.

J. A. Barker, MD

Imaging and Monitoring in the ICU

A comparison of transcutaneous Doppler corrected flow time, b-type natriuretic peptide and central venous pressure as predictors of fluid responsiveness in septic shock: a preliminary evaluation

Sturgess DJ, Pascoe RLS, Scalia G, et al (The Wesley Hosp, Brisbane, Queensland, Australia)
Anaesth Intensive Care 38:336-341, 2010

Aortic corrected flow time (FTc) is easily measured by Doppler techniques. Recent data using transoesophageal Doppler suggest that it may predict fluid responsiveness in critical care. This use of FTc has not previously been evaluated in septic shock, nor have any studies incorporated transcutaneously measured FTc. Furthermore, no comparison has been made between FTc, plasma B-type natriuretic peptide concentration (BNP) or central venous pressure. The aim of this preliminary study was to compare FTc, BNP and central venous pressure as predictors of fluid responsiveness in septic shock patients without cardiac dysrhythmia.

This was a prospective study of 10 consecutive adult septic shock patients (in sinus rhythm; 60% mechanically ventilated) treated with intravenous fluid challenge (4% albumin 250 ml over 15 minutes) in a mixed medical/surgical tertiary intensive care unit.

Mean ± SD Acute Physiological and Chronic Health Evaluation II score was 21.8 ± 12.7. Haemodynamic assessment incorporating transcutaneous aortic Doppler (USCOM®) occurred before and five minutes after fluid challenge. Concurrent with initial assessment, blood samples were collected for BNP assay (ADIVA Centaur®). Four patients demonstrated an increase in stroke volume $\geq 15\%$ (responders). Percent change in stroke volume strongly correlated with baseline FTc (r=−0.81, P=0.004) but not BNP (r=−0.3, P=0.4) or central venous pressure (r=−0.4, P=0.2). Baseline FTc <350 ms discriminated responders from non-responders (P=0.047).

Our data support FTc as a better predictor of fluid responsiveness than either BNP or central venous pressure in septic shock. Transcutaneous aortic Doppler FTc offers promise as a simple, completely non-invasive predictor of fluid responsiveness and should be evaluated further.

▶ This is an exciting noninvasive technique. We continue to search for the holy grail of monitoring to find a technique which will replace guesswork, also known as best clinical judgment! Volume status really is important in critically ill patients. We all agree on that. There is indisputable evidence that too little fluid worsens renal function, which in turn worsens both morbidity and mortality. Alternatively, excess fluid resuscitation clearly worsens acute respiratory distress syndrome.

Pulmonary artery catheters used for monitoring have had negative outcome results. Central venous pressure measurement is a flawed technique in all but the young and healthy.

I found this approach relatively simple and highly desirable in its noninvasive approach. Validation with a larger study is of course now in order.

J. A. Barker, MD

The case against confirmatory tests for determining brain death in adults
Wijdicks EFM (Mayo Clinic, Rochester, MN)
Neurology 75:77-83, 2010

The determination of brain death is based on a comprehensive clinical assessment. A confirmatory test—at least, in adult patients in the United States—is not mandatory, but it typically is used as a safeguard or added when findings on clinical examination are unwontedly incomplete. In other countries, confirmatory tests are mandatory; in many, they are optional. These tests can be divided into those that test the brain's electrical function and those that test cerebral blood flow. A false-positive result (i.e., the test result suggests brain death, but clinically the patient does not meet the criteria) is not common but has been described for tests frequently used to determine brain death. A false-negative result (i.e., the test result suggests intact brain function, but clinically the patient meets the criteria) in one test may result in more confirmatory tests and no resolution when the test results diverge. Also, pathologic studies have shown that considerable areas of viable brain tissue may remain in patients who meet the clinical criteria of brain death, a fact that makes these tests less diagnostic. Confirmatory tests are residua from earlier days of refining

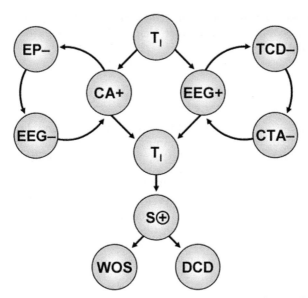

FIGURE 1.—Chaotic approach with confirmatory tests. The chaotic approach uses multiple confirmatory tests when test results do not match the findings on clinical examination. Generally, flow studies are followed by electrical physiologic studies and vice versa. Circles indicate other considered tests. In the worst case scenario, 2–3 tests are used to resolve the discrepancies. CA+ = flow on cerebral angiogram; CTA− = no flow on contrast CT angiogram; DCD = donation after cardiac death criteria met; EEG+ = discernible cortical activity; EP− = absent evoked potentials (brainstem or somatosensory potentials or both); S+ = return of brainstem reflexes (e.g., cough returns); TCD− = no flow identified on transcranial Doppler; T_I = test incomplete or confounded; WOS = withdrawal of support. (Reprinted from Wijdicks EFM. The case against confirmatory tests for determining brain death in adults. *Neurology.* 2010;75:77-83, with permission from AAN Enterprises, Inc.)

comatose states. A comprehensive clinical examination, when performed by skilled examiners, should have perfect diagnostic accuracy (Fig 1).

▶ This is a cogent well-discussed editorial by an authoritative leader in neuro-critical care. I happen to agree with him completely. Performance of unnecessary tests is never helpful and always has the risk of unintended consequences or harmful side effects. The neurologic examination performed by an experienced and competent physician coupled with a simple bedside apnea test is certainly sufficient for this diagnosis. Fig 1 well demonstrates the chaos that can occur when confirmatory tests are added to the mix. I cringe when families ask for an electroencephalogram in an ICU. The chance of electrical interference is so high that electrical silence may not be diagnosed despite its high likelihood.

I appreciate the candor expressed in this well-thought editorial. Bravo, Dr Wijdicks!

J. A. Barker, MD

A Descriptive Comparison of Ultrasound-guided Central Venous Cannulation of the Internal Jugular Vein to Landmark-based Subclavian Vein Cannulation

Theodoro D, Bausano B, Lewis L, et al (Washington Univ School of Medicine, St Louis, MO)
Acad Emerg Med 17:416-422, 2010

Objectives.—The safest site for central venous cannulation (CVC) remains debated. Many emergency physicians (EPs) advocate the ultrasound-guided internal jugular (USIJ) approach because of data supporting its efficiency. However, a number of physicians prefer, and are most comfortable with, the subclavian (SC) vein approach. The purpose of this study was to describe adverse event rates among operators using the USIJ approach, and the landmark SC vein approach without US.

Methods.—This was a prospective observational trial of patients undergoing CVC of the SC or internal jugular veins in the emergency department (ED). Physicians performing the procedures did not undergo standardized training in either technique. The primary outcome was a composite of adverse events defined as hematoma, arterial cannulation, pneumothorax, and failure to cannulate. Physicians recorded the anatomical site of cannulation, US assistance, indications, and acute complications. Variables of interest were collected from the pharmacy and ED record. Physician experience was based on a self-reported survey. The authors followed outcomes of central line insertion until device removal or patient discharge.

Results.—Physicians attempted 236 USIJ and 132 SC cannulations on 333 patients. The overall adverse event rate was 22% with failure to cannulate being the most common. Adverse events occurred in 19% of USIJ attempts, compared to 29% of non–US-guided SC attempts. Among highly experienced operators, CVCs placed at the SC site resulted in more adverse events than those performed using USIJ (relative risk [RR] = 1.89, 95% confidence interval [CI] = 1.05 to 3.39).

Conclusions.—While limited by observational design, our results suggest that the USIJ technique may result in fewer adverse events compared to the landmark SC approach.

▶ The timing of this article is prescient and the utility is high. Obviously, this is not a project that could be done as a randomized controlled double-blinded trial. However, even as a clinical observational study, I find that it has use. This is a real question. Namely, many trainees are learning ultrasound-guided central line placement, which implies that an internal jugular (IJ) or femoral vein cannulation will occur. Yet Centers for Disease Control and Prevention and other bodies recommend subclavian vein site selection because of decreased line complications (perhaps deep vein thrombosis [DVT] and/or blood stream infection [BSI]) in comparison to the other 2 sites. In turn, current technology does not really allow practical usage of ultrasound guidance for subclavian placement. Is it better to place catheters under visualization and have fewer pneumothoraces and arterial punctures or is it better to use the tried and true but unguided method where the catheter seems to have a slightly lower DVT and BSI rate? The results here are unequivocal. In this cohort of patients, even with experienced operators, there are fewer adverse events (AEs) when using the IJ ultrasound approach.

Does this emergency department-based study apply to my own ICU patients? I am not sure. The AE rate is very high as is the mortality rate. Thus, these patients may be even more ill than our usual ICU cohort. Nonetheless, this is a very useful study in answering an important clinical question.

J. A. Barker, MD

Pulmonary Hypertension

A More Aggressive Approach to Emergency Embolectomy for Acute Pulmonary Embolism

Sareyyupoglu B, Greason KL, Suri RM, et al (Mayo Clinic, Rochester, MN)
Mayo Clin Proc 85:785-790, 2010

Objective.—To examine operative outcomes after acute pulmonary embolectomy (APE), a recently adopted, more aggressive surgical approach.

Patients and Methods.—We retrospectively identified patients who underwent surgical APE from April 1, 2001, through March 31, 2009, and reviewed their clinical records for perioperative outcome. Operations were performed with normothermic cardiopulmonary bypass and a beating heart, absent a patent foramen ovale. For completeness, embolectomy was performed via separate incisions in the left and right pulmonary arteries (PAs) in 15 patients.

Results.—Of the 18 patients identified, the mean age was 60 years, and 13 patients (72%) were men. Thirteen patients (72%) had been hospitalized recently or had systemic disease. The preoperative diagnosis was established by echocardiography or computed tomography (or both). The median (range) follow-up time for all surviving patients was 16 months (2-74 months). Indications for APE included cardiogenic shock (n=12; 67%) and severe right ventricular dysfunction as shown by echocardiography (n=5; 28%). Seven patients (39%) had an embolus in transit. Seven patients (39%) experienced cardiopulmonary arrest before APE. Four early deaths (22%) occurred; all 4 of these patients had preoperative cardiopulmonary arrest, and 2 had APE via the main PA only, without branch PA incisions. Two late deaths (11%) occurred. Right ventricular function improved in all survivors.

Conclusion.—The results of emergent APE are encouraging, particularly among patients without cardiopulmonary arrest. It should not be reserved for patients in extremis; rather, it should be considered for patients with right ventricular dysfunction that is an early sign of impending hemodynamic collapse.

▶ Current dogma is that acute operative approach to pulmonary emboli does not change mortality. These authors present data to the contrary. This is important to pulmonary physicians because these patients are often in extremis and outcomes are often poor. In addition, many patients are not candidates for lytic therapy because of recent operations, bleeding, or neurologic lesions.

Obviously, a multicenter prospective study would be the next logical step for this aggressive approach.

J. A. Barker, MD

Trauma Issues

A Massive Pulmonary Embolism Treatment Protocol: How Trauma Performance Improvement Affects Outcome Throughout the Hospital System

Velopulos CG, Zumberg M, McAuliffe P, et al (Univ of Florida, Gainesville)
Am Surg 76:145-148, 2010

Trauma performance improvement is the hallmark of a mature trauma center. If loop closure is to be complete, preventable deaths must result in significant change in management and the establishment of protocol-driven improvements so such an instance does not recur. The trauma performance improvement committee reviewed a case of a massive pulmonary embolus and determined that this was a preventable death. The hospital performance improvement committee then initiated a root cause analysis, which led to creation of a treatment protocol for patients with massive or submassive pulmonary embolism. A focused review of the first 6 months of the implementation of the protocol was undertaken. Four patients over a 6-month period had massive or submassive pulmonary embolus. All four had sudden death or near sudden death and were appropriately resuscitated. All four sustained right heart failure. Two patients were treated by catheter-directed fibrinolysis, one with catheter-directed suction embolectomy, and one by surgical pulmonary embolectomy. All survived with full neurologic function. Trauma performance improvement is the model by which all hospital performance improvement should be done. Preventable deaths can result in change, which can have a future impact on survival in potentially lethal scenarios.

▶ This is a truly provocative article. I think reviewing it is definitely worthwhile. The authors certainly have some right ideas; a rapid cycle real-time performance improvement approach really can effect real and important change. They saved 4 lives here! Likewise, they stress and demonstrate the importance that a closed-loop approach to quality improvement (QI) must happen. So the sequence should be: (1) be vigilant for acute and treatable problems; (2) react as fast as possible to diagnose and then treat the problem; (3) analyze results as they happen; and (4) close the loop—meaning report back the results and then adjust the protocol approach for better results with the next case. In other words, this is a plan, do, study, and act cycle on steroids!

Here, they show how deaths from massive or submassive pulmonary embolism (PE) can be averted or diminished by rapid diagnosis and very aggressive therapy. All 4 patients had some form of acute clot removal: interventional radiologic removal of clot with suction device, catheter-directed fibrinolytics, or acute embolectomy.

Yet I called this provocative rather than excellent. Why? First, the statement "trauma performance improvement is the model by which all hospital performance improvement should be done" is absurd and immodest. There is a huge body of QI literature and work out there. This hospital trauma team did not invent it. Yet we have to give them credit that they are on to something: rapid cycle closed-loop QI is definitely the way to go when risks are so high. Moreover, who can argue that mortality is not a high-risk measure to improve on!

My second criticism of this article is that it is reactive. They aren't preventing PEs but instead are aggressively diagnosing and treating. Odds are that with enough numbers of patients, they will still lose a few once their results reach sufficient power for true analysis. Wouldn't this be more powerful if they worked on the front end to prevent deep vein thrombosis (DVT)/PE? Likewise, current literature does not confirm that the 3 techniques for acute rescue that they are using are truly changing mortality.

I applaud these authors' efforts. Now we need more: a larger study, a second look at DVT/PE prevention in trauma patients, and a challenge to the QI community to speed up processes so as to more quickly effect change that saves lives.

J. A. Barker, MD

Are small hospitals with small intensive care units able to treat patients with severe sepsis?

Reinikainen M, Karlsson S, Varpula T, et al (North Karelia Central Hosp, Tikkamäentie, Joensuu, Finland; Tampere Univ Hosp, Finland; Helsinki Univ Central Hosp, Finland; et al)
Intensive Care Med 36:673-679, 2010

Purpose.—To find out whether mortality from sepsis is influenced by the size of the hospital and of the intensive care unit (ICU).

Methods.—In the Finnsepsis study, 470 patients with severe sepsis were identified. The present study is a retrospective subgroup analysis of the Finnsepsis study. Eighteen patients were excluded because of treatment in more than one ICU. We divided the 24 units into three groups based on hospital size and academic status.

Results.—There were no significant differences between the ICU groups in terms of severity of illness. Overall, the hospital mortality rate was 29.2%. In post-operative patients, the hospital mortality rate was 22.9% for patients treated in large ICUs (including university and large non-university hospital ICUs) but 42.3% for patients treated in small ICUs ($p = 0.045$). In medical patients, no differences in outcomes were found.

Conclusions.—Treatment of surgical patients with severe sepsis in small ICUs was associated with increased mortality. Because of the relatively small sample size, further studies are needed to confirm or refute this association.

▶ Should critical care be regionalized? Is it dangerous to be treated in a small hospital ICU? These are relevant questions in the United States just as they are in Finland. In our hospital system, certainly these are major decision points in terms of planning for hospitals, staffing, and transport, for example.

The small sample sizes of this study certainly mean that large powered studies are needed for more definitive conclusions. However, we certainly glean from this that septic surgical patients are much more likely to survive in tertiary type hospitals.

J. A. Barker, MD

A brief history of shock
Millham FH (Newton Wellesley Hosp, MA)
Surgery 148:1026-1037, 2010

Background.—The term *shock* varies in meaning depending on the context. In hemodynamically unstable patients it indicates a syndrome of hypotension, tachycardia, and mental status alteration caused presumably by inadequate tissue perfusion. Currently shock describes patients in extremis who suffer from various pathophysiologic processes that share the condition of insufficient tissue perfusion as a consequence. The history of shock was traced through its evolution to its present status.

Galen and LeDran Eras.—Galen (CE 129-200) dominated medical thought for 1600 years. He did not speak of shock but viewed the hemorrhaging he treated in gladiators as a condition that could be treated with bloodletting. In 1628 William Harvey corrected Galen's physiologic theory that blood flowed outward in both arteries and veins and showed that blood actually circulated from the heart through the arteries and returned in the veins. He also determined that the liver could not manufacture all the blood needed in the Galenic model and postulated that there was a fixed and likely optimal blood volume that circulated in the human body.

Shock first appeared in the English medical literature in a translation of a French paper on gunshot wounds by Henri-François LeDran in 1743. It was used to describe a syndrome associated with gunshot wounds in which victims are stunned and agitated, indicating a neurologic phenomenon. Based on experiences during the Spanish War of Independence, G.J. Guthrie expanded the concept of shock to include both a stimulus produced by trauma and a physiologic response to extreme injury. Velpeau of France described sequential physiologic decline after gunshot wounds with the first stage being the shock of wounding and affecting particularly the nervous system. The second stage was termed a *reaction* and referred to physiologic recovery after shock.

American Civil War Through 1925.—Little was learned about the physiology of shock during the American Civil War but surgeons did see that it developed in response to more than just gunshot wounds. Symptoms were noted as excessive facial pallor, weak or absent pulse, confused mental state, nausea and/or vomiting, and excessive body prostration. Therapies were designed to stimulate the patient to the state of reaction, as postulated earlier and included early and frequent preoperative administration of coffee and alcohol, wrapping the patient in blankets, and waiting for the reaction to occur.

The common use of the term *shock* to describe a clinical syndrome began after Edwin Morris' *A Practical Treatise on Shock* was published in 1868. Careful laboratory experiments led to several discoveries in the late 19th century, including the concept that the central nervous system operated via the autonomic outflow to adjust and maintain blood pressure and systemic perfusion and the view of shock as a continuum of pathologic conditions ranging from the most severe, which quickly led to death, to a chronic condition similar to what is now termed posttraumatic stress disorder. Development of the sphygmomanometer added hypotension as a characteristic of shock. Pathologic vasoconstriction was suggested as a cause of shock, with spasm of the superficial arterioles being the central culprit. Saline infusion began to be used as a treatment for shock. Two theories of shock also emerged from laboratory studies. In George Crile's theory, vasomotor changes resulting from nervous stimulation played an important role in the pathophysiology of shock. Excessive activity occurred in visceral efferent nerves and created a state of visceral vasodilation that caused hypotension. It was believed that shock could be avoided through adequate sedation and anesthesia. Yandell Henderson believed that pathologic hyperventilation led to shock in his acapneic theory.

In World War I, fat embolism was postulated as a cause of traumatic shock, and "wound shock" was viewed by EM Cowell as resulting from agents in the wound itself that released toxins. Walter Cannon understood that the hypocarbia and tachypnea seen in shock proved the presence of the bicarbonate buffer system. He postulated a "missing blood" theory of shock. Both he and William Bayliss found several intravenous solutions, including synthetic colloid solutions, were efficacious in treating shock. Shock was now seen as having two stages: primary shock, which occurred just after being wounded, and secondary shock, which developed later because of toxins the wound released.

Blalock and Beyond.—Alfred Blalock proposed that shock was a disorder of blood volume in 1927 and listed 10 common causes of clinical shock. He found there was no missing blood or fluid at issue and excluded central nervous system injury as a cause of shock. His classification system grouped different pathologic situations together as conditions of disordered blood volume. The five distinct pathologic settings for shock were hematogenic shock, neurogenic shock, vasogenic shock, cardiogenic shock, and unclassified, which was later dropped. The four-part Blalock classification is still used. Blalock also described the various conditions responsible for shock as a decrease in the ratio of the blood volume in the circulation to the vascular tree's capacity, thus characterizing all shock as the result of a simple but profound ratio.

It was discovered in the mid-20th century that large volumes of isotonic crystalloid solution could be substituted for blood in resuscitative efforts. Success with huge amounts of crystalloid resuscitative fluids for burn patients may have contributed to the use of inappropriately large volumes of crystalloids to resuscitate non-burn trauma patients. More recently, work at the molecular level has shown that histone acetylation has a role in shock, suggesting treatment strategies that manipulate DNA transcription. The Bezold-Jarisch reflex of the central nervous system was also shown to exacerbate hemodynamic collapse in severe hypovolemic shock. Genetic polymorphisms in the autonomic nervous system may affect mortality among trauma patients. Also, the propensity for multiple organ system failure may complicate the course of shock patients.

Conclusions.—Over the years, ideas about the physiology of shock have varied and shock may not yet be fully comprehended. The clinical syndrome itself has remained unchanged, however. Tracing the history of shock reveals much about the physiologic considerations that complicate the current understanding of shock.

▶ This is quite an enjoyable read and highly recommended. The author makes it clear that his context of shock is in relation to the patient undergoing surgery, especially the patient with trauma. I find it useful to look backwards to know how far we have come. I wonder where we will be a century from now. Somehow, it seems unlikely that guns and accidents will be extinct.

J. A. Barker, MD

Ventilator Weaning

A Long-Term Clinical Evaluation of AutoFlow During Assist-Controlled Ventilation: A Randomized Controlled Trial

Lasocki S, Labat F, Plantefeve G, et al (Centre Hospitalier Victor Dupouy, Argenteuil, France)
Anesth Analg 111:915-921, 2010

Background.—Many new mechanical ventilation modes are proposed without any clinical evaluation. "Dual-controlled" modes, such as AutoFlow™, are supposed to improve patient–ventilator interfacing and could lead to fewer alarms. We performed a long-term clinical evaluation of the efficacy and safety of AutoFlow during assist-controlled ventilation, focusing on ventilator alarms.

Methods.—Forty-two adult patients, receiving mechanical ventilation for more than 2 days with a Dräger Evita 4 ventilator were randomized to conventional ($n = 21$) or AutoFlow ($n = 21$) assist-controlled ventilation. Sedation was given using a nurse-driven protocol. Ventilator-generated alarms were exhaustively recorded from the ventilator logbook with a computer. Daily blood gases and ventilation outcome were recorded.

Results.—A total of 403 days of mechanical ventilation were studied and 45,022 alarms were recorded over a period of 8074 hours. The course of respiratory rate, minute ventilation, F_{IO_2}, positive end-expiratory pressure, Pa_{O_2}/F_{IO_2}, Pa_{CO_2}, and pH and doses and duration of sedation did not differ between the 2 groups. Outcome (duration of mechanical ventilation, ventilator-associated pneumonia, course of Sequential Organ Failure Assessment score, or death) was not different between the 2 groups. The number of alarms per hour was lower with AutoFlow assist-controlled ventilation: 3.3 [1.5 to 17] versus 9.1 [5 to 19], $P < 0.0001$ (median [quartile range]). In multivariate analysis, a low alarm rate was associated with activation of AutoFlow and a higher midazolam dose.

Conclusions.—This first long-term clinical evaluation of the AutoFlow mode demonstrated its safety with regard to gas exchange and patient outcome. AutoFlow also allowed a very marked reduction in the number of ventilator alarms.

▶ I found this an informative and helpful article. We need more like this. All too often, we clinicians accept at face value new features on mechanical devices such as the mechanical ventilator AutoFlow evaluated here.

The concept is clear: breathing on a mechanical device with a tube down one's trachea is not natural and is inherently more work than free breathing. Think of the difference in the size of endotracheal tube compared with that of the trachea, for example. Now think of having to suck open valves through that tube to get a breath. AutoFlow is designed to allow asynchronous breaths at any time a patient makes effort on this particular ventilator brand. Ideally, there would then be less work of breathing and improved patient comfort.

The authors did look for possible differences in the 2 groups of patients. The fact is that there were very few. Yes, decreasing ventilator alarms (their primary finding) is good. Hopefully, it equates to improved patient restfulness or even sleep. I had thought that perhaps breath rate would be lower in those on AutoFlow (and it was but not in a statistical sense) or that time on the ventilator would be less (again, it was but not in a statistically significant way).

One item not discussed by the authors is the issue of peak inspiratory pressure measurement. This is clearly always higher with AutoFlow on, rather than off. Is this an important phenomenon? Most respiratory therapists would say no. Some concrete evidence would have been useful here.

J. A. Barker, MD

A proposal of a new model for long-term weaning: Respiratory intensive care unit and weaning center

Carpenè N, Vagheggini G, Panait E, et al (Univ Hosp of Pisa, Italy; Auxilium Vitae, Volterra, Italy)
Respir Med 104:1505-1511, 2010

Background.—Respiratory intermediate care units (RICU) are hospital locations to treat acute and acute on chronic respiratory failure. Dedicated weaning centers (WC) are facilities for long-term weaning.

Aim.—We propose and describe the initial results of a long-term weaning model consisting of sequential activity of a RICU and a WC.

Methods.—We retrospectively analysed characteristics and outcome of tracheostomised difficult-to wean patients admitted to a RICU and, when necessary, to a dedicated WC along a 18-month period.

Results.—Since February 2008 to November 2009, 49 tracheostomised difficult-to wean patients were transferred from ICUs to a University-Hospital RICU after a mean ICU length of stay (LOS) of 32.6 ± 26.6 days. The weaning success rate in RICU was 67.3% with a mean LOS of 16.6 ± 10.9 days. Five patients (10.2%) died either in the RICU or after being transferred to ICU, 10 (20.4%) failed weaning and were transferred to a dedicated WC where 6 of them (60%) were weaned. One of these patients was discharged from WC needing invasive mechanical ventilation for less than 12 h, 2 died in the WC, 1 was transferred to a ICU. The overall weaning success rate of the model was 79.6%, with 16.3% and 4.8% in-hospital and 3-month mortality respectively. The model resulted in an overall 39 845 ± 22 578 € mean cost saving per patient compared to ICU.

Conclusion.—The sequential activity of a RICU and a WC resulted in additive weaning success rate of difficult-to wean patients. The cost-benefit ratio of the program warrants prospective investigations (Fig 1).

▶ These Italian clinician investigators report their results of a sequential system of respiratory care units. Patients actually have 3 stops in this system. They come from another hospital or another ICU within the Pisa hospital to the respiratory intermediate care unit (RICU). Then an attempt to wean is made. If it does not occur quickly, the patients next travel to a weaning center (WC), which appears to be identical to a North American long-term acute care (LTAC) facility. See Fig 1 for results and pathways.

At each step along the way, patients get better and get off ventilators or succumb to their illnesses. The WC has a 30% mortality, so apparently those who don't wean are converted to withdrawal of ventilation at some point.

Acute care ICU to LTAC pathway is common practice in the United States. The length of stay is generally much shorter than reported here. Apparently these patients stayed in their initial ICUs for approximately a month before going to the RICU and then the WC.

I would have preferred more discussion as to the protocol for weaning used at both facilities. It apparently was a combination of pressure support drops and free breathing trials.

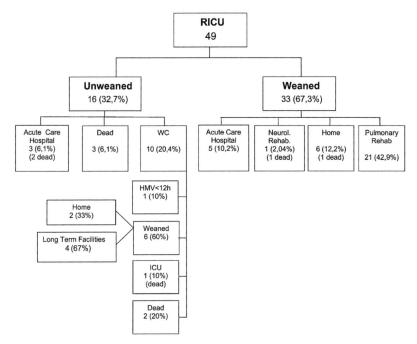

FIGURE 1.—Outcome of patients. (Reprinted from Carpenè N, Vagheggini G, Panait E, et al. A proposal of a new model for long-term weaning: respiratory intensive care unit and weaning center. *Respir Med.* 2010;104:1505-1511, with permission from Elsevier Ltd.)

This study adds further support to the use of protocolized weaning in specialized centers for those patients who remain on mechanical ventilation for prolonged periods of time after an acute illness.

J. A. Barker, MD

Miscellaneous

Reduction in elective delivery at <39 weeks of gestation: comparative effectiveness of 3 approaches to change and the impact on neonatal intensive care admission and stillbirth

Clark SL, Frye DR, Meyers JA, et al (Women's and Children's Clinical Service Group, Nashville, TN)
Am J Obstet Gynecol 203:449.e1-449.e6, 2010

Objective.—No studies exist that have examined the effectiveness of different approaches to a reduction in elective early term deliveries or the effect of such policies on newborn intensive care admissions and stillbirth rates.

Study Design.—We conducted a retrospective cohort study of prospectively collected data and examined outcomes in 27 hospitals before and after implementation of 1 of 3 strategies for the reduction of elective early term deliveries.

Results.—Elective early term delivery was reduced from 9.6-4.3% of deliveries, and the rate of term neonatal intensive care admissions fell by 16%. We observed no increase in still births. The greatest improvement was seen when elective deliveries at <39 weeks were not allowed by hospital personnel.

Conclusion.—Physician education and the adoption of policies backed only by peer review are less effective than "hard stop" hospital policies to prevent this practice. A 5% rate of elective early term delivery would be reasonable as a national quality benchmark.

▶ Elective deliveries before 39 weeks gestation is very common and accounts for up to 15% of all deliveries. Although reasons for their performance vary widely, published practice parameters and research imply that such elective deliveries should not be performed because of the increased newborn morbidity. Opponents of these recommendations suggest that delivery after 39 weeks gestation would promote and increase the number of term stillbirths.

The investigators investigated the comparative effectiveness of 3 types of policies to reduce the number of elective deliveries < 39 weeks gestation. (Separate from this study is that comparative effectiveness research will be emphasized more heavily in the future.) The 3 strategies were (1) a hard stop approach in which a policy prohibiting purely elective inductions and primary and repeat cesarean deliveries < 39 weeks' gestation, (2) a soft stop approach in which these procedures would be allowed but only if determined by an attending physician and further scrutiny through a peer review process, and (3) procedures would be allowed to continue as usual but only education would be provided to discourage these acts.

Strong points to this study include the inclusion of hospitals with wide delivery volumes. Implementation of hard stop and soft stop policies decreased elective deliveries < 39 weeks gestation from 8.2% to 1.7% and 8.4% to 3.3%, respectively. Both policies created statistically significant reductions. On the other hand, only education was inadequate at achieving any statistically significant reductions, although a reduction from 10.9% to 6.0% did occur. Reductions in elective deliveries at < 39 weeks gestation generated a reduction in neonatal ICU admissions by 16%. Although cost analysis was not included in this study, a significant cost saving is obvious.

What is unfortunate about this study is that education alone is insufficient to create significant change, even if the change is rooted in evidence-based medicine. The creation of a quality benchmark measure by the joint commission to be implemented will surely create such change.

S. F. Jones, MD

Unplanned early readmission to the intensive care unit: a case-control study of patient, intensive care and ward-related factors
Makris N, Dulhunty JM, Paratz JD, et al (Royal Brisbane and Women's Hosp, Queensland, Australia)
Anaesth Intensive Care 38:723-731, 2010

The purpose of this study was to identify patient, intensive care and ward-based risk factors for early, unplanned readmission to the intensive care unit. A five-year retrospective case-control study at a tertiary referral teaching hospital of 205 cases readmitted within 72 hours of intensive care unit discharge and 205 controls matched for admission diagnosis and severity of illness was conducted. The rate of unplanned readmissions was 3.1% and cases had significantly higher overall mortality than control patients (odds ratio [OR] 4.7, 95% confidence interval [CI] 2.1 to 10.7). New onset respiratory compromise and sepsis were the most common cause of readmission. Independent risk factors for readmission were chronic respiratory disease (OR 3.7, 95% CI 1.2 to 12, P=0.029), pre-existing anxiety/depression (OR 3.3, 95% CI 1.7 to 6.6, P <0.001), international normalised ratio > 1.3 (OR 2.3, 95% CI 1.1 to 4.9, P=0.024), immobility (OR 2.3, 95% CI 1.4 to 3.6, P=0.001), nasogastric nutrition (OR 2.0, 95% CI 1.0 to 4.0, P=0.041), a white cell count > 15×10^9/l (OR 2.0, 95% CI 1.2 to 3.4, P=0.012) and non-weekend intensive care unit discharge (OR 1.9, 95% CI 1.1 to 3.5, P=0.029). Physiological derangement on the ward (OR 26, 95% CI 8.0 to 81, P <0.001) strongly predicted readmission, although only 20% of patients meeting medical emergency team criteria had a medical emergency team call made. Risk of readmission is associated with both patient and intensive care factors. Physiological derangement on the ward predicts intensive care unit readmission, however, clinical response to this appears suboptimal (Table 2).

▶ Readmission to the hospital within 30 days of discharge is now considered an indicator of poor quality and will not be reimbursed by some insurers. Perhaps worse is the scenario studied here: readmission to the ICU within 3 days of discharge to ward. I had heard that mortality was higher in those patients and now we see that it is indeed.

The authors nicely lay out the data in Table 2. Some risk factors such as chronic lung disease are very predictable. Others such as anxiety or depression are definitely not on my radar screen.

The bed bound category makes one wonder if these aren't a surrogate for palliative care or hospice patients. The surprisingly high rate of hospital acquired systemic inflammatory response syndrome indicates a need for more concentrated hospital quality improvement work (such as central line bundle, ventilator-associated pneumonia bundle, foley catheter checklists, and so on).

TABLE 2.—Demographic Characteristics and Potential Risk Factors for Readmission in Bivariate Analysis

Characteristic	Cases (n=205)	Controls (n=205)	P Value
APACHE II score*, mean ± SD	18±7.1	18±7.0	0.96
Postoperative index admission*	107 (52%)	107 (52%)	1.00
Top index diagnoses (frequency ≥10)*			
Head trauma ± multi-trauma	18 (8.8)	18 (8.8)	1.00
Cranial neoplasm	17 (8.3)	17 (8.3)	1.00
Burns	14 (6.8)	14 (6.8)	1.00
Elective AAA	11 (5.4)	12 (5.9)	1.00
GI neoplasm	10 (4.9)	10 (4.9)	1.00
Subarachnoid haemorrhage	10 (4.9)	10 (4.9)	1.00
Index ICU stay, days, median (IQR)	2.2 (0.92-6.6)	1.7 (0.88-6.2)	0.12
Total ICU stay, days, median (IQR)	7.5 (3.8-14)	2.0 (0.89-6.8)	<0.001
Hospital stay, days, median (IQR)	30 (17-56)	20 (9.2-40)	<0.001
Hospital mortality	37 (18%)	11 (5.4%)	<0.001
Patient-related factors			
Gender, female	85 (41%)	69 (34%)	0.086
Age, mean ± SD	58±19	55±20	0.15
Comorbidity			
Anxiety/depression	43 (21%)	21 (9.3%)	0.001
Respiratory disease	16 (7.8%)	10 (4%)	0.033
Immunocompromised	14 (6.8%)	35 (13%)	0.17
Neoplasm	13 (6.3%)	21 (9.3%)	0.26
Renal disease	9 (4.4%)	10 (4%)	0.81
Heart failure	12 (5.9%)	13 (5%)	1.00
Liver disease	2 (1.0%)	0 (0%)	–
ICU-related factors			
Bed-bound	128 (62%)	94 (46%)	0.001
WCC >15×10⁹/l	55 (27%)	35 (17%)	0.027
HR >110/min	72 (35%)	53 (26%)	0.034
Weekend discharge	28 (14%)	44 (21%)	0.056
Haemoglobin <100 g/l	99 (48%)	81 (40%)	0.063
Nasogastric nutrition	49 (24%)	36 (18%)	0.092
Respiratory rate >20/min	158 (77%)	142 (69%)	0.11
INR >1.3	28 (14%)	17 (8.3%)	0.12
Respiratory failure (SOFA >2)	69 (34%)	55 (27%)	0.13
After hours discharge	40 (20%)	34 (17%)	0.50
Tracheostomy at discharge	28 (14%)	31 (15%)	0.76
Renal failure (SOFA >2)	12 (5.9%)	10 (4.9%)	0.82
CVC at discharge	91 (44%)	90 (44%)	1.00
Cardiovascular failure (SOFA >2)	9 (4.4%)	9 (4.4%)	1.00
Colonised with resistant organism	7 (3.4%)	6 (2.9%)	1.00
Coagulation failure (SOFA >2)	4 (2.0%)	4 (2.0%)	1.00
Liver failure (SOFA >2)	2 (1.0%)	1 (0.49%)	1.00
Ward-related factors			
MET criteria	113 (55%)	15 (7.3%)	<0.001
SIRS criteria	141 (69%)	86 (42%)	<0.001
Sepsis	71 (35%)	28 (14%)	<0.001
Non-treating team consult	128 (62%)	36 (18%)	<0.001

APACHE=Acute Physiology and Chronic Health Evaluation, AAA=abdominal aortic aneurysm, GI=gastrointestinal, ICU=intensive care unit, IQR=interquartile range, WCC=white cell count, HR=heart rate, INR=international normalised ratio, SOFA=sequential organ failure assessment, CVC=central venous catheter, MET=medical emergency team, SIRS=systemic inflammatory response syndrome. Significance tested by paired samples t-test and McNemar's test.
*Matched variable. Potential risk factors with P <0.15 identified in bold.

This article provides a nice baseline for a common problem. The how and why of reducing ICU readmission is the new frontier before us.

J. A. Barker, MD

Prognostic factors in critically ill patients with solid tumours admitted to an oncological intensive care unit

Ñamendys-Silva SA, Texcocano-Becerra J, Herrera-Gómez A (Natl Cancer Inst, Mexico)
Anaesth Intensive Care 38:317-324, 2010

The mortality and prognostic factors for patients admitted to the intensive care unit (ICU) with solid tumours are unclear. The aim of this study was to describe demographic, clinical and survival data and to identify factors associated with mortality in critically ill patients with solid tumours. A prospective observational cohort study of 177 critically ill patients with solid tumours admitted to a medical-surgical oncological ICU was undertaken. There were no interventions. Among the admissions, 66% were surgical, 79.7% required mechanical ventilation during their stay in the ICU and 31.6% presented with severe sepsis or septic shock. In a multivariate analysis, independent prognostic factors for in-ICU death were the need for vasopressors (OR: 22.66, 95% confidence interval: 6.09 to 82.22, P <0.001) and the acute physiology and chronic health evaluation (APACHE) II score (OR: 1.92, 95% confidence interval: 1.43 to 2.58, P <0.001). Cox multivariate analysis identified the length of stay in the ICU, Charlson comorbidity index score greater than 2, and the need for vasopressors as independent predictors of death after ICU discharge. The mortality rate in the ICU was 21.4%. Improved outcomes in critically ill cancer patients extended to the subgroup of patients with solid tumours. Independent prognostic factors for in-ICU death were the

TABLE 3.—Univariate Analyses Risk Factors for Mortality in the ICU

Variables	Odds Ratio	95% CI	P
Age, y	0.99	0.97-1.01	0.407
Female gender	0.83	0.40-1.76	0.643
Need for MV	12.45	1.64-94.13	0.015
Length of MV (days)	1.02	0.94-1.11	0.505
PEEP	1.35	1.12-1.51	<0.001
ARDS	11.61	4.69-28.70	<0.001
Sepsis	4.24	2.0-9.0	<0.001
Need for vasopressors	26.94	7.84-92.5	<0.001
Creatinine >93 μmg/l	3.46	1.67-7.32	<0.001
Haemoglobin <10.0 g/dl	1.51	0.72-3.17	0.265
Platelets <150×10^9/l	2.52	1.21-5.25	0.013
TB >18 μmg/l	2.32	1.10-4.87	0.025
Albumin <20 g/l	2.87	1.32-6.25	0.008
Length of stay in ICU (days)	0.95	0.88-1.03	0.277
APACHE II score (per 1-point increase)	2.00	1.55-2.58	<0.001
SOFA score (per 1-point increase)	1.48	1.31-1.69	<0.001
Chemotherapy (yes)	0.32	0.15-0.682	0.003
CCI >2	2.23	0.86-55.74	0.096

ICU=intensive care unit, MV=mechanical ventilation, PEEP=positive end-expiratory pressure, ARDS=acute respiratory distress syndrome, TB=total bilirubin, APACHE= acute physiology and chronic health evaluation, SOFA=sequential organ failure assessment, CCI=Charlson comorbidity index, CI=confidence interval.

need for vasopressors and the APACHE II score, while the length of stay in the ICU, Charlson comorbidity index score >2, and the need for vasopressors were independent predictors of death after ICU discharge (Table 3).

▶ I like it when an article challenges my personal biases. I have always felt that patients with solid tumors did extremely poorly if admitted to an ICU. However, this mortality rate of 21% is surprisingly low. The data of 3-organ failure leading to > 80% mortality are quite helpful as well in anticipation of family conferences and need for prognostication. This is nicely illustrated in Table 3. Need for pressors is another important splitter, although a significant percentage of these patients survived septic shock.

Clearly, critical care results will reflect improvements in cancer therapy, and these appear to reflect that.

J. A. Barker, MD

A survey of intensive care unit visiting policies in the United Kingdom
Hunter JD, Goddard C, Rothwell M, et al (Macclesfield District General Hosp, UK)
Anaesthesia 65:1101-1105, 2010

Admission to an intensive care unit is a highly stressful event for both patients and their relatives. Feelings of anxiety, pain, fear and a sense of isolation are often reported by survivors of a critical illness, whilst the majority of relatives report symptoms of anxiety or depression while their relative was in the intensive care unit. Traditionally, infection control concerns and a belief that liberal visiting by patients' relatives interferes with the provision of patient care have led many units to impose restricted visiting policies. However, recent studies suggest that an open visiting policy with unrestricted visiting hours improve visitors' satisfaction and reduces anxiety. In order to determine current visiting practice and provision for relatives within intensive care units, a questionnaire was sent to the principal nurse in all units within the United Kingdom. A total of 206 hospitals out of 271 completed the survey (76%). We found that 165 (80.1%) of responding units still impose restricted visiting policies, with wide variations in the facilities available to patients' relatives.

▶ I suspect that practice in the United States is similar to this. Even though we espouse and embrace patient centeredness, we live in the past, at least in the case of ICU visitation. The authors had an excellent response to their survey about visiting hours for ICUs in the United Kingdom. Only 20% had open visiting hours. Just 22% list visiting in their operational policies (a surrogate for importance!). Not surprisingly, a visit to dying patients is always liberalized; 12% of those surveyed had no visitation policy at all.

Children were allowed to visit in all but 4% of the ICUs. Almost all units limited visitor numbers to 2 or fewer at a time. Only 1.5% allowed unlimited visitors.

Several reports have shown improved patient outcomes and experiences when families are involved in care. These are summarized nicely in the discussion part of this article.

I think this article points out the need for a move from theory to reality for all of us who wish to practice in a patient-centered, high-quality, highly reliable fashion. We need to re-examine current practice (which is often just based on history—"we do it this way, because this is how we do it"), eliminate workarounds (which is what all these unofficial modifications to policy are), and make patient-centered/family-centered care a reality. The best way to do it is to formalize it!

J. A. Barker, MD

Article Index

Chapter 1: Asthma and Cystic Fibrosis

Chapter 2: Chronic Obstructive Pulmonary Disease

Chapter 3: Lung Cancer

Chapter 4: Pleural, Interstitial Lung, and Pulmonary Vascular Disease

Chapter 5: Community-Acquired Pneumonia

Chapter 6: Lung Transplantation

Chapter 7: Sleep Disorders

Chapter 8: Critical Care Medicine

Author Index

Printed and bound by CPI Group (UK) Ltd, Croydon, CR0 4YY

08/05/2025

01864677-0003